M000116485

WITHDRAWN

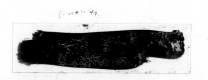

NOV 21 1989

CHILDREN AT RISK

Children at Risk

In the Web of Parental Mental Illness

RONALD A. FELDMAN
ARLENE RUBIN STIFFMAN
KENNETH G. JUNG

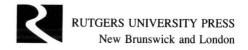

RUTGERS UNIVERSITY PRESS
New Brunswick and London

Grateful acknowledgment is made to the University Press of New England
for permission to reproduce Figure 3.2 from "Vulnerability to
Schizophrenic Episodes and Their Prevention in Adults," by B. Spring
and J. Zubin, in *The Issues: An Overview of Primary Prevention*, edited
by G. W. Albee and J. M. Joffe (1977).

Library of Congress Cataloging-in-Publication Data

Feldman, Ronald A.
Children at risk.

Bibliography: p.
Includes index.
1. Children of mentally ill.   2. Mentally ill
children—Family relationships.   3. Adjustment
(Psychology)   4. Mental illness—Prevention.
I. Stiffman, Arlene Rubin, 1941–   . II. Jung,
Kenneth G., 1957–   . III. Title.
RJ507.M44F45   1987   362.2′088054   86-10203
ISBN 0-8135-1192-5

British Cataloguing-in-Publication Information Available

Copyright © 1987 by Rutgers, the State University
All Rights Reserved
Manufactured in the United States of America

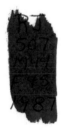

*This book
is dedicated to our families, who surround us with a web of
love and support.*

Our Parents:
The late David Feldman
Clara Feldman
Dr. Samuel and Rina Rubin
Vernon and Gertrude Jung

Our Spouses:
Dina Feldman
Rabbi Jeffrey Stiffman
Barbara Rose-Jung

Our Children:
Daniel, Deborah, and Darrah Feldman
Michael, Marti, and Cheryl Stiffman

HOLYOKE COMMUNITY COLLEGE LIBRARY

CONTENTS

LIST OF FIGURES   ix

LIST OF TABLES   xi

PREFACE   xiii

1   Introduction   1

2   Parental Mental Illness and Childhood Risk   4

3   Current Conceptions of the Invulnerable Child   34

4   A Social Interaction Model   56

5   Methods, Measures, and Data Analysis Procedures   75

6   The Children   95

7   The Parents   106

8   Family Relationships   119

9   Family Support Networks   143

10 Life Events of At-Risk Children   159

11 Living Arrangements of At-Risk Children   172

12 Coping Skills of At-Risk Children   186

13 A Multivariate Perspective   203

14 High-Risk Children versus Low-Risk Children   214

15 An Integrated Perspective   234

      APPENDIX: RESEARCH INSTRUMENTS   253

      BIBLIOGRAPHY   277

      INDEX   293

FIGURES

3.1 Child's Mental Health Status   43

3.2 Relationship between Vulnerability and Life Event
       Stressors   48

4.1 Net Environmental Protectors and Stressors, Personal
       Coping Skills, and Childhood Vulnerability to Mental
       Illness   59

6.1 Frequency Distributions of CBCL Scores for a General
       Population of Children and for the Web Children   96

12.1 Frequency Distributions of Social Competence Scores
       for a General Population of Children and for the Web
       Children   188

13.1 Behavior Problem Scores as a Function of Activity
       Competence Scores for Subjects with High, Medium, or
       Low Proportions of Mentally Ill Family Members   209

TABLES

6.1	Age Distribution of Web Subjects	98
7.1	Associations between Mean CBCL Scores and Current Living Arrangement	107
7.2	Associations between Mean CBCL Scores and Selected Parental Characteristics	110
7.3	Frequency Distribution of Parental Diagnosis	113
7.4	Distribution of Mental Illness among Parents of At-Risk Children	114
7.5	Associations between Mean CBCL Scores and Proportion of Mentally Ill Parents	115
8.1	Correlations between Children's CBCL Scores and Selected Family Variables	122
8.2	Hierarchical Multiple Regression Analysis Assessing the Effects of Sex of Mentally Ill Parents and Sex of Child on CBCL Scores, Families with Only One Ill Parent	124
8.3	Product-Moment Correlations among Seven Measures of Discord in Family Relationships	128
8.4	Associations between Proportion of Mentally Ill Parents in Family and Selected Types of Parent-Reported Discord, Two-Parent Families Only	132
8.5	Correlations between Parent-Reported Family Discord and Selected Family Variables	135
8.6	Correlations between CBCL Scores and Selected Measures of Discord in Family Relationships	135
8.7	Simultaneous Multiple Regression Analysis Assessing the Effects of Mother-Child Discord and Father-Child Discord on CBCL Scores, Two-Parent Families Only	139
8.8	Simultaneous Multiple Regression Analysis Assessing the Effects of Mother-Child Discord, Family Discord, and Proportion of Mentally Ill Family Members on CBCL Scores	141
9.1	Family Problems during the Past Year	146
9.2	Sources of Family Support	149
11.1	Current Living Arrangements, Residential Change Patterns, and Mean CBCL Scores	178
11.2	Hierarchical Multiple Regression for the Association	

between Current Living Arrangements and CBCL Scores,
Controlling for Proportion of Mentally Ill Persons in
Family and Frequency of Mother-Child Discord   181

11.3   Mean Proportion of Mentally Ill Persons in the Family,
Mean Frequency of Mother-Child Discord, and Mean
CBCL Scores, by Current Living Arrangement   182

12.1   Mean Values for Selected Coping Skills, by Current
Living Arrangments of the At-Risk Child   191

12.2   Mean Values for Selected Coping Skills, by Race of
the At-Risk Child   193

12.3   Associations among Selected Coping Skills, Age, and
Socioeconomic Status of the At-Risk Child   194

12.4   Mean Values for Selected Coping Skills, by Physical
Health of Parents   197

12.5   Associations among Selected Coping Skills and Types
of Discord   197

13.1   Multiple Regression Analysis of the Cumulative and
Interactive Associations among Important
Environmental Factors, Coping Skills, and Children's
Behavior   206

14.1   Frequency Distribution of the Current Living
Arrangements of Web Subjects and Comparison
Subjects   217

14.2   Frequency of Selected Types of Discord for Web
Subjects and Comparison Subjects   219

14.3   Mean CBCL Scores and Selected Coping Skill Scores
Web Subjects and Comparison Subjects   221

14.4   Product-Moment Correlations of CBCL Scores with
Discordant Family Relationships and Subjects' Coping
Skills   226

PREFACE

T HE STUDY REPORTED HERE IS PART OF A LARGER RESEARCH
project that has sought to investigate the efficacy of various preventive
intervention programs for children who are at high risk for mental illness.
The subjects' risk status was determined by the fact that they had one or more
mentally ill parents at the time of the study. During the course of the research
we found extremely large numbers of high-risk youngsters with severe behavior problems, despite their relatively young age.

In conjunction with the research we were able to identify children who appeared to be either victimized by the exposure to their parents' mental illness, vulnerable but not yet victimized by it, or seemingly invincible. In a
very basic sense, all were enmeshed to a greater or lesser extent in a web of
mental illness associated with their parents' dysfunction. Yet, as we continued to learn about the young participants in our study, we realized that the
behavioral outcomes of at-risk children depended essentially upon the mutual
interplay between particular combinations of individual coping skills and environmental forces.

The web of mental illness appeared, in fact, to constitute a shifting and
multifaceted phenomenon that must be clearly understood before one can ascertain whether a particular at-risk child will succumb or not to a behavior
disorder. Given the paucity of large-scale studies that had attempted to examine this phenomenon, or even to accept our basic premise about the continuous interplay between individual coping skills and environmental forces, we
deemed it timely to launch the investigation reported here. Throughout the
study, a social interaction model of childhood vulnerability is employed to
examine the web of mental illness.

For purposes of brevity, we frequently refer to the present research as the
Web study. The research was funded by a generous grant from the National
Institute of Mental Health, Office of Prevention (MH35033). We wish to express our heartfelt appreciation to this agency and our project officer, Irma
Lann, for their support. In addition, funds were received from the Administration for Children, Youth and Families, Youth Development Bureau
(90PD86517). Joan Gaffney, Donald Swicord, and Edward Bradford, in particular, facilitated our work. Without the assistance of these parties the Web
Study could never have been performed. By the same token, the research

could not have come to fruition without the full support and assistance of the executive officers and staff of the Jewish Community Centers Association, St. Louis, Missouri. This agency served as the field site for the Web study. We especially wish to acknowledge the guidance and help of Martin Kraar, Aubrey Herman, Stanley Ferdman, Buddy Sapolsky, Lee Onkeles, Robert Gummers, and the late Mortimer Goodman.

A special tribute also is in order for the many members of the research team who helped to implement all aspects of the research. Deborah Evans, John Orme, and Phoebe Keeney provided crucial assistance with respect to such varied activities as research design, methodology, computerization, data collection and analysis, and staff training. A large number of research students also helped with interviewing, coding, and data analysis. Our particular thanks for assistance with these activities are expressed to Nancy Bristol, Doris Bryant, Consuela De Prada, Cynthia Egyed, Ruth Ehresman, Catherine Hirner, Evelyn Irving, Gloria Jourdan, Anthony King, Suzanne Mays, Mary North, Patricia Rizzo, Cheri Sinnot, Maria Sutera, Susan Vlcek, and Julie Wolff. Cynthia Jones provided invaluable assistance with scheduling, word processing, and other aspects of the research. In addition, Marlie Wasserman, of Rutgers University Press, along with Joel Milner and an anonymous reviewer, contributed greatly to our efforts to refine this volume.

Last, but perhaps foremost, we wish to express our sincere appreciation to the hundreds of children and parents who participated in the Web study. They enabled us to acquire a fuller understanding about the web of mental illness and about our own capacity to elude its debilitating effects. In doing so, they also helped us to appreciate even more deeply our own families, to whom this book is dedicated.

R.A.F.
A.R.S.
K.G.J.

CHILDREN AT RISK

1 Introduction

WHY DO SOME CHILDREN WHO HAVE MENTALLY ILL PARents suffer from emotional or behavioral disorders while others do not? Why do some youngsters fall "victim" to their parents' mental illness while others, who appear to be equally susceptible, remain "invincible"? This question is of paramount importance not only for mental health professionals but also for parents, school teachers, law enforcement officials, policy makers, and many others. If it can be answered meaningfully, the prospects will be greatly enhanced for creating programs of intervention to avert or prevent behavior problems or mental illness on the part of many high-risk youngsters. Accordingly, this book describes a study that examines how children respond differentially to mental illness on the part of their parents. The study represents a systematic effort to understand how children are positioned in an intricate ecological web which, in large part, determines their susceptibility to mental illness. However, while knowledge about a child's position in the "web of mental illness" is necessary to predict his or her mental health, it is far from sufficient. Hence, the study also examines a broad array of psychological and behavioral factors which, in conjunction with a child's position in the web, influences his or her likelihood of developing behavioral problems.

From the outset, we wish to emphasize that youngsters cannot be regarded simply as "victims" of mental illness, on the one hand, or as "invincibles," on the other. Rather, a third group of youngsters also can be identified, those who do not fall neatly into either of the two foregoing categories. These youngsters appear to be "vulnerable" to mental illness. While they do not display clear evidence of mental illness, neither are they free of symptoms that portend their possible emotional or behavioral disorder. In the present volume, therefore, we examine children who are at high risk for mental illness and who may be characterized, respectively, as "victims," "vulnerables," or "invincibles."

The realization that children differ in their response to a parent's mental illness reflects, in part, the fact that some youngsters are far more capable or stress-resistant than others. Likewise, it partially reflects the fact that youngsters are enmeshed in different ways, and to varying degrees, in social systems that can either generate disorders or offer protection against them.

All youngsters are enmeshed in social "webs" that tend to enhance their respective likelihood of being either a victim, a vulnerable, or an invincible. These webs consist of a myriad of social, demographic, environmental, and behavioral factors that interact in a complex fashion. Therefore, the dominant objective of this book is to distinguish among the essential features of the social webs that either promote or deter behavior problems on the part of high-risk children.

Recent advances in the social sciences and the mental health professions have placed researchers on the threshold of major breakthroughs in preventive intervention for children who are at risk for mental illness. Whether or not such breakthroughs will occur, however, depends essentially on which of several possible pathways are followed in research and experimentation. As demonstrated in the following chapters, an especially promising research route inheres in the systematic study of children who do *not* develop behavior problems even though they are exposed to risk factors that induce some youngsters in similar circumstances to do so. Children tend to be at high risk for behavior disorders, for instance, if one or both of their parents are mentally ill. More than other youngsters, they are susceptible due to a variety of factors—genetic, biochemical, environmental, social, behavioral, or a combination thereof. Yet, even though some of these youngsters are deeply enmeshed in social systems that tend to promote or sustain behavior disorders, they exhibit the ability to resist the potent forces that contribute to such disturbance on the part of others. Both groups of youngsters are assaulted by insidious forces, but some fall victim while others remain impervious. Are the former youngsters somehow weaker or less capable than the latter?

Many observers contend that children who thrive in the midst of adversity are, indeed, superior. Purportedly, they possess unique competencies and attributes which, in large part, are reflected in the labels used to describe them. Thus, such youths have been called superphrenics (Anthony and Koupernik 1978), superkids (Pines 1979), and invulnerables (Garmezy 1974a). However, as we demonstrate in chapter 3, the available research about such youths is fragmentary. As a result, intervention programs based upon these findings are of limited value. To formulate effective prevention and rehabilitation programs in the mental health realm, it is necessary to consider the complex forces that either shape or maintain particular patterns of human behavior. This can be accomplished only if one's perspective expands from univariate to multivariate analysis, from cross-sectional to longitudinal assessment, and from idiographic to nomothetic or ecological investigation.

Drawing upon these perspectives, the present research seeks to examine why some youngsters escape the effects of their parent's mental illness while others are victimized by it. Accordingly, many specific questions are posed. Do children who remain healthy despite their parents' mental illness differ in attributes or behaviors from children who become mentally ill? Do either or both types of children differ appreciably from youngsters who seem vulnerable to mental illness but who do not exhibit behavioral patterns that clearly identify them as either a victim or an invincible? How can children be reliably labeled as victims, vulnerables, or invincibles in view of their shared high-risk status? What social and demographic factors are associated differentially with the onset of behavior disorders or with effective resistance against them? What are the respective effects of one's family, peer group, neighborhood, and social support networks upon resistance to behavior problems? And, ultimately, how do such factors interact to cause children either to withstand or fall prey to mental illness? These are but a few of the key questions posed during the course of our investigation. In scrutinizing the lives of participants in the Web study, the at-risk child is viewed *in situ* rather than *in vacuo*. Hence, we blend the research and practice perspectives of social psychology, community psychology, social psychiatry, and social group work.

In the early sections of the volume we examine the interrelationships among risk status, human development, and mental illness, and we review the associations between parental mental illness and childhood risk in detail. By employing an ecological perspective to explicate the web construct pervading the study, we devote particular attention to the features of a social interaction model of childhood vulnerability to mental illness. Next, we set forth the design, methods, and sampling features of the research. Operational distinctions are made among the child subjects who are regarded, respectively, as either victims, vulnerables, or invincibles. Subsequently, we systematically examine key characteristics of the "web of mental illness": the at-risk children and their parents, family systems, peers, and support networks. We also examine the life events, living arrangements, and coping skills of the high-risk children. The interrelationships among these variables are investigated throughout the subjects' life course. In the final sections of the volume we view the research findings in multivariate fashion and then examine a comparison sample of low-risk children. The web model is then revised and refined to better depict the intricate interplay among the numerous factors that determine whether a particular child is likely to become a victim, a vulnerable, or an invincible. As the research findings are synthesized and summarized, we highlight their implications for preventive mental health programs for children and adolescents.

2 Parental
Mental Illness and Childhood
Risk

GENERALLY IT IS ASSUMED THAT CHILDREN WITH MEN-tally ill parents are more prone to behavioral disturbance than children with "normal" parents. However, the available research does not clearly demonstrate whether the level and nature of a child's risk varies in accord with the particular type of disorder manifested by the parent. Moreover, it is not altogether clear whether or not the effects of parental mental illness are mitigated or mediated by factors such as the at-risk child's siblings, peers, family relationships, or personal capabilities. Such information is necessary, however, to formulate an explanatory model that enables one to fully comprehend the dynamics of childhood vulnerability to parental mental illness. To lay the groundwork for such a model we will examine the pertinent literature for the four types of mental health disorders most prevalent among parents who participated in the Web study: schizophrenic disorders, affective and depressive disorders, antisocial personality disorders, and substance abuse disorders.

SCHIZOPHRENIC DISORDERS AND CHILDHOOD RISK

A substantial body of research has focused on the behavioral outcomes of children who have schizophrenic parents. Although the reported level of risk varies from study to study, children of schizophrenics usually manifest higher rates of disturbed behavior than the children of normal parents. Cowie (1961a, 1961b), who found no differences in the prevalence of neurotic symptoms between the children of psychotic in-patients ($n = 132$) and a matched group of subjects with normal parents, reports the sole exception to this trend. One of the best ways to ascertain the effects of parental schizophrenia is to examine behavioral variations among children reared by schizophrenic parents, on the one hand, and the children of schizophrenics reared away from their mentally ill parents, on the other hand.

4

Children Reared by Schizophrenic Parents

One of the first studies that compared psychotic parents and their at-risk children was performed by Canavan and Clark (1923a, 1923b). These investigators found that 9.5% of children who had parents with a diagnosis of dementia praecox ($n = 463$) manifested conduct disorders while the corresponding prevalence for children with normal parents ($n = 581$) was only 1.6%. Unfortunately, however, this early study did not distinguish clearly between adult offspring and younger offspring. A half century later, Bleuler (1974) conducted a classic study in Switzerland regarding the offspring of psychotic parents. After following 184 children of schizophrenic parents over a twenty-year period, he found that only 10 were definitely schizophrenic. While this yielded a prevalence of 5%, Bleuler noted that the average expectancy rate in other studies was $13.7\% \pm 1$. The maximum was 16.9%, and the minimum was 7%. The children of schizophrenics were almost ten times as vulnerable to schizophrenia as the children of nonschizophrenics, but, importantly, the former children were no more likely to develop other types of psychoses than youngsters in the general population. Bleuler found that 18% of the older offspring (that is, above twenty years of age) of schizophrenics exhibited "unfavorable personality developments" or "eccentricities." The comparable figure for two control groups was only 5%.

Five children in Bleuler's sample were raised by two schizophrenic parents. Although none of these children developed schizophrenia, one was a schizoid psychopath, a second was extremely neurotic, and the other three behaved normally. Though this subsample is small, Bleuler concluded that "even long-term upbringing by two schizophrenic parents does not foredoom a child to become a schizophrenic, or even abnormal" (99). He asserted trenchantly—but somewhat prematurely in our opinion—that close home contact with schizophrenic parents cannot have any important or decisive causal significance in the onset of psychosis in the offspring of schizophrenics (103). Interestingly, the children of male schizophrenics in his family more often spent their entire childhood with both parents than did the children of female schizophrenics. This suggests that families are more susceptible to disruption or break-up when the mother is schizophrenic than when the father is schizophrenic.

Whereas Bleuler's work was conducted from a highly clinical perspective, more recent investigations have been of an epidemiological nature. One of the most widely-cited examples of the latter approach is a series of studies conducted in Denmark (and elsewhere) by Mednick and Schulsinger. For example, Schulsinger (1976), compared 207 high-risk subjects who had severely schizophrenic mothers with a matched group of 104 low-risk subjects whose parents and grandparents were not mentally ill. The subjects were followed for a ten-year period beginning in 1972; they were between eighteen and thirty years of age at the time of the follow-up assessment. Hence, they were examined before the onset of illness and were followed through a major part of the known risk period for schizophrenia. All eight subjects who died during the study were from the high-risk group, including four suicides, one probable suicide, two accidents, and one pulmonary embolism. Of the high-risk group 9% manifested schizophrenia, and another 32% displayed borderline states such as schizoid and paranoid personality disorders. For the low-risk group, the comparable incidences were only 1% and 4%. Only 15% of the high-risk subjects had no mental disorder, while 30% of the low-risk subjects had no disorder. Dysfunctions found in the remaining subjects include psychopathy, neuroses, nonspecific conditions, and "other conditions" such as affective and paranoid psychoses.

In a related study, Orvaschel, Mednick, Schulsinger, and Rolf (1979) examined 216 preadolescent and early adolescent children in Denmark. They found that children with a psychiatrically disturbed parent, despite the type of disturbance, exhibited fundamentally different modes of perception and behavior than children whose parents had no psychiatric disorder. In particular, the former children demonstrated greater tactile sensitivity and a greater degree of clumsy and awkward behavior. Regardless of the parent's sex, the offspring of schizophrenic parents were more prone to neurological dysfunctions in motor persistence, posture, and gait. In a study of much younger subjects, Gamer, Gallant, Grunebaum, and Cohler (1977) compared three-year-old children of psychotic mothers ($n = 21$) with children of well mothers ($n = 21$) on the Embedded Figures Test and the Peabody Picture Vocabulary Test. Because the high-risk children performed less ably than the low-risk children on the former test but did not differ on the latter, these results were interpreted as showing greater impairment of attention among children of psychotic mothers than among children of well mothers.

In another study of young children, Sameroff and Seifer (1981) found that the offspring of schizophrenic mothers and of neurotic depressive mothers showed relatively high degrees of social-emotional dysfunction at thirty months of age on the Rochester Adaptive Behavior Inventory (RABI). In contrast, the children of parents with personality disorders or without mental illness displayed lesser degrees of dysfunction. The severity of the mother's mental illness was a better predictor of low RABI scores than was the type of mental illness. While the data show that the offspring of schizophrenic mothers had high levels of illness, fearfulness, sadness, retardation, and social maladaptiveness, they do *not* render them different from the offspring of women with other severe or chronic mental disorders or, even, from the children of psychiatrically normal women of lower socioeconomic status. In part, this finding led Sameroff and Seifer to conclude that "caretaking environments in which high levels of stress exist, whether through economic or emotional instability, produce young children with high levels of incompetent behavior" (277).

Beisser, Glasser, and Grant (1967) also conducted a long-range study of schizophrenia and family behavior. These investigators examined 101 children of schizophrenic mothers, 45 children of psychoneurotic mothers, and 78 children of "normal" mothers. The subjects ranged in age from five through twelve years. Mothers with a schizophrenic history reported a greater number of behavioral deviations in their children than mothers with no such history. The schizophrenic and control children differed significantly from the children of schizophrenic mothers in temper tantrums, sibling conflict, and sleep interruption. Children of psychoneurotic mothers scored in the middle on these variables, not significantly different from the other categories of subjects. Although stealing and destructiveness were infrequent, they occurred significantly more often among the offspring of schizophrenic mothers. Therefore, the researchers concluded that greater maladjustment tends to occur in the children of schizophrenic mothers than in the children of mothers with no psychiatric history. However, the former children did not exhibit more behavioral deviations than the children of psychoneurotic mothers. Indeed, many children of schizophrenic mothers seemed to fall within the well-adjusted range. These findings clearly suggest that the factors which lead to health in children may be present in all families despite the presence of severe parental psychopathology. The investigators noted that the lack of observed differences between the children of schizophrenic and psychoneurotic mothers may be due to the comparable severity of the parents' psychopathology. This was inferred from the fact that all the mothers had been required to undergo hospitalization regardless of the type of mental illness manifested.

Schizophrenia is not the only risk to which the children of schizophrenic parents are vulnerable. Higgins (1976) found that 75% of children at risk for schizophrenia exhibit one type of psychiatric disturbance or another even though only a distinct minority are schizophrenic. Other evidence suggests, however, that the behavioral differences between the offspring of schizophrenics and other youths may be rather negligible. In a fifteen-year follow-up study, for instance, Miller, Challas, and Gee (1972) contrasted the behavioral records of children of schizophrenic mothers with those of the offspring of welfare mothers. The two groups were similar in economic status. These researchers concluded that the children of schizophrenic mothers exhibited fewer school problems and a less serious deviance than the children of either welfare mothers or matched controls. Instead, variables such as race, residential transience, welfare status, and childrearing in a foster or adoptive family were the key predictors of behavior problems.

Somewhat similarly, Weintraub, Prinz, and Neale (1978) employed a Pupil Evaluation Inventory to study 75 children of schizophrenic mothers, 57 children of depressed mothers, and 153 controls. Both the male and female children of schizophrenics were viewed as more deviant than the controls on aggression and unhappiness-withdrawal factors. However, there were no obvious differences between the children of the schizophrenics and the children of depressives; in fact, children from both categories were considered low in social competence. These findings are consistent with Rutter's (1980) conclusion that parental diagnosis, on the whole, is not a crucial variable in childhood mental illness. Neither a close nor an immutable association seems to exist between a parent's specific diagnosis and the child's particular kind of behavior.

Sameroff, Seifer, and Zax (1982) concluded that the offspring of schizophrenic women have many developmental problems, but not as the simple result of maternal schizophrenia. In general, a major difficulty with studies of schizophrenia is the fact that subjects are not followed throughout the peak risk period for this illness; only inferential conclusions can be drawn about etiology. Furthermore, sample sizes tend to be limited because of the small number of schizophrenic adults who have children, the inherent difficulties in differential diagnosis, and the instability of families with schizophrenia. Most studies that report a tenfold greater risk for the offspring of schizophrenics were conducted during the first half of this century. Today, the amount and quality of social interaction between schizophrenics and their children may be greatly enhanced by briefer hospitalizations, more frequent use of outpatient programs, and the application of antipsychotic medications. By diminishing the need for a traumatic separation between the schizophrenic parent and his or her child, it now is more possible to avert one of the main factors that Mednick, Schulsinger, and Cudeck (1980) deem predictive of childhood disorder—early institutionalization of the child in a foster care facility.

Children Reared by Nonschizophrenic Parents

Useful information about the relationship between parental mental illness and children's behavior can be acquired by examining children born to schizophrenic parents but not reared by them. MacCrimmon, Cleghorn, Asarnow, and Steffy (1980) have provided data about this relationship by studying adolescents reared in foster homes following their birth to a schizophrenic mother. Nine such children were contrasted with ten children of nonschizophrenic mothers who had been reared in foster homes. These two groups of subjects were compared with ten "average" youths from a public school. None of the high-risk subjects manifested major psychotic symptomatology. Nevertheless, the investigators found that the high-risk adolescents, more isolated socially, exhibited greater difficulty in the student role, elevated total symptom scores on a Psychiatric Status Schedule, and elevated schizophrenic scale scores on the Minnesota Multiphasic Personality Inventory. Half of the high-risk subjects demonstrated significant impairment on a battery of attention-demanding tasks.

Genetic influences clearly are not the sole determinants of the transmission of mental illness from parent to child. Relevant social and environmental factors must also be considered. Sobel (1961), for instance, studied seven infants born to families in which both parents were schizophrenic. Four of the subjects were placed in foster homes. After eighteen months, none manifested any overt psychopathology. In contrast, the three children reared by ill mothers showed somber mood, irritability, lack of spontaneity, hypoactivity, and motor retardation. Because their mothers interacted with them rarely and with little positive feeling, Sobel assumed that either these children learned maladaptive responses from their ill parents or they were so seldom reinforced by them that adaptive learning was delayed. Despite such striking results, however, the small size of Sobel's sample militates against definitive conclusions.

In contrast, Heston (1966) studied the psychosocial adjustment of forty-seven adults born to schizophrenic mothers. Comparative data were acquired for fifty control adults. All subjects had been separated from their natural mothers in the first few days of life. Schizophrenic and sociopathic personality disorders were found in excess of chance (p. < .05) among the subjects born to schizophrenic parents. Of the forty-seven persons in this category five were schizophrenic, whereas no cases of schizophrenia were found in the fifty control subjects. Thus, Heston concluded that the results provide ample evidence of a genetic predisposition toward schizophrenia. Weinberg and Weinberg (1982) argue, in contrast, that direct hereditary or biogenetic influences are minimal in the onset of transient schizophrenia. Instead, they assert that stressful family influences are the key determinants of schizophrenic onset. These are associated especially with the relationship between the mother and child. Modal family processes pertinent to the onset of schizophrenia include unstable family relationships, maternal dominance, and negative reactions toward the at-risk child. Mothers with schizophrenic children are characterized by behavioral inconsistency, communication of unrealistic versions of the social world, and behavior that diminishes their children's self-esteem and initiative.

One of the most frequent queries in the mental health literature pertains to whether or not there are sex-based linkages between parental mental illness and the behavior of at-risk children. To examine this question, Gardner (1967a, 1967b) studied child guidance clinic records regarding psychopathology exhibited by the mothers of 165 young patients. Of these children, 108 were later hospitalized for schizophrenia, while 57 achieved adequate adjustment in work and interpersonal relationships. The girls who became schizophrenic were more likely to have severely disturbed mothers than those who achieved adequate adjustment. In contrast, the relationship between the severity of maternal psychopathology and the child's later status was not significant for boys. Consequently, Gardner regarded sex role identification as a crucial factor in the etiology of schizophrenia. Similarly, Prinz, Weintraub, and Neale (1975) found that girls with a schizophrenic mother were somewhat more deviant than girls with a schizophrenic father. In contrast, boys with a schizophrenic father were more deviant than boys with a schizophrenic mother. In a later study, Weintraub, Prinz, and Neale (1978) reported clear differences only between the older daughters of schizophrenic and depressed women. This finding may be partially attributable to the fact that the subjects were rapidly approaching the age of peak risk for schizophrenia.

Erlenmeyer-Kimling (1977) investigated the purported linkage between maternal schizophrenia and children's mental illness by reviewing the results of major studies. The risk for the offspring of schizophrenic women seldom exceeded the risk for the offspring of schizophrenic men, as long as the other parent was psychiatrically normal. Age-correlated risk estimates for definite schizophrenia, excluding borderline and questionable diagnoses, ranged from 6.8% to 19.4%, with a mean of 11.6%. When both parents were schizophrenic, the range varied from 32% to 55.3%, with a mean of 36%. Children with one schizophrenic parent, regardless of the sex of that parent, had a risk for schizophrenic psychosis that was some 7% to 19% higher than the schizophrenic risk of the population at large. However, risk increased if a second parent was psychiatrically disturbed, rising to nearly 40% when both parents were overtly schizophrenic. Separation from the schizophrenic parent did not reduce the risk of disturbance in the offspring.

AFFECTIVE DISORDERS AND CHILDHOOD RISK

Depressive or affective disorders, the most prevalent of the major illnesses, are the leading cause of hospital admissions for mental illness in the United States. A series of American studies, using criteria outlined in the Diagnostic and Statistical Manual (DSM-III) of Mental Disorders (American Psychiatric Association 1980) reports that 5% to 9% of females and 2% to 4% of males in the adult population have had a major depressive disorder (Robins, Helzer, Weissman, Orvaschel, Gruenberg, Burke, and Regier, 1984). Weissman, Myers, and Harding (1978) posit that 25% of the United States population will experience at least one significant depression in their lifetime. In stark contrast, however, Erlenmeyer-Kimling (1977) reports a relatively low incidence of affective disorders in the general population, ranging between 0.4% and 2%. Such variations are attributable in part to the difficulties entailed in record-keeping and differential diagnosis.

Somewhat akin to the case with schizophrenia, family studies show an increased prevalence of affective disorders among biological relatives. For children who have one parent with an affective disorder, the risk varies between 6% and 24.1% (President's Commission on Mental Health 1978). These figures rise considerably if "doubtful cases" and "suicides" are regarded as affective disorders. In absolute numbers, therefore, many more children are subjected to the consequences of parental affective disorders than to parental schizophrenia. Cox and his colleagues have shown that mothers with recurrent or chronic depressive disorders tend to be less involved with their children, less likely to sustain positive interactions, less able to put their children's experiences into a personal context, and more often involved in unsuccessful attempts to control their children (Mills, Puckering, Pound, and Cox 1984; Pound, Cox, Puckering, and Mills 1985).

Gammon (1983) reported that the children of depressed parents appeared to have a threefold higher risk than normals for manifesting an emotional disturbance. When compared with children of normal parents, they were far more likely to experience major depression. They also suffered more frequently than the control group from attention-deficit disorders, separation anxiety, and conduct disorders; furthermore, they abused alcohol and other substances more frequently. The child's risk was higher when both parents suffered from depression. Thus, the rate of major depression was 8% for children with one depressed parent, 12% for children with two depressed parents, and nil when neither parent was ill. The rates for any kind of psychiatric disturbance were 17% for children with one ill parent, 23% for children with two ill parents, and 10% when neither parent was ill. Many of the study variables—parent's age, sex, and social class, the child's age and sex, number of children, history of childhood psychiatric disorder, separation from a parent in childhood, living arrangement, current social support, and life event history—did not have an effect on the child's risk for emotional problems. The parental factors that appear most influential are early age of depression onset, number of close relatives with depression or another type of psychiatric illness, and marital status.

Weissman, Paykel, and Klerman (1972) investigated the parental role behavior of 35 depressed women. They found that such women were less involved with their children, suffered from impaired communication, and manifested greater guilt, resentment, lack of affection, and friction when ill. They also displayed overprotection, irritability, preoccupation, and withdrawn and rejecting behavior toward their offspring. Although 58% of the 109 children of these depressed mothers exhibited some degree of disturbed functioning, the type of problem shown by their children varied widely. Besides depression, there were school problems, enuresis, and such forms of acting-out behavior as hyperactivity, truancy, and delinquency.

Many studies demonstrate an especially high rate of impairment in at-risk children when both parents are mentally ill. Gershon and associates (1982) found, for instance, that risk increases almost threefold for affective disorders in offspring when both parents have an affective illness. Beardslee, Bemporad, Keller, and Klerman (1983) have reported similar findings. In a related vein, Quinton, Rutter, and Rowlands (1976) and Wallerstein and Kelly (1980) contend that the marital discord and acrimony which can result from parental depression often adversely affect the mental health of the at-risk child. Yet, many studies suggest that there is not an especially direct relationship between parental diagnosis and a specific type of childhood behavior disorder. Thus, Rolf and Garmezy (1974) found that the children of depressed parents tend to be socially isolated, withdrawn, and shy rather than depressed. Weintraub, Neale, and Liebert (1975) reported a greater degree of acting-out behavior in the classroom, inattention, and disrespectful and defiant behavior.

One of the most recent and comprehensive literature reviews concerning the children of parents with a major affective disorder was performed by Beardslee and colleagues (1983). Their survey of cross-sectional ($n = 11$) and longitudinal ($n = 10$) studies found considerable risk and impairment on the part of children whose parents have a major affective disorder. The pertinent studies revealed rates of psychiatric diagnosis in children of affectively disturbed parents that vary from 40% to 45%. A variety of symptoms were evident, including neurotic illness, neurotic behavior disturbance, mixed behavior disturbances, and conduct disturbance. Other symptoms were indicative of personality disorders, adjustment reactions, hyperkinetic syndromes, and affective disorders. Some of the reviewed studies also reported drug problems, sociopathy, and trouble with the law.

Of the studies reviewed, the reported rates of depression among at-risk children varied widely, from 7% to 75%. During the school age period (that is, six through twelve years), high-risk children displayed excessive rivalry for attention with peers and siblings, feelings of isolation or depression, hyperactivity, school problems, and enuresis. They also were comparatively low in social competence and social compliance. During adolescence they were more likely to be defiant, rebellious and withdrawn. Some studies suggest that at-risk children do not differ from control subjects at ages nine through eleven but that they become more impaired as they proceed through high school. When impairment occurs, it is regarded as longstanding and major rather than transitory. Pending further studies, Beardslee and his colleagues concluded that factors such as the degree and duration of parental impairment, speed of recovery from the mental illness, and difficulties in family communication may be more powerful predictors of childhood disorder than the parent's diagnostic category. Also, certain attributes of the child—intelligence, the presence or absence of learning disabilities, and the quality of the child's coping skills—may mediate the impact of the ill parent.

In a later report, Beardslee (1984) again emphasized that the psychosocial impact on children of parents with major affective disorders may derive not from the specific nature of the affective diagnosis itself but from the accumulated life stress due to parental unavailability and impairment. Alternatively, however, a specific psychosocial impact can follow from the parent's depression through such mechanisms as the youngster imitating the parent's behavior, learning over time to view and react to the world as the parent does, or through a specific factor in the interaction between the depressed parent and the child, such as parental withdrawal or devaluation of the child's actions.

CONTRASTS BETWEEN THE EFFECTS OF SCHIZOPHRENIC AND AFFECTIVE DISORDERS

At this juncture, it is informative to review some of the similarities and differences between children of either schizophrenic parents or parents who suffer from an affective disorder. These comparisons are possible because a considerable number of studies have included subjects of both types. The relative profusion of such studies is due primarily to the prevalence and severity of these two types of parental disorders.

In one investigation, Worland, Lander, and Hesselbrock (1979) evaluated the children of parents who were either schizophrenic or manic-depressive. They employed the Wechsler Intelligence Scale, Thematic Apperception Test, Rorschach Inkblot Test, Beery-Buktenica Developmental Form Sequence, figure drawings, and blind clinical disturbance ratings from the test batteries. Children of psychiatrically ill parents were found to be more disturbed than children of nonpsychotic parents. The children of schizophrenic and manic-depressive parents differed from one another and from controls on two measures. In the aggressive content of their TAT stories, children with a schizophrenic parent showed less aggression than normals; children with a manic-depressive parent showed more aggression than normals. On the Rorschach test, children of schizophrenics gave more primitive responses than children of manic-depressives; the children of normal parents gave an intermediate number of such responses. Otherwise, the children of schizophrenics and the children of manic-depressives exhibited a similar degree of clinical psychopathology. The investigators concluded that "parental psychosis, rather than parental schizophrenia, is associated with the clinical disturbance of offspring" (21).

In a related study, Weintraub, Neale, and Liebert (1975) reported that elementary school teachers of children with either schizophrenic or depressed mothers were unable to distinguish key differences in the children's behavior on a variety of scales. In contrast with a control group of children with normal parents, however, both groups were rated higher on classroom disturbance, impatience, disrespect-defiance, and inattentiveness-withdrawal and rated lower on comprehension, creative initiative, and relatedness to the teacher. The investigators unfortunately do not report how their findings vary by the subjects' age. This datum is important because the subjects ranged from kindergarten through the ninth grade. In a later report, Weintraub and Neale (1984) found that children with a schizophrenic parent differed from children with normal parents on almost every variable assessed, including aggressiveness, withdrawal, relatedness to the teacher, distractibility, conceptual skills, and cognitive factors. They also differed from children with a depressed parent on certain variables, such as cognitive slippage. For the most part, however, children with a depressed parent showed similar patterns of incompetence, even on supposedly schizophrenia-specific variables.

One of the most comprehensive studies regarding parents with various types of psychiatric disorder was conducted by Rutter (1966). In a London hospital he examined 137 children who had a psychiatrically ill parent and 592 children whose parents did not have a psychiatric illness. Among other things, he found that children with a psychiatric disorder were placed more frequently than other children with stepparents, foster parents, or in other settings that separated them from their natural parents. Children with a mentally ill parent manifested certain symptoms at a significantly higher incidence than did comparison children. These included anxiety, disobedience, aggression, temper tantrums, disturbed relationships with the mother and siblings, hyperactivity, gratification and tension habits, and sleep disorders. However, delinquency on the child's part was not associated with parental mental illness. Rutter concluded that these symptoms are closely linked with disharmony between the parent and child. One-third of the subjects with mentally ill parents had siblings who also manifested a psychiatric disorder; this contrasts sharply with only one in seven of the children from the comparison group (p<.0001). It was common for several children to be adversely affected in families with a mentally ill parent, but, when the parents were well, only one child usually manifested a disorder. Difficulties in interpersonal relationships—as reflected by a diagnosis of personality disorder—were considered an important determinant of children's adjustment.

Like other investigators, Rutter found few similarities between the specific psychiatric diagnosis for a mentally ill parent and the diagnosis of his or her mentally ill child. Nearly 75% of the ill children from homes "broken" because of a parent's mental illness suffered from conduct disorders or mixed behavior disorders rather than neurotic illnesses or neurotic behavior disorders. With the exception of suicidal parents, broken homes were most frequent when one or both of the ill parents had a personality disorder rather than schizophrenia, depression, or neurosis. Rutter's data also indicate that children who remained well despite their parent's mental illness tended to be either very young (that is, two years or less) or well into adolescence at the onset of their parent's illness. Subjects between these ages were at the highest risk, suggesting that children are least vulnerable to a parent's mental illness when they are either too young to be aware of it or are relatively well-stabilized in their personality development. Rutter's data further indicate that disorders in children tend to be associated with disorders in the parent of the same sex. He suggests this may be due to the oft-reported finding that parents are somewhat more affectionate and lenient with a child of the opposite sex and more reserved and strict with one of their own sex.

Subsequently, Rutter, Quinton, and Yule (1977) conducted a four-year prospective study of adult patients who had children of school age or younger. Compared with classroom controls, nearly twice as many of the patients' children had persistent emotional or behavioral difficulties. Childhood problems were especially likely if the parent had a personality disorder or if persistent marital discord existed. As in many of the previously cited studies, the clinical type or severity of the parental illness was not a strong predictor. Instead, the child's risk was greatest when the parent's disorder exerted a marked social impact or was associated with "gross irritability" toward the child.

In somewhat similar fashion, Clausen and Huffine (1979) performed a longitudinal study of two distinct cohorts of children with mentally ill parents. Fifty-seven subjects had a schizophrenic parent, while twenty-two had a parent with an "other" diagnosis, usually an affective disorder. One of the main variables examined was the educational attainment of the subjects. Parental social status was the most potent influence on a child's school performance. The children of middle-class mental patients were far more likely to graduate from high school than were the children of working-class patients. When the effects of socioeconomic status (SES) were controlled, the children of patients with a diagnosis of affective psychosis or psychoneurosis clearly exceeded the children of schizophrenics in educational attainment. Problems of parent-child communication were reported more often in the families of schizophrenics than in the families of patients with other diagnoses. Furthermore, these problems appeared to be sex-linked. They were most acute in families where the mother was the patient and the child was a male. Serious emotional problems were reported more frequently among the offspring of schizophrenic female patients than for any other category. Unlike others of the above cited studies, Clausen and Huffine found that the most serious emotional problems occurred among children who were two to six years old at the time of the mother's first hospitalization.

Although these data are illuminating, they must be regarded cautiously. First, the modest size of the sample yielded cells too small for second-order analyses. Second, the researchers combined two cohorts of subjects who were examined after substantially different follow-up periods (one of approximately twenty years and another of less than five years); nowhere do they report variations that might be attributable to differences in history or in the length of the follow-up periods. Third, Clausen and Huffine do not clearly describe the types of diagnoses constituting the "other" category. While it is obvious that affective disorders were predominant, it is unclear to what extent this is so, or to what extent the remaining diagnoses were of lesser severity. And, fourth, many of the "emotional disorders" that they deemed "serious" are of dubious status—for example, "psychiatric treatment," "other evidence of nonpsychotic disturbance," and "illegitimate pregnancy."

More recently, a study by Sameroff, Seifer, and Zax (1982) found that a specific maternal diagnosis of schizophrenia had the least impact on children's cognitive, psychomotor, social, and emotional assessments. However, this may be due in part, to the fact that the children in their study had not yet entered the peak risk period for schizophrenia. Neurotic-depressive mothers had children with more serious developmental problems than either schizophrenic or personality-disordered mothers. The children of more severely or chronically ill mothers and of lower-SES black mothers performed most poorly. Sameroff and his colleagues concluded, among other things, that infants from single-child families do better because they engage in more interaction with their mother than do infants from families with two or more children. Blacks had fewer one-child families, while high-SES whites had the highest proportion of one-child families. The infants of others with neurotic depression demonstrated especially poor responsivity to people in the laboratory. In the investigators' opinion, "if one were to choose a diagnostic group where children were most at risk, it would be neurotic depression rather than schizophrenia" (58). Unlike schizophrenia, the impact of maternal depression seemed to remain constant throughout the first few years of the child's life. This is noteworthy because the schizophrenic mothers were more severely ill, on the average, than were the depressed mothers. Yet, as Kokes, Harder, Fisher, and Strauss (1980) suggest, incompetence in school-age children may be related to symptoms of depression and withdrawal in their mother regardless of whether she has been diagnosed as either schizophrenic or depressive.

Unlike the case with schizophrenia, numerous studies of affective disorders also posit a major causal role for socioenvironmental factors. Pearlin and Johnson (1977) suggest, for instance, that depression is explained largely by such life strains as economic hardship, lack of social support, and emotional pressures associated with the responsibility of raising young children. Studies by Holmes and Rahe (1967), Uhlenhuth, Lipman, and Balter (1974), and Warheit (1979) have demonstrated a link between environmental stresses and depressive disorders. An association between depression in parents and their children is likely to the extent that both are victimized by such stresses or are adversely affected by their reciprocal responses to them.

The National Institute of Mental Health (NIMH) Laboratory of Developmental Psychology conducted a particularly important study in this respect. Comparisons of families with either normal or depressive parents showed that 87% of the five-to-eight-year-old children of lower-class depressed mothers, 40% of the children of middle-class depressed mothers, and 33% of the children of middle-class normal mothers had been subjected to a psychiatric diagnosis (Fishman 1982). In the lower economic group, a depressive disorder was diagnosed in 71% of the cases; in the middle-class, in only 29% of the cases. For the children of depressed middle-class parents, depressive items on the Achenbach scale reflected self-criticism, guilt, and concerns with perfection. For lower-class children, they indicated ambivalence, dependency, and despair. Furthermore, there was a significant relationship between aggression and depression in the children of depressed mothers.

A comprehensive review by Teuting, Koslow, and Hirschfeld (1981) further illustrates the role of socioenvironmental factors in the development of depression. They found that epidemiological studies revealed depression to be more common among women than men and more prevalent in lower socioeconomic groups than higher ones. Similarly, studies by Ilfeld (1977), Markush and Favero (1974) and Paykel and associates (1969) have demonstrated that depression is related to stressful life events. Evidence for a socioenvironmental model also appears in an excellent intergenerational study of child neglect by Polansky, Chalmos, Buttenweiser, and Williams (1981). These investigators found that neglectful mothers tend to suffer from an "apathy-futility" syndrome, characterized by a pervasive condition of futility, emotional numbness, loneliness, and crippled problem-solving. This leads to neglectful childrearing which, in turn, leads to children who manifest an apathy-futility syndrome or other form of mental illness. When the children later become parents, their own offspring are likely to be neglected and, therefore, to suffer from the apathy-futility syndrome, further perpetuating and prolonging the vicious cycle. Although maladaptive behavior is transmitted from parent to child, the dynamic mechanism is not necessarily genetic but rather behavioral—that is, patterns established between the ill mother and her at-risk child.

Similarly Rutter, Yule, Quinton, Rowlands, Yule, and Berger (1975) found the factors most strongly associated with psychiatric disturbance in children are parental personality disorder, prolonged marital discord, and the social impact of the parent's irritability and hostility toward the child. More recently, Rutter and Quinton (1984) reported the findings of a four-year prospective study of 137 psychiatric patients who had children under fifteen years of age at home. The children's risk was greatest in the case of parental personality disorders associated with high levels of hostile behavior toward the child. Again, the parent's relationship with the child was a better predictor of the child's behavioral outcomes than was the particular diagnosis of the parent. They concluded, for the most part, that "parental mental disorder does not give rise to an increased risk for the children that is independent of the family's psychosocial circumstances as a whole. Rather, it should be seen as one of several psychosocial risk factors that are more damaging in combination than in isolation" (866). The overall pattern of their findings demonstrated that the main risk to a child did not stem from the parent's illness itself; rather, it derived from the associated psychosocial disturbance in the family, especially as manifested in terms of marital discord, parental hostility, irritability, aggression, and violence. In their opinion, family discord and hostility constitute the chief mediating variables between parental mental disorder and children's psychiatric disturbance.

Following a superb review of the available literature, Rutter (1980) concluded that a link exists between mental disorders in parents and psychiatric problems in their children. Although chronic disorders and conditions associated with personality abnormalities seem to carry a greater risk for children, parental diagnosis itself does not appear to be a crucial variable. Disorders in children do not follow any particular pattern, and there is little evidence of a close and consistent connection between parental diagnosis and specific types of children's disorders. Again, parental mental disorder is often associated with marital discord and disharmony, conflict over childrearing, irritability or hostility toward the children, and impaired family communication. Since family discord is associated more directly with problems in the children of mentally ill parents, youngsters may be at risk primarily because of the accompanying family disturbances and marital problems. Thus, as Rutter notes, the risk to children is not an inevitable consequence of the parental illness; it results from the involvement of these children in abnormal parental behavior and the association between parental mental illness on the one hand, and family discord, maladaptive communication, and impaired parent-child interaction on the other. These findings lead us inexorably toward a social interaction model of childhood vulnerability to mental illness.

ANTISOCIAL PERSONALITY DISORDERS AND CHILDHOOD RISK

Relevant information about the relationship between parental deviance and children's maladaptive behavior can also be gleaned by reviewing the literature about parental criminality and juvenile delinquency. The latter form of childhood behavior typically falls within the DSM-III designation of "antisocial personality disorder." In a seminal investigation regarding this topic, Joan and William McCord (1957) found that 87% of youths with two criminal parents subsequently became delinquent. Similarly, Robins and Lewis (1966) found a clear relationship between parents' criminality (as indicated by formal police records) and their sons' delinquency and/or failure to com-

plete high school. More recently, Robins (1975) examined arrests and delinquency in multiple generations of families in St. Louis, Missouri. It is assumed that deviance is linked across generations, but she found that little
is known about the particular conditions under which such linkage occurs,
whether children reflect specific parental behaviors, and whether a general
tendency toward intergenerational deviance exists. Her research shows that
criminal parents tend to produce disproportionately larger numbers of disturbed children, but that some of their children nonetheless appear to be normal. Moreover, disturbances in the former children do not always take the
form of delinquent behavior.

In a study of 145 black males, Robins, West, and Herjanic (1975) found
that delinquent male and female offspring tend to have delinquent mothers
(that is, mothers known to the juvenile courts or to the police for nontraffic
offenses before their seventeenth birthday). Delinquent boys tended to have
delinquent fathers, but the difference fell slightly short of significance; there
was no association between delinquent daughters and their fathers. As with
other forms of parental disorder (cf. Rutter 1966), maternal delinquency had
a much stronger effect than paternal delinquency, especially for the daughters
of parents who had been delinquents during their childhood. When the parents' adult arrest records were examined, almost half of the boys with an arrested father were delinquent (45%), compared with only 9% of boys whose
fathers had not been arrested. Among girls, 24% were delinquent if they had
an arrested father, and none was delinquent if the father had not been arrested.

Regardless of the child's sex, arrests of both parents were associated with
higher risk than having only one parent arrested, and as Robins and her colleagues note, it was rare for a mother to be arrested if her spouse had not also
been arrested. Consequently, it is difficult to ascertain if the children's outcomes are due to a "double dose of parental influence" or merely to the adverse effects of having one's mother arrested. If the mother had been a delinquent half the youths became delinquent, but if the father had also been a
delinquent, the rate increased to 56%. If the mother had a delinquent record
as well as an adult offense, the rate increased to 60%. And, if both parents
had delinquent records plus adult offenses, it increased to 67%. This clearly
suggests that children are at greater risk when both parents have a sustained
history of deviant behavior. Nevertheless, it is important to note that one-
third of the children in the Robins study did *not* become delinquent even
when both parents had been delinquent and arrested as adults.

An extensive review by Rutter and Madge (1976) likewise shows that parental criminality tends to be associated with delinquency on the part of their

children. Studies in Scandinavia (Jonsson 1967) and Britain (West and Farrington 1973) demonstrate that the rate of delinquency in children increases
two or threefold when the parent is a criminal, and even more if both parents
are criminals. From a mental health perspective, it is pertinent to note that
studies of the general population in London and the Isle of Wight (Rutter,
Yule, Quinton, Rowlands, Yule, and Berger 1975) have found, through interviews and behavioral deviance observed at school, that paternal criminality is associated with a twofold increase of psychiatric disorder in children.
In conjunction with these studies, and varying somewhat from his earlier reports, Rutter (1977) concluded that identification with the same-sex parent is
an insufficient explanation for the transmission of deviance. The link with parental criminality appears to be equally strong among both boys and girls.

SUBSTANCE ABUSE DISORDERS AND CHILDHOOD RISK

Like the above-cited disorders, parental substance abuse is also presumed to
exert an adverse impact upon at-risk children. However, a key distinction obtains between either schizophrenia, affective disorders, or antisocial personality disorders and substance abuse. A greater element of choice is attributed
to the behavior of the abusing individual. Furthermore, unlike the case with
either schizophrenia or affective disorders, peers are presumed to play a major role in the etiology of substance abuse and conduct disorders. The present
review reflects both the available literature and the distribution of subjects in
our study by concentrating primarily upon parental alcohol abuse rather than
drug abuse. It should be recognized, however, that many studies reveal a
high degree of association among drinking, use of cannabis, and the use of
other drugs (cf., for instance, Gibbs 1982; Potvin and Lee 1980). Major
studies of this topic have focused largely upon genetic relationships, behavioral influences, and family dynamics.

Genetic Relationships

As with the above cited disorders, some investigators posit a genetic factor in
the development of drinking patterns; however, this appears to be much more
pronounced among males than females. Cotton (1979), for example, pub-
lished an extensive review of findings about alcoholism incidences. She summarized the results of thirty-nine studies that included 6,251 alcoholics and
4,083 nonalcoholics. Regardless of the nature of the nonalcoholic population, an alcoholic was more likely than a nonalcoholic to have a father,
mother, or more distant relative who was an alcoholic. In one of the only

studies on alcoholism in half-siblings, Schuckit, Goodwin, and Winokur (1972) found that significantly more alcoholic (62%) than nonalcoholic (20%) half-siblings had alcoholic biological parents. Half-siblings who shared their childhood with an alcoholic proband showed a high incidence of alcoholism only if they had an alcoholic biological parent.

In a series of Danish studies, Goodwin and his colleagues (1973, 1974, 1977a, 1977b) compared the incidence of alcoholism for adopted sons (mean age=thirty years) and daughters (mean age=thirty-seven years) of alcoholic biological parents with the incidence for adoptees having nonalcoholic biological parents. The subjects were matched for age and circumstances of adoption. They found that sons of alcoholics were four times more likely to develop alcoholism than were sons of nonalcoholics. Respectively, the rates were 18% and 5%, as opposed to 3% to 5% for males in the general population. The fourfold increase was the same whether the sons were raised by nonalcoholic foster parents or by their own biological parents. However, there were no differences in the incidence of alcoholism between the adopted daughters of alcoholic parents and those with nonalcoholic parents. Importantly, the daughters of alcoholics raised by their biological parents manifested twice the frequency of depression as did their adopted sisters. Hence, as with other disorders, the effects of parental alcohol abuse may be manifested in the form of a different disorder, such as depression, on the child's part. As with problems concerning the investigation of schizophrenia, it is often difficult to gauge incidences of alcohol abuse among women, in particular, because their peak risk period is approximately forty years of age. The peak age for males is only in the mid to late twenties (Russell, Henderson, and Blume 1985).

As noted previously, depression seems to be one of the major symptoms in children of alcoholics. In a clinical and genetic study of male alcoholics, Amark (1951) found psychogenic depression to be the most common form of disorder among the relatives of alcoholics. In a study of 259 alcoholic probands, Winokur, Reich, Rimmer, and Pitts (1970) found that male relatives clearly exhibit more alcoholism and sociopathy while females manifest more affective disorders. A study of the adopted-out daughters of alcoholics suggests the origins of depression are more behavioral than genetic. Goodwin et al. (1977a) compared forty-nine daughters of alcoholics with forty-seven daughters of nonalcoholics; both groups had been adopted by nonrelatives early in life. The daughters of the alcoholics had no more depression than the controls, indicating that alcoholism in the biological parents did not increase the risk of depression in daughters raised by foster parents. The daughters of the alcoholics did not differ from the daughters of nonalcoholics with regard to problem drinking, depression, or other psychiatric disorders. Winokur and colleagues suggest that genetic factors may outweigh environmental factors in producing alcoholism in men but that the opposite may be true in women. Goodwin et al. (1977b) report a similar overlap in alcoholism and depression among women. Daughters of alcoholics raised by their alcoholic parents, for instance, had a history of depression significantly more often than did nonadopted census controls, respectively, 27% and 7% (p<.02).

Behavioral Influences

Haberman (1966) conducted a study of respondents who were identified either as alcoholics, persons with chronic stomach trouble, or persons with neither type of pathology. Women in the alcoholic and comparison groups were asked a series of childhood symptom questions about their offspring. More symptomatology was reported for the children of alcoholics, corroborating prior observations about the detrimental effects of parental alcoholism on children. In comparison with the control subjects, the children of alcoholics were more likely to manifest stuttering or stammering, unreasonable fears, frequent temper tantrums, constant fighting with other children, bedwetting, and frequent school troubles because of bad conduct or truancy. Haberman concluded, therefore, that parental alcoholism frequently involves harmful interpersonal behavior reflected in their children's symptoms.

Jacob, Favorini, Meisel, and Anderson (1978) reported that available studies show a number of related problems on the part of children of alcoholics—problems in identity formation, personality development, role performance, and the ability to form relationships. The inconsistency and unpredictability of parental support and expectations in alcoholic families seems to affect the child's sense of trust, security, self-esteem, and confidence in others. In fact, the role model provided by the alcoholic parent may distort the child's socialization process. For instance, if the alcoholic parent has difficulty in accepting society's rules and demands, a poor model is provided for the child's development of internalized rules and respect for authority. On the other hand, if the alcoholic parent is not held responsible for his or her own behavior while drinking, the child may intentionally or unintentionally adopt this mode of coping. Furthermore, family breakdown and disorganization may create maladaptive parenting patterns and adverse outcomes for the child.

Family Dynamics

Chafetz, Blane, and Hill (1971) compared demographic and clinical data regarding one hundred children of alcoholics and one hundred children of psychiatrically disturbed nonalcoholics. The family conditions of the two samples differed considerably. The alcoholics' families had significantly higher rates of instability, as indicated by marital problems and separation. Although the children of alcoholics were similar in most ways to the children of nonalcoholics, they were significantly more likely to have had a serious illness or accident, school problems, and problems with police or the courts. Moreover, only 10.5% of the children with alcoholic parents had a "good" relationship with their parents, contrasted with 40.3% of the children from nonalcoholic families (p<.001). Altogether 60.5% of the former children had a poor relationship with their parent, while only 18.2% of the latter had a poor relationship. These investigators contend that distinct and deleterious social consequences occur in conjunction with being the child of an alcoholic; however, it is not entirely clear whether these consequences result from the alcoholism itself or from higher incidences of family instability. Similarly, Fine and associates reported significantly greater emotional detachment, dependency, and social aggression in the children of alcoholics than in the children of nonalcoholics (cited in Jacob, Favorini, Meisel, and Anderson 1978).

In a small pilot study, Mik (1970) found that the sons of alcoholics often came from broken homes and reported negative attitudes toward authority, their fathers, and drinking. Similarly, Becker and Miller (1976) found that alcoholics' children ($n = 147$) were more likely than nonalcoholics' children ($n = 112$) to encounter serious developmental problems; be reared in unstable or broken homes; be removed from their homes; be runaways or juvenile delinquents; not graduate from high school; drop out of school to marry, have a baby, or join the military; be expelled from school; experience psychological problems in school and receive counseling for these problems; and, as adults, fail in their marriages and jobs. Aronson and Gilbert (1963) compared forty-one sons of male alcoholics with normal controls and found that the former scored significantly higher in ratings of "dependency" and "evading unpleasantness." Kammeier (1971) studied sixty-five children of untreated alcoholics and sixty-five same-aged normal controls in a Roman Catholic high school. Her findings revealed a significantly higher rate of separation and divorce in families with problem drinkers but no significant differences in emotional characteristics, social relationships, or school performance except for ninth- and tenth-grade girls who were the daughters of problem drinkers.

McLachlan, Walderman, and Thomas (1973) compared fifty-four children of treated alcoholics and fifty-four normal controls. Unlike the above investigators, they found no significant differences in school performance, alcohol and drug use, or other measures of personality disturbance; rather, the major difference between the groups was in family relationships. The former children rated their families significantly lower in family harmony and reported a significantly more disturbed relationship with the alcoholic parent.

Rouse, Waller, and Ewing (1973) found significantly higher rates of depression and broken homes in children of heavy drinkers than in the children of moderate drinkers or abstainers. O'Gorman (1975), in a similar study, found that the children of unrecovered alcoholics were rated significantly lower on self-esteem, perceived paternal affection, and attention but higher on external locus of control. A study of fifty children of alcoholics by Lindbeck (cited in Jacob, Favorini, Meisel, and Anderson 1978) revealed a broad range of significant problems, including emotional neglect by parents (64%), parental conflict (58%), parent-child conflict and verbal abuse by the parent (26%), nonfulfillment of parental responsibilities (22%), depression (20%), personal delinquency (15%), and child abuse by the parents (10%). The subjects also reported high rates of broken homes and childhood feelings of guilt, embarrassment, and resentment. Although most of the children were under thirty years of age, 16% misused alcohol and nearly 50% of those who were married had a spouse with a drinking problem. Following their review of this study and fifteen others, Jacob and his associates (1978) concluded that there is "modest-to-moderate support for the view that children of alcoholics exhibit significant difficulties in psychological, social, and family functioning" (1242).

As Russell, Henderson, and Blume (1985) point out, many studies of alcoholism have revealed that an alcoholic family history is associated with increased familial incidence of other psychiatric disorders. These disorders occur as multiple syndromes in the same individual or in different members of the same family more often than expected by chance. Miller and Jang (1977), for instance, studied 160 children of alcoholic parents matched to 160 children from nonalcoholic families. They stated that the extraordinarily high rates of intergenerational alcoholism within families cannot be explained completely or satisfactorily by a genetic interpretation since not all children of alcoholics become heavy drinkers. Instead, they posit that parental alcoholism creates conditions in the family, varying both in severity and timing, that shape a child's later adult adjustment. Consequently, a good socialization experience for a child can mitigate a history of parental alcoholism and, similarly, a bad socialization experience can vitiate a good history of no alcoholism on the parent's part. Their formulation recognizes that alcoholism is not the only possible deviant behavior that can develop among the adult children of alcoholics; substance abuse, criminality, or mental illness are other possibilities. In short, then, alcoholism leads to poor parenting and, consequently, to a bad socialization experience for the child. The severity and impact of poor parenting affects the child's later adult behavior and self-concept, which may be manifested in individually destructive coping behavior, such as drinking, mental illness, or criminal activity.

The subjects in the Miller and Jang study were more heavily involved in drinking than subjects from the general population. The investigators attribute this in part to their low socioeconomic status. About 33% of the sons who were heavy drinkers did not have an alcoholic parent; in contrast, 41% had an alcoholic father, 29% had an alcoholic mother, and 54% had two alcoholic parents. Among heavy-drinking daughters, 17% had no alcoholic parents, 24% had an alcoholic mother, and 36% had two alcoholic parents. In general, more sons were heavy drinkers than daughters, irrespective of the parents' alcoholism. However, when only the mother was an alcoholic, more daughters than sons were found to be heavy drinkers. The mother's parenting role seems especially crucial, therefore, in determining the drinking patterns of her daughter.

More central to the investigators' hypotheses were their findings about family problems. Vis-à-vis the children of nonalcoholics, the children of alcoholics had experienced one or more major crises in the family (for example, a parent's arrest, incarceration, absence, or hospitalization for a behavior disorder), a broken or unstable home, parental neglect, removal from the home, being on welfare, delinquent behavior, or a runaway episode. Thus, as might be expected, the children in these families were also significantly more likely to receive social and legal services in their developmental years. Although all the subjects were from poor urban multiproblem families, the findings confirmed several hypotheses: children of alcoholic parents had greater socialization difficulties than children of nonalcoholic parents; the greater the degree of parental alcoholism, the greater the negative impact on the children both in their developmental and adult years; if both parents were alcoholics, the adult subject fared the worst; and the negative impact of an alcoholic mother was greater than that of an alcoholic father. Hence, whatever else was wrong with these multiproblem families, an alcoholic parent increased the degree of misery for the children. Children who grew up in a home with an alcoholic parent were much more likely than children from similar multiproblem families to encounter large numbers of serious problems, be concerned about the impact of alcoholism on the family, develop concerns about mental health problems, engage in suicidal acts, and have severe marital difficulties.

Wilson and Orford (1978) conducted a detailed study of eleven families in which one parent was alcoholic. They, too, concluded that marital separation and marital conflict may be crucial intervening variables for the association between parental alcoholism and ill effects on the at-risk child. Few children in their study reported that "drinking" or "drunkenness" were their main concerns; instead, marital conflict, violence, parental hospitalization, and maladaptive parent-child relationships were of greater concern. In addition, they found that the children of alcoholics lacked close relationships with peers. Their literature review also demonstrates that the children of alcoholics may suffer from a broad variety of behavior problems: a higher incidence of school problems; difficulty in concentrating; conduct problems and truancy from school; poor school attendance and performance; elevated rates of emotional problems such as anxiety and depression; developmental disorders; higher rates of arrest and involvement with police or courts; and greater misuse of drugs. Moreover, as noted by Rouse, Waller, and Ewing (1973), children of alcoholic fathers may show less variety in their coping behavior than controls. They resort to solitary activities (for example, cigarette smoking and trying to forget) whereas children of abstainers are more likely to cope with stress by talking with friends and relatives. Furthermore, Wilson and Orford comment that the nondrinking parent's role can be crucial in helping the child to cope. If the at-risk child resides with a single alcoholic parent, however, the prospects for this form of palliation are minimal. Similar findings have been reported by Nardi (1981). His literature review suggests that the impact of severe parental disturbance on children is often mediated by social and cultural factors. Since not every child is affected by the alcoholic parent in the same way, social and psychological mediating forces come into play. In particular, Nardi contends that the children of alcoholics are confronted by confused and inconsistent parental expectations.

Benson (1980) studied 240 students and women employees at a major university. The daughters of alcoholics reported more neurotic symptoms and scored higher on a measure of acting-out pathology than did daughters of normal fathers. However, a similar elevation of neurotic symptoms was found among the daughters of psychiatrically disturbed fathers. While the daughters of alcoholic fathers had a very high rate of alcoholism, it was not significantly different from the alcoholism rates found among other groups of subjects. Family climate and social support variables were found to be more powerful predictors of the daughter's current adjustment than her father's history of alcoholism or psychiatric illness.

Cork (1969) interviewed 115 middle-class and upper-class children aged ten to sixteen years. More than 90% expressed a lack of self-confidence and feelings of being unloved and rejected by one or both parents, and more than 50% reported anger toward and disrespect for the alcoholic parent and resentment toward the nonalcoholic parent. They perceived the latter as responsible for the alcoholic parent's drinking and neglectful of their own needs. Similarly, Wilson and Orford (1978) found that the extreme tension and argumentativeness in alcoholic families was more upsetting to the child than parental drinking itself. When youths in such families compared their families to those of friends, they frequently reported that theirs was not a "real family:" they were less likely to do things together and to have fun as a family unit. Morehouse (1979) found that at-risk children were confused by the different types of drinking behavior and parental moods exhibited when their alcoholic parent fluctuated between sobriety and drunkeness. The children tended to blame themselves for the parent's drinking and to equate the drinking problem with being unloved. Finally, in one of the most recent and comprehensive literature reviews, Russell, Henderson, and Blume (1985) concluded that family dynamics may play a more crucial role than parental modeling in the development of drinking patterns among children. They suggest that the major sources of stress in alcoholic families are poor communication, permissiveness and undersocialization of the children, familial role ambivalance, a family environment of tension, violence, and neglect, and broken homes.

Alcoholism and Affective Disorders

After an extensive review of the available literature, Lord (1983) noted that "alcoholism" is treated as an independent variable in most studies even though it can represent a conglomerate of conditions. A number of factors are often associated with parental alcoholism, including family disunity, depletion of finances, and maternal deprivation or overprotection. Therefore, it is necessary to separate parental "alcoholism" from moderating variables that might influence the mental health of offspring. Furthermore, alcoholism may be associated with such maladies as depression (Russell, Henderson, and Blume 1985). Schuckit (1982) cites four studies which found that as many as one-third to one-half of alcoholics display depressive symptoms at some time during the course of their illness. Likewise, Weissman (1984) found a consistent pattern, for both sexes and all ages, in which depression is associated with alcoholism. However, it is difficult to isolate the causal relationship between these two phenomena. Cloninger, Reich, and Wetzel (1979) have reported that alcoholism and depression not only coexist in individuals but aggregate in the same families. Schuckit (1982) suggests that this is due in part to assortative mating. That is, alcoholic men may tend to be attracted to and marry depressed women, or vice versa, and the increased risk for these two disorders may then be passed on to their children. In one study, Schuckit and Chiles (1978) found that alcoholic or antisocial behavior on the part of parents was associated with depression in 37% of offspring. Finally, in this regard, several longitudinal studies have found that depressive symptomatology and self-derogation tend to precede drug use (cf. Kandel 1978; Kaplan 1980; Kaplan and Pokorny 1976; Kaplan, Lander, Weinhold, and Shenker 1984).

Alcoholism and Antisocial Personality Disorders

Antisocial personality disorder, or sociopathy, like depression, is found more often than expected by chance in individuals who are alcoholic or who are reared in alcoholic families. As Solomon and Hanson (1982) note, many of the behaviors and patterns characteristic of antisocial personality disorders also apply to the alcohol abuser. The longitudinal research of Robins, Bates, and O'Neal (1962) found that children referred to a clinic for antisocial behavior developed more alcoholism as adults than a control group. These adult alcoholics resembled adult sociopaths not only in their childhood behavior problems but also in their family background—they had a pronounced history of broken homes and behaviorally disturbed siblings. Frances, Timms, and Bucky (1980) likewise report that alcoholics from families with extensive drinking exhibit more antisocial behavior. And, following a prospective study of 456 boys, Vaillant (1983) concluded that alcoholism may lead to sociopathy more often than vice versa.

Herjanic, Herjanic, Penick, Tomellein, and Armbruster (1977) studied the incidence of behavior problems and psychiatric disorders in eighty-two children of alcoholics and sixty-seven control children of nonalcoholics who were patients in a pediatric clinic. In the adolescent group, the children of alcoholics showed significantly more deviant behavior and were twice as likely to receive a psychiatric diagnosis as controls. The children of alcoholics evidenced more problems at home, antisocial behavior, alcohol and drug use, and suspension from school; they were also the only group of children in whom a diagnosis of conduct disorder could be made. More recently, Gibbs (1982) studied forty-eight delinquent females. She found that patterns of substance abuse vary by delinquent personality type, with antisocial personalities exhibiting the greatest alcohol and drug abuse. Drug-abusing subjects, in particular, manifested more frequent self-mutilating behavior, sexual promiscuity, hostile feelings, sarcastic affect, defiant behavior, running away, and fighting. Similar findings also have been reported in a review by El-Guebaly and Offord (1977).

In sum, it is evident that substance-abusing parents often exert potent adverse effects on their at-risk children. While large numbers of at-risk youngsters may become substance abusers, they may also manifest other psychosocial pathologies, as exemplified by the results of a study by Schuckit and Chiles (1978). Psychiatric diagnostic patterns were examined in two different samples of adolescents, one a group of psychiatric inpatients and the other apprehended by the law for alcohol-related difficulties. Parental affective disorders were most closely correlated with a similar patient diagnosis or constellation of depressive-type symptoms in both samples. Parental antisocial personality, alcohol abuse, and drug problems correlated most closely with high levels of similar difficulties in individuals in the two study groups. However, antisocial, alcohol, or drug problems of a mild degree were present in all subgroups of the two samples, perhaps representing a nonspecific reaction to parental illness or to the occurrence of a broken home. Subjects who experienced broken homes demonstrated a consistently higher level of antisocial problems even when parental diagnosis was controlled. These findings differ little from those which report that the severity of a parent's disturbance is more predictive of schizophrenia in the child than is the particular type of disturbance (cf. Waring and Ricks 1965).

SUMMARY AND DISCUSSION

Although a number of clear trends appear in the literature, it is obvious that conclusions about the relationship between parental mental illness and childhood risk must be couched in guarded terms, due to both methodological weaknesses of the literature and a plethora of fragmentary and inconsistent findings. From a methodological perspective, the extant research concerning parental mental illness and childhood risk remains in a relatively primitive state of development. Very few studies examine the systematic interrelationships among genetic and environmental factors, and the handful that do are rudimentary. Key variables usually are defined in nominal—and often dichotomous—terms such as "fostered-away" versus "raised with biological parents," "schizophrenic parents" versus "other parents," "ill parents" versus "well parents," "delinquent" versus "nondelinquent," and so forth. Ordinal and interval classifications would be more useful for purposes of research, clinical diagnosis, and practical intervention. Moreover, only a handful of prospective studies, limited in size and representativeness, appear in the available literature. The analytic procedures employed in the extant studies tend to be univariate and cross-sectional. Many studies do not utilize control groups, comparison groups, or standardized procedures for assessing at-risk children and their relationships with parents, siblings, and peers.

For the most part, the available data indicate that the children of mentally ill parents are at far greater risk for some types of disorders than are children in the general population. However, several qualifications must be noted. Although biological influences, genetic predispositions, and stress-diathesis formulations can be invoked to account for childhood risk, it is obvious that socioenvironmental factors play a major, if not prepotent, role in the onset of childhood behavior disorders. Children of parents with a major psychiatric disorder (for example, schizophrenia, an affective or depressive disorder, antisocial personality disorder, or substance abuse disorder) are at comparatively higher risk for that particular type of disorder than are other children. Nevertheless, the parent's illness is not necessarily the foremost cause of disturbance in the child. Peak risk periods vary from one kind of disorder to another. Thus, the peak risk period for the onset of schizophrenia ranges from eighteen through forty-five years of age, while the peak risk periods for affective disorders and conduct disorders begin at much younger ages. Not all children of mentally ill parents manifest a behavior disorder, nor do all children react similarly to their parent's mental illness. Only a minority of high-risk children are likely to have the same type of psychiatric illness exhibited by their parent. Nevertheless, the available data suggest that a substantial majority of high-risk children are likely to have *some* kind of major or minor sociobehavioral or psychiatric disorder as they progress toward adulthood. It cannot be stated conclusively, however, that the incidences for these latter forms of disorder are significantly higher than the ones for children who do *not* have psychiatrically ill parents.

A child's risk appears to increase according to the proportion of mentally ill "significant others" who regularly interact with him or her. Specifically, risk is increased if two parents, rather than one, are mentally ill, and it increases in accord with the number of mentally ill siblings in the family. Indeed, higher risk seems to be associated with the total number of siblings in a family, regardless of their particular mental health status. For many kinds of childhood mental illness, risk status seems to be associated with such variables as the type of parental mental illness, duration of parental hospitalization, length of time since onset of a parent's illness, socioeconomic status, race, family size, marital discord, removal of the child from hospitalized or separated parents, residential mobility, and the absence of community supports for the family and the at-risk child. The effects of these variables seem to be mediated in a complex fashion by their interactions with other factors. Consequently, their effects are not uniform in all circumstances. While such variables typically are studied *in vacuo* and in a univariate manner, it is essential to recognize that they usually interact with one another. Consequently, future studies must attempt to examine their interactive and longitudinal relationships.

Although up to 85% of children with schizophrenic parents may have some type of major or minor sociobehavioral disorder, the same apparently can be said for up to 70% of children with "normal" parents. Moreover, the former children evidently are not at significantly higher risk than the latter for nonschizophrenic psychoses or psychoneuroses. Although there are clear differences between the symptomatologies of schizophrenic and depressive parents, the symptomatologies of the majority of their children tend to have a great deal in common. Consequently, it is difficult, if not impossible, to distinguish the preponderance of high-risk children from one another merely on the basis of their parent's diagnosis. Childhood conduct disorders and juvenile delinquency tend to be associated with delinquency or criminality on the part of parents. Yet, they can also be linked with other types of parental mental illness. The majority of children with criminal parents are at high-risk for delinquent behavior or conduct disorders. However, factors such as marital discord and inconsistent patterns of childrearing are even better predictors of childhood conduct disorder than are parental criminology itself.

Despite some evidence to the contrary, the chronicity and severity of parental mental illness appear to be better predictors of childhood disorder than the parent's specific diagnostic label. The parent's effects upon the at-risk child are related most directly to the ways in which the child is involved in the parent's symptomatology, the modes of social interaction that the parent establishes and maintains with the child, and the quality of complementary or alternative care available to the child and the family. Little consensus exists about the peak periods of vulnerability for high-risk children. Some studies suggest that the peak period occurs before two or three years of age; others posit that the peak risk period occurs between two years of age and adolescence, while even others suggest that the peak ages are from five to six years and eleven to twelve years. In all likelihood, the peak risk periods for childhood mental illness cannot be derived solely from knowledge about a parent's diagnosis or the onset of the parent's mental illness. These periods are variable. They can be best understood by examining the longitudinal interplay among many factors, including the modes of behavior directed toward the child by his or her parent, the availability of a healthy parent or parental surrogate in the family, and the presence of formal or informal support systems.

Similarly, little consensus exists regarding whether or not the relationship between parental mental illness and childhood behavior disorder is sex-linked. In many instances, the mother seems to be the more influential parent in the transmission of mental illness, especially for conduct disorders, regardless of whether the child is male or female. For other types of parental disorders, however, it is neither absolutely nor consistently clear how sex linkages are manifested, if at all, between mentally ill parents and their offspring. Comprehension of this phenomenon tends to be obscured by a variety of confounding factors including assortative mating, one-parent families, and serial changes of one parent or another due to separation, remarriage, or liaisons among parents and caregivers.

Despite the presence of a number of clear trends, the interrelationships among parental mental illness and childhood risk are complex, multifaceted, and changeable over time. The webs in which children are enmeshed are intricate. Yet, not all children necessarily are victimized by them. Rigorous research concerning these factors—based upon a social and ecological perspective which examines the child within the total environment—must become increasingly multivariate, interactive, and longitudinal. However imperfectly applied, this is the basic approach we shall pursue throughout the present volume. Its results will shed light upon some of the unresolved issues we have discussed in this literature review.

3 Current Conceptions of the Invulnerable Child

IN THEIR REVIEW OF THE MANY FORCES THAT SHAPE children's behavior, Julius Segal and Herbert Yahraes (1978, 1) have posed many of the same questions that guide the present research:

> What determines the course of a child's mental health? Is it accidents of heredity—the roulette wheel of genes and chromosomes—or the child-rearing strategies of parents? Is it the impact of friends, the quality of family life, the stresses of our society, or is a child, as psychologists strongly believed just a few decades ago, simply "born that way"? What is it that causes one child to be aggressive and another passive, withdrawn or friendly, depressed or optimistic, focused on goals and achievements or mired in self-depreciation and defeat? Moreover, why do some children, although beset by massive trauma, bend but never break, while others appear to crumble in the face of apparently far lesser stress?

Simply, what makes one child especially vulnerable to adverse life stresses while another remains seemingly invincible? To inform our consideration of these questions and others, it is essential to understand why invulnerable children have become of interest to researchers during the last decade or so.

As Clausen (1968) observed nearly two decades ago, evaluations of an individual's behavior must deal with positive performance as well as symptoms and improvements. Comprehensive assessments are necessary to determine the overall functioning of an individual and to promote effective treatment planning. Traditionally, however, helping professionals have restricted their diagnoses to the pathologies, dysfunctions, and behavioral problems of clients. Thus, as Garmezy (1974a) has commented, diagnoses focus primarily upon disorder and not on adaptation, on breakdown under stress and not on the elements of "rally" in the face of adversity. Likewise, they concentrate on individual stimulus and response rather than environmental cause and reaction. Only in the last decade have investigators sought to analyze the longitudinal interactions among these important sets of variables.

Even more, mental health professionals frequently diagnose malfunctioning individuals *in vacuo*, especially in traditional forms of therapy where *psycho*pathology is predominant. Many theoretical formulations about human maladaptation and professional intervention ignore key environmental variables that influence behavior, such as the family, peer group, school, and neighborhood. Only a small minority of helping professionals identify themselves as *social* psychiatrists, *social* psychologists, or *social* group workers.

In their zeal to discover the causes and cures of individual dysfunction, researchers and helping professionals have greatly neglected those human beings who manage to function well despite prolonged exposure to formidable stressors. Clinicians and researchers strive to learn about human behavior by studying individuals who fall victim to stressors rather than by studying persons who are invincible to them; this bias severely hampers our ability to learn how human beings cope with stress. Furthermore, most mental health professionals have adopted a "medical model" of human behavior that permeates not only their conceptions of "vulnerability" but also their views of "invulnerability." For instance, some investigators have sought doggedly to discover an "innoculation" against mental illness, but such an approach is based upon a simplistic interpretation of the dynamics that underlie mental health and mental illness.

Efforts to learn about children's invulnerability to mental illness have been hindered by a number of factors. In large part, the social sciences and the helping professions have failed to coordinate or integrate their efforts to understand childhood invulnerability. Their research literatures, operational arenas, and professional associations tend to be insulated and isolated from one another. As a result, few mechanisms exist for ongoing collegial interchange about shared problems of research and practice.

Nevertheless, in recent years there has been increasing appreciation of the need to study "invulnerable," as well as "vulnerable," children. In large part, this follows significant conceptual and methodological advances in the social sciences and the helping professions, especially in epidemiological, longitudinal, and ecological research. These studies have revealed important associations between parental mental illness and childhood mental health (see chapter 2) and also between childhood mental health and adult risk; they have dramatized the utility of assessing individuals' adaptive as well as maladaptive behavioral patterns. Moreover, recent research has shown the value of assessing subjects in natural social settings such as families, schools, peer groups, and neighborhoods. Also, advances in multivariate and interactive analyses have enabled researchers to investigate the complex interrelationships among key determinants and correlates of mental health.

Concomitant with such advances, important organizational and associational changes have occurred within the social sciences and the helping professions. For example, the young field of developmental psychopathology has brought together a growing number of psychologists interested in the epidemiology of mental illness and mental health (see Cicchetti 1984) and in the complex interactions among variables that affect mental health (Rolf and Read 1984; Sroufe and Rutter 1984). These trends have renewed interest in the psychological and social factors that conduce toward invulnerability.

In the wake of such advances, we must take stock of the resulting knowledge. It is essential to consider what is known about children vulnerable to mental illness and, even more importantly, invulnerable to it. Accordingly, it is germane to examine the linkages between the scientific conceptions and empirical data that serve either to inform or to becloud our efforts to learn about such children.

VULNERABLE OR INVULNERABLE?

Rigorous empirical studies about invulnerable children have appeared in the research literature during the past two decades. Although the accretion of pertinent research is obvious, the resultant knowledge has not yet attained a critical mass because, in part, the literature is characterized by much definitional and semantic confusion. This is typical in the early developmental phases of any field. Marked progress usually does not occur until a consensus emerges among key investigators about basic definitions and measurement procedures. Unfortunately, such consensus does not yet exist among the handful of investigators who study invulnerable children.

Many, if not most, problems in research about vulnerability stem from uncertainties about the very definition of this construct. These problems appear in several forms: first, definitions of vulnerability are framed primarily in terms of risk status; second, while the concepts of vulnerability and invulnerability should constitute polar opposites, they usually are framed in terms that do not reflect this understanding; and third, researchers have used many different descriptors to denote an essentially unitary construct. We must examine each issue to understand the vast potential, as well as the unfulfilled promise, of research concerning invulnerable children.

Vulnerability and Risk Status

A major problem inheres in the literature about childhood mental health. That is, vulnerable is sometimes employed synonymously with high-risk, but at other times it modifies this construct. Goldston (1977, 20), for instance, asserts that primary prevention "encompasses activities directed toward specifically identified vulnerable high risk groups within the community who have not been labeled psychiatrically ill and for whom measures can be undertaken to avoid the onset of emotional disturbance and/or to enhance their level of positive mental health." Such language substantially obscures the relationship between vulnerability and risk status. Should an individual's vulnerability and high-risk status be considered equivalents of one another? Or, alternatively, is vulnerability deemed orthogonal to risk status, thereby implying that high-risk individuals may be either vulnerable or invulnerable? If the latter, what specific meanings are to be attached to vulnerability?

What criteria should be applied to define a vulnerable child? In mental health research, the usual practice is to denote a child's risk status in terms of his or her parents' mental health. As explicated in chapter 2, most researchers consider a child to be at high risk if one of the child's parents has had a history of mental illness. The extent of risk varies in accord with such considerations as the type and duration of parental illness and age of onset. In virtually all forms of mental illness, a child's risk status increases markedly if both parents are ill. Thus, risk status is usually defined by a rudimentary exogenous variable (that is, which resides in the external environment of the child), namely, the presence or absence of mental illness on the part of a parent.

While this approach to defining vulnerability may be of some predictive value, it is seriously flawed in two major respects. First, the determination of the child's risk status is univariate. Even though a parent's mental health may be a reasonable predictor of a child's future well-being, it explains only a small portion of the pertinent variance. Clinical experience shows that other exogenous variables, as well as important endogenous factors (that is, those characteristic of the individual child himself or herself), also account for a child's mental health. Second, this criterion takes no cognizance of the child's unique strengths and weaknesses. All children who have parents with a given mental health profile are assumed to be at relatively equal risk. But the child's vulnerability results from complex interactions among a broad range of exogenous and endogenous variables that influence mental health.

Invulnerability and Risk Status

A fundamental paradox is evident in the literature about childhood mental health. Vulnerability is typically defined in terms of exogenous variables, such as parents' mental health, but invulnerability is usually defined in terms of endogenous variables, such as the child's coping skills. Yet, the preponderance of research concerning childhood mental health suffers from a pronounced psychological determinism that pervades current conceptions of pathology. Unfortunately, however, this mode of determinism also shapes contemporary views of adaptive behavior. While the main source of vulnerability is deemed external to the child, the youngster's *in*vulnerability is thought to stem almost exclusively from internal sources. Hence, invulnerable children are thought to possess extraordinary coping skills that enable them to withstand severe stresses which might adversely affect lesser human beings. Little recognition is accorded to the many extraindividual factors that enable a child to resist stress.

Invulnerable or Invincible? Superkid or Superphrenic?

Many criteria have been employed to define childhood vulnerability to mental illness. However, the most evident feature of the literature about invulnerable children is its emphasis upon putative coping skills. Invulnerable children are deemed extraordinarily capable of caring for themselves in the midst of adversity; indeed, they often seem to thrive in the face of misfortune. Thus, following his well-known study of the offspring of schizophrenic parents, Bleuler (1974, 106) remarked that "one is left with the impression that pain and suffering can have a steeling—a hardening—effect on some children, rendering them capable of mastering life with all its obstacles, just to spite their inherent disadvantages." Furthermore, he suggests, "it would be instructive for future investigators to keep as careful watch on the favorable development of the majority of these children as they do on the progressive deterioration of the sick minority."

Unfortunately, however, the literature reveals that a wide array of labels is used to describe such children. Among other things, these remarkable youngsters have been called invulnerables, invincibles, superkids, superphrenics, and stress-resistant children. To advance research in this crucial area, it is essential to understand both the manifest and the latent distinctions among such terms and, even more, to devise labels that promote rather than hinder systematic study.

INVULNERABLE CHILDREN

The research literature about invulnerable children has been shaped substantially by the germinal work of several well-known scholars who merit special attention. Their contributions are the foundation for important, later studies by researchers from a variety of disciplines.

Contributions of E. James Anthony

Anthony's work regarding invulnerability has evolved, interestingly, from investigations that focused initially upon children considered at high risk for mental illness. In 1968 he initiated a longitudinal study of 141 children who had at least one schizophrenic or manic-depressive parent. In the course of this research, Anthony and his colleagues discovered that highly vulnerable children could be identified on the basis of close involvement and identification with the psychotic parent and, also, in conjunction with such personality traits as submissiveness and suggestibility. In their judgment, these attributes often led a youngster to internalize the distorted perceptual and cognitive world of the psychotic parent.

In the course of a subsequent study, Anthony and his associates identified nineteen High Vulnerable children and twenty-one Low Vulnerable children. The former attained scores of five or more on a vulnerability rating scale, while the latter had scores of zero or one. High scores depended on the child's identification with the sick parent, credulity about parental delusions, influence of parental illness on the child, undue submissiveness, undue suggestibility, and involvement with the ill parent (indicated by the child's expressed desire to live with that parent and by inclusion of the parent in the child's wishes and dreams). Analyses showed that 62% of the Low Vulnerables were well-adjusted children, but only 10% of the High Vulnerables were well-adjusted.

The investigators found several factors instrumental in protecting the Low Vulnerables from the impact of a parent's mental illness. Among these were the child's ability to "stand away" psychologically from the sick parent and to defend against submissive involvements that could lead to the adoption of disturbed thought processes. Confidence and a "healthy skepticism" also helped to protect these high-risk children (Anthony 1975; Lander, Anthony, Cass, Franklin, and Bass 1978). As a result of his work with the children of psychotic parents, Anthony (1974) formulated a model in which the commonly encountered childhood risks and chronic stresses were grouped under several major headings — genetic, reproductive, constitutional, developmental, physical, environmental, and traumatic. Each subtype was evaluated separately along seven dimensions of risk, and vulnerability was measured by the degree of involvement with the psychotic parent. Standardized tests and psychiatric interviews were employed in the investigations.

In related work, Anthony and his colleagues also attended to the family's role in shaping childhood mental illness (cf., for example, Anthony and Koupernik 1978). But, while their studies greatly expanded our knowledge about the ecological and environmental forces that shape vulnerability, Anthony and his associates construed *in*vulnerability in much narrower terms, namely, the unique personal strengths of the at-risk child. Although this perspective occurs frequently in the early stages of research or conceptualization, it nevertheless remains limiting. Moreover, some of Anthony's important contributions to the literature have been obscured because he employs different labels in his studies of childhood behavior. Thus, the distinctions among vulnerable, invulnerable, high vulnerable, low vulnerable, and superphrenic children are not always clear.

Contributions of Norman Garmezy

Utilizing a somewhat different perspective, Garmezy and Nuechterlein (1972) examined childhood risk by reviewing the literature on competent, but economically disadvantaged, youngsters. Such children were deemed to be "healthy children who live in an unhealthy setting" (Garmezy 1971). As stated succinctly by Garmezy (1974b, 107):

> These children possess social skills; they are friendly and well liked by peers in contrast to less adaptive children of comparable social status who are often lethargic, tense, sullen, and restless; these are children of interpersonal ease who are capable of relating to adults as well as to their peers in the course of play and social exchange. Such children also show self-regard rather than self-derogation; they see positive attributes in themselves and sense a quality of personal power for influencing events in their environment in contrast to the powerlessness that permeates the self-perceptions of less adequate peers; they are intellectually competent, tending to perform well in school; they bring to their test behavior an appropriate sense of caution which may relate to an important criterion of maturity, namely, "impulse control" and "reflectivity." They are children who are highly motivated to perform well; "apathy" is not a way of life for them. Their families are not necessarily intact; father absence is not an uncommon feature, but there is order to their homes in the sense that an organization is imposed not only on the physical environment but on time itself.

Despite extreme economic impoverishment, the parents of such children are considered by Garmezy to be "competence-inducing." As Elder (1974) has shown in a sophisticated longitudinal study, it is indeed true that economic impoverishment need not result in mentally ill or incompetent children as long as their parents are healthy enough to help the family cope with its economic plight. But, since Garmezy and Nuechterlein studied families in which the parents were well-adjusted, albeit financially stressed, one wonders if their findings would have been the same if the parents had been mentally ill?

Garmezy was one of the first to assert that studies of high-risk children must distinguish clearly between youngsters who behave maladaptively and those who behave adaptively. As he has noted, the preponderant research emphasizes "failures of adaptation because that is our literature." Yet, "it is equally, if not more, important that we be able to identify and study the stress-resistant children among our risk populations" (1974, 108). Indeed, the long-term benefits of studying invulnerable children may be much more meaningful for society than efforts that aim merely to remediate youngsters who have already succumbed to environmental stressors.

In similar fashion, Garmezy has urged investigators to distinguish between "high-risk adaptive" children and "high-risk maladaptive" children. Simple as this distinction may seem, it represents an important step in the elaboration of a useful mental health lexicon. It is based upon an important pair of assumptions: risk status derives mainly from external stressors which impinge upon a child, and adaptation refers to personal coping skills which enable the child to withstand stress. With several important extensions, these distinctions provide the basis for the model of childhood vulnerability that appears in chapter 4.

Garmezy has referred to invulnerable children as youngsters who "bear the visible indices that are hallmarks of competence: good peer relations, academic achievement, commitment to education and to purposeful life goals, early and successful work histories" (1971, 114). Although one cannot quarrel with his indicators of competence—except, perhaps, to cite certain omissions—Garmezy here introduces an emphasis that characterizes most mental health literature. He understates the reciprocal interplay between personal coping skills and environmental stressors by couching his definition of invulnerability primarily in personal terms. Analogously, he considers invulnerable children to be individuals who "are seemingly immunized against disorganization." Here, too, he defines a child's status essentially in terms of the personal ability to withstand stress, but it is obvious that protective factors within children's environments must also contribute to their invulnerability.

In accord with this mode of analysis, Garmezy has proposed that the prevention of mental illness be achieved by "innoculating" children against disorder (1974b, 109). He suggests that youngsters be trained in mastery techniques that might be able to sustain them in times of adversity. This conception has provided the framework for a well-known program of preventive intervention by Spivack and Shure (1977). But, as noted earlier, such an innovation strategy is predicated upon a "medical model" that may not be altogether valid for vulnerable children because the ultimate responsibility for preventing stress is imposed upon the vulnerable child. Little cognizance is taken of the preventive or supportive assistance that can be provided by families, peers, teachers, and other relevant parties.

More recently, the title of one of Garmezy's key research programs, namely, Project Competence, reflects a continuing emphasis upon the individual determinants of invulnerability (Garmezy, Masten, and Tellegen 1984). In this program, the main criteria of childhood competence include the following:

1. Effectiveness in work, play, and love; satisfactory educational and occupational progress; peer regard and friendships.
2. Healthy expectancies and the belief that "good outcomes" will follow from the imposition of effort and initiative; an orientation to success rather than the anticipation of failure in performing tasks; a realistic level of aspiration unbeclouded by unrealistically high or low goal-setting behaviors.
3. Self-esteem, feelings of personal worthiness, a proper evaluation set toward self and a sense of "fate control," that is, the belief that one can control events in one's environment rather than being a passive victim of them (an internal as opposed to external locus of control).
4. Control and regulation of impulsive drives; the ability to adopt a reflective as opposed to an impulsive style in coping with problem situations.
5. The ability to think abstractly; to approach new situations flexibly and to be able to attempt alternate solutions to a problem. (Garmezy, 1974a, 86)

In Project Competence, Garmezy further conceptualizes invulnerability in terms of the interaction between two variables central to the present study—stress and adaptation. Using these variables, he elaborates a simple 2×2 matrix that delineates four separate childhood statuses (see figure 3.1). Invulnerable, or stress-resistant, children, who adapt well although exposed to severe situational stresses (see cell 1), are characterized by high stress and high adaptation. In contrast, children denoted by cell 2 live in low-stress situations and adapt well. Regardless of whether this set of circumstances is normative in American society, it is certainly the preferred one. Garmezy's vulnerable children, depicted by cell 3, live under high stress and adapt poorly.

Figure 3.1.
Child's Mental Health Status (Adapted from Garmezy 1981, 253)

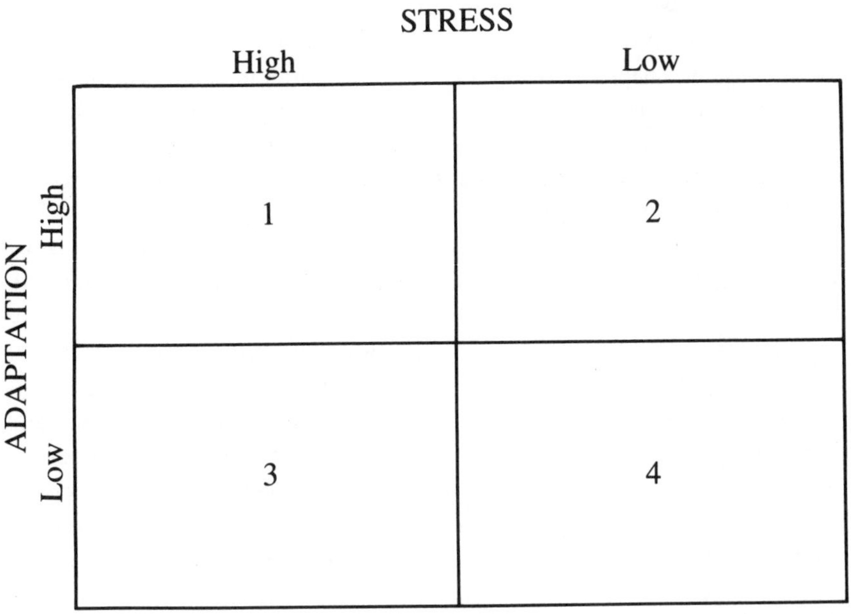

STRESS

Finally, the children depicted in cell 4 have "an even lower threshold of vulnerability, as signaled by their adaptive failure despite relatively low levels of environmental stress" (1981, 253).

Although this model of vulnerability proceeds far beyond Garmezy's earlier psychological determinism, it remains deficient in several key respects. It is likely, for instance, that the children depicted by cell 3 are not only vulnerable to mental illness but, more important, will fall victim to it. By definition, they are subjected to high stress while their coping skills are deficient; hence, they are unlikely to resist such stressors for very long. Their vulnerable status is bound to deteriorate rapidly in view of the marked imbalance between environmental stressors and personal coping skills. A child's triumph over such circumstances is more likely due to significant environmental protectors or social supports than to exceptional coping skills. Furthermore, unlike Garmezy we regard the children in cell 1 as vulnerable —rather than invulnerable—to mental illness. Even though their adaptive skills are strong, these children are threatened by formidable stressors. Given the tenuous balance between their stressors and personal coping skills, it is unwarranted to assume they are truly invulnerable.

For similar reasons, we consider the children depicted by cell 4 to be vulnerable to mental illness. Since their low-stress situation is offset by coping skills that are even weaker than the extant stressors (weak as the latter may be) these children clearly are vulnerable to mental illness. Finally, using the terminology in chapter 4, we posit that the children in cell 2 will be invincible to mental illness. These youngsters have strong coping skills, but they are unlikely to need them given their weak environmental stressors.

In some of his most recent work, Garmezy explicitly considers the role of several exogenous factors that help children remain invulnerable to stress. Although he still emphasizes the high-risk child's personal ability to resist stress, greater attention is paid to environmental variables. Consistent with his earlier conception, Garmezy asserts that children who cope well usually have high self-esteem and a sense of control. They are especially confident when dealing with others and are highly intelligent, as denoted by their reflectivity, problem-solving abilities, social awareness, creative thinking, and sense of humor. However, he also emphasizes the crucial role of a supportive family environment. Garmezy points out, for instance, that invulnerable children frequently have at least one parent or a relative who looks out for their interests or who allows them autonomy in the performance of everyday tasks. In addition, an external support system is crucial since invulnerable children tend to be encouraged and strengthened by social networks that inculcate positive values (*Alcohol, Drug Abuse and Mental Health News*, 16 May 1983).

Garmezy's recent work (1981) also recognizes the interactive effects of environmental stressors and personal coping skills upon vulnerability. It emphasizes two major aspects of children's lives: (1) the presence of sustained and intense life stresses and (2) the maintenance of mastery and competence despite stress exposure. Accordingly, he recognizes the two major sets of factors that determine childhood vulnerability to mental illness. By considering the juxtaposition of these factors, Garmezy lays the groundwork for recognizing the importance of the "ordinary," as opposed to the "extraordinary," nature of invulnerable children. While some vulnerable youngsters may become superachievers despite environmental stress, they obviously are a minority. Luminaries such as Ludwig von Beethoven, Thomas Edison, Helen Keller, Franz Kafka, and T. E. Lawrence—disadvantaged as they were during childhood—are distinct exceptions. Indeed, as Garmezy rightly comments, a "focus on eminence, whether from the viewpoint of the cradle or the rocking chair, can cause us to lose sight of the many children and adults who lead ordinary lives and who are not destined for greatness, but whose very 'ordinariness' can be an accomplishment when placed against the highly traumatizing backgrounds out of which they have come" (1981, 216).

In sum, Garmezy's research has greatly stimulated the study of invulnerable children, but shifting definitions of invulnerability and childhood risk have obscured some of his major contributions to this vital area of study. Nevertheless his work has progressed steadily toward an ecological and interactive perspective. Using Garmezy's work as a point of departure, we posit that childhood behavioral outcomes should be conceptualized in the form of a continuum that ranges from the status of "victim" to the status of "invincible." Even more, we contend that vulnerability is determined by the *relative balance* between environmental stressors and personal coping skills.

Contributions of Michael Rutter

Although a psychiatrist by training, Rutter's research about invulnerable children has been well-informed for many years by an epidemiological perspective. More than a decade ago, he noted properly that much research about vulnerable children was concerned merely with establishing statistical associations for a variety of risk factors. Delinquency, for example, had been associated with broken homes, educational problems with low socioeconomic status, and mental retardation with perinatal complications; however, such associations do little to guide the clinician. An association merely indicates probabilities for the practitioner, but it does not reveal why the association exists or how the pertinent risk factors operate. As Rutter has commented, clinicians need to know about the mechanisms that activate statistical associations and about the factors that modify them or ameliorate the effects of risk factors. In short, a clinician "must know why some children succumb and some escape and what he can do to alter the balance of probabilities in the child's favor" (1974, 168).

Drawing upon extensive field research, Rutter (1974) has delineated five epidemiological strategies that can shed light upon the dynamics of childhood invulnerability. First, and most common, high-risk populations can be defined by means of pertinent background variables, such as parental mental illness. Second, they can be defined by means of factors that refer to the child, such as the presence of organic brain pathology. Third, studies of the general population can be performed to determine patterned variations in vulnerability or invulnerability. A fourth strategy involves the comparison of two populations or areas that differ in their rates of disorder, and a fifth entails the implementation of cross-generational studies. As several findings from Rutter's research illustrate, these differing approaches extend our conception of invulnerability from one that is narrowly psychiatric to one that is interactive, contextual, and ecological.

In one study, Rutter examined all of the families in a London borough who had a child under fifteen years of age plus a parent who had been referred to a psychiatric clinic for a mental health disorder. Unlike many investigators, Rutter was interested less in the fact that certain children are at high risk for psychiatric disorder than in the factors which account for some children succumbing and others escaping from the adverse effects of their risk status. He found that separation from both parents for a period of at least one continuous month is associated with behavioral disturbance in high-risk children from homes characterized by marital discord. The same association was not found among children from harmonious homes. Hence, the particular reason for a separation—rather than separation itself—appears to be the crucial variable in accounting for childhood disorder.

Related analyses demonstrated that parental separation had no ill effects if it were due to a prolonged holiday away from the family or to hospitalization because of a physical illness. In contrast, if a separation were due to family discord or parental mental illness, it clearly exerted an adverse impact upon the child. That is, family discord did more damage to high-risk children than separation, which was "incidental or at most contributory" (169). Moreover, the disorders of high-risk children were largely restricted to conduct disorders rather than emotional or neurotic disturbances. In effect, then, careful epidemiological analysis highlighted the role of subtle second- and third-order relationships.

Rutter also attempted to identify a number of mediating variables that enable invulnerable children to resist stress. Some of these pertain directly to the child's family; for instance, a good relationship with one parent was found to be an important mediating factor. Even among children in discordant and quarrelsome families, those who had one good relationship with a parent were somewhat protected from disorder. While such a relationship did not wholly eliminate the adverse effects of family discord, it clearly weakened them. A second mediating factor was a change to a happier home situation, which did not undo previous damage but at least ameliorated it. Hence, Rutter concluded that the early years of childhood, while influential in generating disordered behavior, are not as critical as had previously been supposed.

Besides identifying family-related mediating factors, Rutter also delineated modifying factors among high-risk children themselves. One is the child's sex. Put simply, boys were much more susceptible than girls to the effects of family discord (Rutter 1970). Similarly, temperamental features in early childhood were predictive of later behavioral disturbance. The most susceptible children were highly irregular in sleeping and eating patterns, nonfastidious, and nonmalleable. Such children presumably found it difficult to adapt to the needs of a changing environment and, perhaps as a result, tended to be the targets of parental criticism. Hence, a child's undesirable characteristics influence parental behavior, which, in turn, may shape psychiatric disorder on the child's part.

In a comparative study of two different populations (namely, all the ten-year-olds in an inner London borough and all the ten-year-olds on the Isle of Wight), Rutter found four sets of factors associated with childhood psychiatric disorder. Each was more prevalent in London than on the Isle of Wight. Respectively, these are family discord and disruption, various forms of parental deviance, social disadvantage (due to such factors as large family size and overcrowded homes), and attendance in schools characterized by high rates of both teacher and pupil turnover. As in the earlier cited studies, family breakup was found in both settings. However, broken homes in London were associated with behavioral deviance, while this seldom was the case on the Isle of Wight. Again, further analyses revealed factors associated differentially with these findings. On the Isle of Wight, for example, a higher proportion of family breakup was due to adoption or parental death (as opposed to separation or divorce). Single mothers in London were less likely to remarry, thus leaving their children with an unsupported parent. Also, remarried parents in London were more likely to have their second marriage result in discord or disharmony. In short, Rutter's findings once again led to the conclusion "that it is not separation as such which is most crucial, but rather it is the circumstances leading to separation, present during separation, and operating after separation which are most important" (1974, 176). These findings and others encouraged subsequent investigators to concentrate increasingly upon the epidemiology of childhood vulnerability and upon the environmental factors that both shape, and are shaped by, the child's coping skills.

Contributions of Spring and Zubin

In the past decade, the contributions of Anthony, Garmezy, and Rutter have been extended substantially by a number of other investigators. By focusing on the vulnerability of adults to schizophrenic episodes, Spring and Zubin (1977), for instance, have advanced a conception of vulnerability that has greatly influenced our own formulation of this important phenomenon. Three

Figure 3.2.

Relationship between Vulnerability and Life Event Stressors
(From Spring and Zubin 1977, 265)

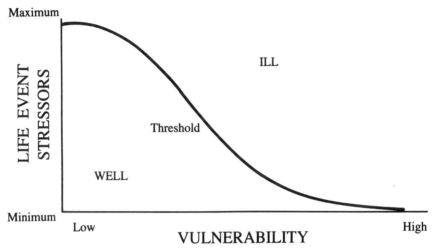

variables are central to their discussion—life event stressors, vulnerability, and competence. In brief, Spring and Zubin define vulnerability in terms of "the constitutional factors (internal) that set the threshold at which stressful life events will catapult an individual into an episode of mental illness" (276). Vulnerability is regarded as an enduring trait that entails "the ability to withstand the stresses induced by life events" (278). Their model of the interrelationships among life event stressors, vulnerability, and a person's mental illness or well-being is depicted succinctly in figure 3.2. In their view, so long as one's stressors remain below a "threshold of vulnerability," the individual will respond in a flexible manner and remain within the limits of normality. But, when stress exceeds the threshold, an individual is likely to experience a psychopathological episode.

Central to this model is the assumption that schizophrenia is an episodic phenomenon rather than a chronic state. Episodes are elicited when life-event stressors surpass the threshold determined by an individual's characteristic level of vulnerability. Hence, Spring and Zubin regard the schizophrenic not as a permanently sick individual, but as "a permanently vulnerable one" (277). By emphasizing life-event stressors as a determinant of risk status, their perspective is congruent with the one we articulate in chapter 4. And, by regarding an individual's ability to withstand stress as an important determinant of outcomes, their model even further approximates our own. Unlike most investigators, Spring and Zubin contend it is improper to presume that the same skills and dispositions which promote competence also are sources of invulnerability to mental illness. In fact, they reject the notion that competence and invulnerability are equivalents; rather they hypothesize that competence is orthogonal to vulnerability. Thus, "highly competent individuals can have all grades of vulnerability, and relatively incompetent folk can be highly vulnerable or quite immune to mental illness" (269).

Their rationales for the foregoing distinction are compelling. First, pending the systematic collection of conclusive data about the interrelationships between these two variables, it is best to assume the null hypothesis and to "avoid incorporating unsubstantiated dogma into the literature" (269). Second, there is a small pool of evidence which suggests that the two variables may, in fact, be independent dimensions. Third, measures of competence and vulnerability appear to have distinctly different uses in psychopathology research. Whereas indicators of vulnerability "measure the likelihood that an individual will succumb" to an episode of mental illness, "a sharp dip in a patient's characteristic level of competence permits us to detect the episode's onset, and a return to the premorbid baseline signals the episode's end" (269).

Spring and Zubin contend that research findings about the relationship between competence and vulnerability are difficult to assess because few studies have unambiguously measured either variable. But they note:

> In considering the relationship between stresses induced by life event stressors and competence, we must not assume that stressful life events are found more often in those of low competence and hence that we should expect the occurrence of episodes more frequently in the low competence groups. Only if the low competence individual is also highly vulnerable will an episode be elicited; and whether high vulnerability occurs more often in those of low competence is not established. It is possible that because the highly vulnerable tend to have more episodes, their competence may wear thin even if it was high to begin with. This downward drift of initially competent patients may contribute to the appearance of a relationship between low competence and high frequency of episodes (1977, 272).

The distinction between vulnerability and competence is welcome since it addresses a badly neglected issue in the mental health literature. Also, the inclusion of environmental stressors and individual competencies in the model represents a distinct advance beyond previous formulations. Most important, perhaps, Spring and Zubin are among the few investigators who articulate a model of vulnerability predicated explicitly upon the relative balance between an individual's environmental stressors and his or her personal coping skills. The major flaws in their exposition inhere in sometimes employing vulnerability as an equivalent of personal coping skills and simultaneously regarding it as an enduring trait. These deficiencies are acceptable ones, however, in view of the fact that their model clearly operationalizes vulnerability in terms of the relative contributions of environmental stressors and personal coping skills.

Contributions of Werner and Smith

Finally, it is germane to mention a noteworthy program of field research by Werner and Smith (1982). One of their studies has substantially foreshadowed our own approach toward the investigation of childhood behavior disorders. Known as the Kauai (Hawaii) Longitudinal Study, it is unique in its examination of all pregnancies and births which occurred in an entire community and across a wide socioeconomic and ethnic spectrum. They followed more than 600 subjects for nearly two decades. The title of their report, *Vulnerable But Invincible: A Study of Resilient Children*, succinctly summarizes its major emphases. The Kauai study is the only one to our knowledge that clearly distinguishes between two concepts especially central to our own research—vulnerability and invincibility. Although Werner and Smith do not explicitly define either concept, they propose a research model that readily permits one to infer the basic distinctions between them.

In brief, they regard vulnerable children as youngsters who have been exposed to major risk factors such as chronic poverty, uneducated mothers, moderate to severe perinatal complications, developmental delays or irregularities, genetic abnormalities, and parental psychopathology. Invincible children are those who, despite such exposure, develop into competent and autonomous young adults who "work well, play well, love well, and expect well" (3). Vulnerability, in their view, is shaped by major environmental stressors (prolonged separation from a primary caretaker, chronic family discord, change of schools), protective factors within the child (birth order, responsiveness to people, autonomy, self-help skills), and key sources of support (the availability of kin and neighbors, close peer friends, access to social services). These variables mediate the effects of major risk factors and thereby shape a child's vulnerability to mental illness; in turn, as some investigators fail to acknowledge, they are partially shaped by the child's shifting vulnerability. Again, however, a key protective factor within the child is his or her coping skills, or adaptation in the face of challenges, frustrations, threats, and other difficult circumstances.

In Werner and Smith's model, the foregoing factors yield a broad range of probable developmental outcomes for any particular child. At the one extreme, a child's outcomes may be adaptive; this is likely when there are few stressful events and many protective factors within the child or the caregiving environment. At the other extreme, a child's outcomes may be maladaptive; this is likely when there are greater numbers of stressful events and fewer protective factors. Hence, their model incorporates the major sets of variables that inevitably influence childhood outcomes, namely, environmental stressors, environmental supports, and protective factors that flow from the child's personal abilities. In addition, the model assumes variations in outcomes that range from adaptive to maladaptive. Importantly, it defines vulnerability in terms of the relationship between environmental stressors and personal coping skills. Yet, invincibility is defined in terms of the actual behavioral outcomes experienced by a given youngster. Finally, the model adopts an ecological perspective that enables the investigators to examine interactions among many different variables influencing childhood outcomes. But, while Werner and Smith have laid a firm foundation for the model of childhood vulnerability that appears in chapter 4, others have propounded labels that tend to obscure the interrelationships among the key determinants of childhood mental illness.

SUPERKIDS

In 1979, Maya Pines introduced the term "superkids" to the mental health literature. This term refers to children "who thrive where others break" (53). Throughout her discussion, however, Pines merely regards superkids as exceptionally invulnerable children. In this regard, she departs markedly from Garmezy's focus upon youngsters whose mere "ordinariness" is remarkable in the face of traumatic circumstances. Although the superkid label lends drama and flair to this area of study, its emphasis upon extraordinary individual coping reflects a pronounced psychological determinism.

In describing the attributes of superkids, Pines reiterates the basic characteristics usually ascribed to invulnerables: they are at exceptional ease in social situations; they know how to attract and use the support of adults; despite major difficulties they actively master their environments and have a sense of their own power; they think for themselves and develop a high degree of autonomy early in life; and they are achievers who generally do well at most tasks they undertake. Pines suggests that several distinct conditions conduce toward superkid status. For instance, prospective superkids must have a good relationship with at least one adult, particularly during the first few years of life. In our view, however, the popularized superkids label merely heightens the conceptual and semantic confusion pertaining to childhood invulnerability. Its referents differ hardly, if at all, from those of invulnerable children.

Nonetheless, one particular investigation that employs the superkids label is worthy of special consideration. Kauffman, Grunebaum, Cohler, and Gamer (1979) conducted a follow-up study of thirty mentally ill women (eighteen with a diagnosis of schizophrenia and twelve with bipolar or unipolar affective psychosis) and their children. The mothers received intensive home nursing aftercare subsequent to their discharge from a psychiatric hospital. In addition, a comparison group of twenty-two well mothers was studied. The children's competence was examined by means of Anthony's six-point scale: (1) psychopathology, (2) peer relationships, (3) academic functioning, (4) hobbies and areas of interest or expertise, (5) cognitive development and deployment of attention, and (6) behavior exhibited during testing, interview, or observation. The children were rank-ordered by means of a summary competence score. The six subjects who were ranked most and least competent in both the ill-parent and well-parent groups were selected for more detailed study. The investigators labeled the "most competent" children in the high-risk group as superkids; of these children, three had schizophrenic mothers, two had schizo-affective mothers, and one had a depressed mother. In the "least competent" group of high-risk children, five had depressed mothers.

Among the high-risk subjects, the six least competent children had mothers who received the lowest scores on a level-of-functioning scale. In contrast, the mothers of the most competent children showed more frequent social contacts, higher efficiency in working outside the home, and greater ability to meet their own needs than the mothers of the least competent children. Also, they had more satisfying social relationships and fewer symptoms characteristic of psychiatric illness. All of the children in the most competent group had received caring attention from their mothers during the seven years that preceded the study, but such attention was absent in the histories of the least competent children. The mothers of the latter children were regarded by the research staff as unresponsive, vague, abrupt, and intrusive. Five of the six most competent children reported extensive contacts with an adult outside the family, while none of the least competent children had such relationships. Furthermore, four of the six most competent youngsters had at least one very close friend, while four of the six least competent children reported no special friendships. Interestingly, the most competent children from the well families were neither as outstanding nor as creative as those from the most competent high-risk families.

Besides reaffirming the importance of the child-mother relationship, these data suggest that a child can be made less vulnerable by exposing him or her to well-functioning individuals outside the family, thereby reducing the "density" of the child's association with malfunctioning individuals or role models. Hence, the at-risk child is not viewed *in vacuo*. While a designation of "maternal mental illness" may establish that a child is at high risk, it is *not* sufficient to foredoom a child to mental illness. Kauffman and his associates report that serious psychopathology does not necessarily diminish a mother's ability to become involved with her child in a warm and supportive manner. A child's vulnerability or invulnerability depends essentially on how the mother's illness is manifested, her social, psychological, and behavioral resources, and the extent to which the child's coping skills can offset the adverse effects of maternal malfunctioning and other stressors.

The Kauffman, Grunebaum, Cohler, and Gamer data indicate that severe maternal depression exerts a stronger adverse impact on a child than maternal schizophrenia. As a result, these investigators suggest that the apathy and lethargy of severely distressed mothers has a more deleterious effect than the alterations of mood and cognitive disturbance characteristic of schizophrenic mothers. Furthermore, they posit that socially isolated women, whose impaired functioning provides a poor model for the child, are more likely than others to have low-competence children. Also, the mother's isolation tends to restrict the child's social ties and prevent the development of extensive and intensive social relations. Indeed, as a mother becomes isolated from social ties, she may depend increasingly on her child for support, thus creating a symbiotic relationship that represents a form of *folie à deux*. Furthermore, the frequent hospitalizations of such mothers are likely to disrupt their children's development. Unlike Anthony's "superphrenic" children, these superkids maintain important relationships with peers and adults. Their success does not occur at the expense of close and satisfying relationships with others; instead, they have many friends, high self-esteem, and an impressive array of talents. Nevertheless, because their brothers and sisters appear to be far less successful, they may have unique personality characteristics that enable them to resist stress. Alternatively, they may be differentially exposed to extrafamilial sources of support that heighten their ability to withstand stress.

Although the findings of Kauffman and his associates are informative, their sample is very small. Moreover, the subjects' ages do not appear in their report. Yet, the importance of adequate social relationships with one's family, peers, and other adults is vividly demonstrated by their research. Even though a child's status as a superkid may depend basically upon his or her individual competencies, the influential role of relevant others is evident. Unfortunately, however, while this study distinguishes clearly between environmental stressors and individual abilities, its focus is restricted solely to extraordinary youngsters. Little attention is accorded to children whose ordinariness is remarkable in the face of traumatic circumstances.

SUPERPHRENICS

In contrast with the foregoing labels, a handful of investigators have employed the term "superphrenic" to describe invulnerable children. Like superkids, this label usually connotes that an at-risk child is functioning not only at an adequate level but, in fact, at a superior level. Karlsson (1968), for example, reported in an Icelandic genealogical study that many gifted scholars, political figures, and community leaders had psychotic relatives. He labeled the gifted individuals as "superphrenics." Similarly, Anthony (1972) used this term to describe "outstanding" children—9% of his high-risk sample—born into schizophrenic households. They were regarded as "supernormal" youngsters who developed "remarkable capacities to adapt to the corrosive pressure of mental illness among their parents." In contrast, 12% of Anthony's subjects were "average" or "well-adjusted"; about 32% were somewhat maladjusted or neurotic, albeit of a mild and transient nature; another 31% were "shy, seclusive, sensitive, or apathetic"; and 16% were regarded as odd, queer, peculiar, strange, or "crazy."

In retrospect, the proliferation of terms such as invulnerable, superkid, and superphrenic has hindered, rather than facilitated, systematic research about childhood mental illness. Contradictory and inconsistent criteria have been employed to study invulnerable children. Conceptual and semantic difficulties are exacerbated when a multitude of labels are applied in ambiguous, inappropriate, or inconsistent ways. A sound ecological, longitudinal, and interactive model of childhood invulnerability must consider the interrelationships among a child's environmental stressors and individual coping skills in a logical, systematic, and consistent fashion. Most important, the model's labels must be derived from a coherent theoretical framework and operationalized in a manner consistent with that framework.

SUMMARY

This chapter reviewed pertinent conceptions and research findings about invulnerable children in order to lay the groundwork for the social interaction model of childhood vulnerability articulated in chapter 4. Concomitantly, this chapter explored the manifestations and causes of current conceptual, semantic, and measurement problems regarding childhood invulnerability. Common denotations such as invulnerable, superkid, and superphrenic were examined to ascertain their similarities and differences. The review demonstrates that a myriad of meanings is ascribed to the foregoing constructs. In some instances definitions are redundant; in others, a single construct is subjected to a variety of inconsistent or incompatible interpretations. Nonetheless, it is evident that progress has been made in studies that examine how high-risk children avoid mental illness. Most important, perhaps, the review indicates that the relative contributions of environmental stressors and individual coping skills must be systematically recognized in forthcoming models of childhood invulnerability.

4 A Social Interaction Model

THE LITERATURE REVIEW IN THE PRECEDING CHAPTERS shows that a variety of factors determine whether or not a high-risk child will experience a behavior disorder at some point during the life course. As explained in chapter 3, many investigators contend that the key factor which enables a child to withstand mental illness is his or her personal capabilities or traits—termed variously as coping skills, behavioral competencies, and stress-resistance. In brief, such investigators invoke a *trait model* of childhood disorder deeply grounded in the disciplines of psychiatry and psychology. Because these are the leading clinical professions, the trait model has dominated theoretical and practical conceptions of mental health until today. In contrast, other investigators assume that environmental stressors are the key variables that determine whether or not a child will become mentally ill. They employ a situational or *environmental model* of childhood disorder essentially grounded in the disciplines of sociology and human ecology. In conjunction with research and methodological advances in the latter disciplines, the environmental model has gained considerable credence during the past two decades. Yet, to date, this perspective has been integrated only minimally into the intervention repertoires of the helping professions.

In our judgment, both perspectives must be considered in formulating a viable model of vulnerability to mental illness or behavior disorder. By itself, neither is sufficiently inclusive to explain the complexities of childhood resistance to parental mental illness. In this chapter, therefore, we propose that childhood behavior disorders are a consequence of the interaction and relative balance between stressful or protective environments and strong or weak personal coping skills. We posit that all environments can vary along a continuum that ranges from decidedly protective, on the one hand, to decidedly stressful, on the other; likewise, we posit that personal coping skills can range along a continuum that varies from decidedly strong to decidedly weak. Hence, we introduce a *social interaction* model of vulnerability to parental mental illness grounded essentially in social psychology. In clinical practice, this model has been employed most frequently by professionals who specialize in social group work or social psychiatry. Eventually, the helping professions are bound to adopt such a model as they strive to establish realistic, multivariate, and cost-effective intervention programs for children at high risk for behavior problems.

With few exceptions (see, for instance, Bell and Pearl 1982), most predictive models of childhood behavior disorders are static and univariate. Moreover, as noted previously, little consensus exists among investigators regarding the preferred definitions, referents, and operationalizations of such key terms as invulnerable, invincible, superkid, and superphrenic. Clinicians and researchers typically have defined childhood vulnerability solely in terms of a given child's coping skills. Yet, if it is true that an invulnerable youngster is a "healthy child in an unhealthy setting" (Garmezy 1974a), it is also obvious that a child's environment must play a crucial role in the definition of his or her mental health status. Unfortunately, however, most conceptions of unhealthy childhood settings are quite rudimentary. Usually, it is assumed that a child's environmental setting is unhealthy, or high-risk, if either or both of the child's parents are mentally ill. However, this conception ignores the previously documented fact that most children who reside in such settings are free of diagnosable or observable mental illness. Indeed, such settings are high-risk only when they are contrasted with other settings in which neither parent is mentally ill. For the most part, they are distinctly low-risk settings for the youngsters who reside in them.

Neither the trait model nor the environmental model enables one to fully comprehend the true dynamics of childhood risk. Even though they are the predominant models in the literature, they are relatively sterile for predictive and clinical purposes. Consequently, we contend that childhood risk status must be defined primarily on the basis of the mutual interaction and relative balance between environmental stressors or protectors and a child's ability to cope. Given such desiderata, a child's risk status is likely to be reflected in his or her behavioral outcomes or, in other words, by the presence or absence of a discernible behavior disorder. According to such a model, a child exposed to a stressful environment is *not* necessarily considered at high risk so long as he or she has exceptionally strong coping skills. Conversely, a child with weak coping skills is not necessarily at high risk so long as his or her environment is a protective one in which the extant environmental protectors are stronger than the extant environmental stressors. Such a model is relative and interactive rather than absolute and static.

BEHAVIOR DISORDERS, ENVIRONMENTAL STRESSORS AND PROTECTORS, AND PERSONAL COPING SKILLS

Three sets of variables are of central importance for the model of childhood vulnerability posited here: childhood behavior disorders, environmental stressors and protectors, and personal coping skills. The interplay among the latter two variables determines the nature of the former; that is, whether a particular child will be vulnerable to parental mental illness, a victim of it, or invincible to it. Figure 4.1 succinctly summarizes the model that provides the foundation for our research.

Childhood Behavior Disorders

The current research focuses on the presence or absence of serious behavior disorders in a sample of high-risk children ($n = 306$) who range in age from six through sixteen years. The research attempts to identify the key similarities and differences that exist among three types of children who have mentally ill parents: (1) children who have fallen victim to their parents' mental illness, (2) children who are vulnerable to their parents' mental illness but have not yet fallen victim to it, and (3) children who seemingly are invincible to their parents' mental illness. To distinguish among these children it is necessary to employ a measurement system that can differentiate discretely and reliably among large numbers of youngsters characterized, to various degrees, by either the presence or the absence of severe behavioral problems.

   In the present study, we employ a recently developed diagnostic instrument that attempts to gauge childhood behavior disorders in interval form. The Child Behavior Checklist (CBCL), devised by Thomas Achenbach and Craig Edelbrock (1981), is utilized to assess the presence or absence of a broad range of behavior problems on the part of children who participated in the research. The CBCL is a parent-report checklist that yields a comprehensive profile of any particular child's problem behaviors. A T-score, ranging from 0 to 100, can be calculated for any child on the basis of parental judgements regarding whether or not each of 118 problem behaviors is characteristic of the child. Information regarding normative scores for the CBCL and their utilization in the present research is provided in chapter 5.

   Achenbach and Edelbrock report that T-scores of 63 or above are indicative of a clinically-significant behavior disorder on the part of a child. Typically, children with such scores can be regarded as "victims" of mental illness. This criterion corresponds to the 90th percentile for a sample of youths from the general population (Achenbach and Edelbrock 1981); that is, only 10% of the children in the general population can be expected to register a

Figure 4.1.

Net Environmental Protectors and Stressors, Personal Coping Skills, and Childhood Vulnerability to Mental Illness

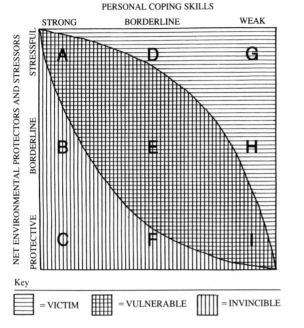

FIELD CHARACTERISTICS

A. Stressful Environment Strong Coping Skills
B. Borderline Environment Strong Coping Skills
C. Protective Environment Strong Coping Skills
D. Stressful Environment Borderline Coping Skills
E. Borderline Environment Borderline Coping Skills
F. Protective Environment Borderline Coping Skills
G. Stressful Environment Weak Coping Skills
H. Borderline Environment Weak Coping Skills
I. Protective Environment Weak Coping Skills

CBCL T-score of 63 or above. Children with CBCL T-scores in the lowest 10% of the general population have T-scores that range from 0 through 37. Since they seldom exhibit discernible behavior problems they can be regarded as invincibles. In contrast, most children have T-scores that fall between these two points—37 and 63. Although these children are not definitively free of behavioral problems, neither do they manifest clinically-significant problem behaviors. Hence, such children can be regarded as vulnerables. Approximately 40% of a parametric sample of children from the general population can be expected to manifest scores within this range.

As with all clinical diagnoses, it is imperative to emphasize that any behavioral label necessarily must be limited by time and context. Thus, while a particular child may have been invincible to mental illness when the CBCL was first administered, this designation should not connote an unchangeable mental health status. Depending on the interplay of environmental factors, personal coping skills, and other desiderata, one's mental health and behavior can change dramatically at any point in the life cycle. This caveat also applies to the victim and vulnerable labels. Indeed, it pertains to all clinical classifications, including delinquent, schizophrenic, and, even, mentally retarded. As we have discussed elsewhere (Feldman 1978), it is essential for diagnostic lexicons and labels to be devised in a logical and systematic fashion. Moreover, it is necessary to examine them at periodic intervals so that behavioral changes can be detected quickly and pertinent labels revised accordingly.

Environmental Stressors and Protectors

The risk factors that shape childhood behavior disorders are legion. Despite —or, perhaps, because of—this profusion, the vast majority of investigators heretofore have simply deemed children to be at high risk whenever one or both of their parents are mentally ill. Important as this criterion may be, however, it is only one among a large array of potential risk factors. It is evident that children who fall victim to parental mental illness are adversely affected by a myriad of factors that act concurrently and interactively.

Chapter 3 notes some of the environmental stressors that constitute key risk factors for children including parental unemployment, low socioeconomic status, frequent geographic mobility, marital discord, and large family size. While most investigators assume that such variables are either additive or exponential in their effects, the validity of this assumption remains virtually unexamined from the perspective of systematic empirical research. Obviously, any particular individual can be exposed to risk factors that range along a continuum in terms of their number and/or the stress they engender. Moreover, such factors undoubtedly vary over time, being at high levels during acute crises and at lower levels after such crises have subsided.

It is important to recognize that any particular individual can be aided by environmental protectors which provide insulation from factors that can adversely affect mental health. These, too, can vary along a continuum in terms of their quantity and/or the amount of protection that they afford. Examples include parental employment, high socioeconomic status, happily married parents, supportive peer groups, and accessible social services.

We submit that it is the net balance between pertinent environmental stressors and environmental protectors that essentially determines whether or not a child will develop a behavior disorder. Importantly, this conception suggests that an environment characterized by strong protectors need not necessarily be a "protective" environment. Likewise, an environment characterized by formidable environmental stressors is not necessarily a "stressful" environment. Rather, it is the *net balance* between stressors and protectors which determines whether a particular environment can be regarded as healthy or unhealthy or, more specifically, as protective or stressful. We view a stressful environment, then, as one in which the extant stressors clearly exceed the extant protectors; conversely, we regard a protective environment as one in which the extant protectors exceed the extant stressors. And a borderline environment is one in which the pertinent stressors and protectors are approximately equal in strength; that is, since neither set of factors clearly surpasses the other in strength, a highly fluid situation results.

In terms of this conception, environments can be arrayed along a continuum which, for heuristic purposes, varies from "protective" to "borderline" to "stressful." All other things being equal, it is posited that a decided surfeit of environmental stressors (vis-à-vis protectors) results in a high likelihood of behavior disorder on the part of a child. Likewise, a relatively equal balance between environmental stressors and protectors presupposes a moderate likelihood of disorder while a decided surfeit of environmental protectors (vis-à-vis stressors) suggests a low likelihood of disorder. We recognize, of course, that all stressors and protectors cannot be accorded equal weight in terms of their influence on childhood behavioral outcomes. Nor can it typically be assumed that all factors are truly equal in the real world. Nevertheless, for heuristic purposes it is helpful in the initial stages of model construction to accord relatively equal weight to the key factors under consideration. In the last section of this volume we will employ empirical data to ascertain the differential predictive potency of a large array of environmental stressors and protectors.

Personal Coping Skills

Many researchers define invulnerable youngsters solely in terms of their stress-resistance, suggesting, of course, that such children possess unique skills or competencies that enable them to cope satisfactorily with the environmental stressors impinging upon them. However, because most studies do not quantify pertinent environmental stressors, research concerning both vulnerable and invulnerable children tends to view them *in vacuo*. Definitions of children's mental health are based solely upon their coping skills. Little attention is paid to the extent of environmental stress or protection that affects the high-risk child nor, in turn, to the resulting demands placed on the child's repertoire of coping skills.

In the present discussion, coping skills refer to the unique personal abilities that enable a child to resist significant environmental stressors. Examples include the child's cognitive and problem-solving abilities, perceptual acuity, persistence, assertiveness, ability to make and sustain friendships, and related competencies. Like environmental stressors and protectors, these skills may expand or deteriorate over time. Coping skills, too, can be arrayed along a continuum which, for heuristic purposes, varies from strong to borderline to weak. All things being equal, it is posited that children with weak coping skills will have a relatively high likelihood of disordered behavior, whereas children with borderline coping skills will have a moderate likelihood of disordered behavior. Since their behavioral strengths will clearly exceed their deficits, children with strong coping skills will have only a low likelihood of disordered behavior. In the present study, however, all other variables are not, in fact, held equal. Rather, all key factors are presumed to vary along a bipolar continuum.

VICTIMS, VULNERABLES, AND INVINCIBLES: A PRELIMINARY MODEL

In the course of their comprehensive longitudinal study of vulnerability, coping, and growth among infants, Lois Murphy and Alice Moriarity (1976, 201) posed a rather fundamental question: does "normality" on a child's part necessarily imply "invulnerability"? Because certain babies in their study seemed to possess important coping skills, they were judged to be at low-risk for behavior problems. In fact, all of the infants in their research had been selected as subjects precisely because they were judged to be "normal." All had demonstrated superior intelligence and strong coping skills. Yet, several of the subjects clearly needed some sort of professional help or therapy before they reached midadolescence. During the critical prepubertal phase, moreover, a majority also exhibited discernible speech problems. Obviously, then, strong coping skills alone were not sufficient to assure the well-being of children who appeared to be normal or even superior when they had been infants.

Unlike the vast majority of investigators, we do not regard a child as invincible simply because he or she has superior, or even extraordinary, coping skills. Such skills undoubtedly ought to serve a youngster in good stead whenever he or she is confronted with weak, or even moderate, environmental stressors that conduce toward disordered behavior. But they are likely to be of little help when a child is faced with environmental stressors overwhelming in quantity or severity. Conversely, we do not necessarily regard a child as invincible if he or she is confronted with only negligible environmental stressors. While most children would be quite secure in such circumstances, others would be highly vulnerable if their coping skills are weak. Hence, we base the determination of any child's vulnerability or invulnerability on the relative balance between that child's coping skills and the net environmental stressors or protectors to which the child is exposed.

The main features of this model of childhood vulnerability are set forth in figure 4.1. As indicated, coping skills are arrayed here along a continuum ranging from strong to borderline to weak. Likewise, the social environments that confront any child are arrayed along a continuum ranging from stressful to borderline to protective. Somewhat similarly, a child's potential vulnerability to a behavior disorder or mental illness also is deemed to vary along a continuum that encompasses, respectively, the statuses of victim, vulnerable, and invincible. The model should not imply that the relationships among these variables are static; rather, as the at-risk child develops, the variables are dynamic, constantly shaping one another in a reciprocal and interactive fashion.

In brief, the model posits that a child is likely to fall victim to a behavior disorder or mental illness when his or her coping skills are significantly weaker than the net environmental stressors and protectors to which the child is exposed. Conversely, a child is likely to be invincible to a behavior disorder or mental illness if his or her coping skills are significantly stronger than the net environmental stressors and protectors encountered. A child is likely to remain vulnerable to a behavior disorder or mental illness, in contrast, if his or her coping skills are neither significantly stronger nor significantly weaker than the net environmental stressors and protectors. In such instances, it is neither altogether evident that the child has sufficient coping skills to prevail against the extant stressors and protectors, nor is it clear that these factors will overwhelm the child's coping abilities.

The research and interventive implications of this model of childhood vulnerability are manifold. For example, various combinations of these factors can differentially affect a child's vulnerability (see figure 4.1). These can be determined on the basis of the mutual interactions among stressful, borderline, or protective environments and strong, borderline, or weak coping skills. The distribution of probable victims, vulnerables, and invincibles in figure 4.1 follows from the fact that the two main predictors (personal coping skills and net environmental protectors and stressors) are conceptualized as continua. For purposes of illustration and discussion, this distribution can be arrayed in terms of nine overlapping "fields" that portray the juxtaposition of the two main predictors. In three of these fields, the net environmental stress clearly exceeds the child's coping skills; therefore, children located within these fields are likely to be victims of a behavior disorder or mental illness.

In three other fields, the child's coping skills clearly exceed the net environmental stress; these children are likely to be invincibles. And, in the three other instances, the child's coping skills and net environmental stressors and protectors are approximately equal in strength; such children are vulnerables. Nonetheless, there are unique differences among victims, vulnerables, and invincibles of considerable importance for practice and research.

Vulnerable Children

In figure 4.1, children depicted by fields A, E, and I of the model (the cross-hatched areas) tend to be quite similar to one another in an important respect: they are all clearly susceptible to behavior disorders, thus resulting in their designation as vulnerable children. However, these children differ markedly from each other when one examines the interrelationships among their respective coping skills and net environmental stressors and protectors. Contrary to popular expectation, perhaps, the children in field A exhibit strong coping skills. Yet, they are vulnerable because, on balance, they are also exposed to a stressful environment that can neutralize their available coping skills. When one encounters extreme stress, even superior coping skills cannot assure that a behavior disorder will be averted.

Children depicted by field I of the model are also considered to be vulnerable. Here, however, the vulnerable child is faced with a relatively protective environment. While most children are likely to remain healthy in such circumstances, the youngsters in field I are vulnerable because they possess weak coping skills. Indeed, as suggested by fields G and H, such children are likely to become victims of a behavior disorder or mental illness if they subsequently are confronted by either a borderline or a stressful environment.

The model also postulates a third genre of vulnerable child—one whose borderline coping skills are threatened by a borderline environment (that is, an environment in which the pertinent stressors and protectors are equipotent). This probably represents one of the more common childhood conditions, albeit one that is, we hope, less prevalent than the circumstances depicted in fields D, G, or H. Because of the unstable situation entailed by their vulnerability, the children in field E are likely to drift toward invincible status if there is either a slight improvement in their coping skills (field B) or a slight reduction in net environmental stress (field F). Conversely, they are likely to drift toward victim status if there is a gain in net environmental stress (field D) or if their coping skills should deteriorate (field H).

Systematic empirical investigation eventually ought to be able to determine which of these three sets of presenting conditions is most prevalent among children of varying ages and social backgrounds. Is it possible, for instance, that the majority of vulnerable youngsters have strong coping skills neutralized by stressful environments? Or, alternatively, are they confronted by borderline or protective environments that nonetheless prove to be crippling given inadequate coping skills on their part? The model suggests even further that the kinds of vulnerable children depicted in field A can be helped best—and, perhaps, only—when mental health interventions are directed toward key environmental stressors and protectors rather than toward their personal coping skills. Traditional clinical therapies are likely to be of little use for such youngsters because their coping skills are already at high levels. Instead, it would seem more productive for intervention agents to weaken the environmental stressors that impinge upon such youngsters or to strengthen pertinent environmental protectors. For the children depicted in field I, conversely, the preferred modes of intervention would be more traditional since these children's environmental protectors are relatively strong. Little should be done to strengthen them further; however, in view of their weak coping skills, it would seem fruitful to help such youngsters develop competencies enabling them to avert behavioral problems. Thus, as noted previously, one could attempt to strengthen their problem-solving skills, assertiveness, frustration tolerance, and related social skills. In contrast, the vulnerable children depicted by field E would benefit most from a multipronged intervention strategy aimed to reduce environmental stressors and strengthen environmental protectors while concurrently enhancing personal coping skills. If successful, such a strategy would enable these youngsters to progress from the status of vulnerable to invincible.

Case Illustration: Meeting a Vulnerable Child. During the course of our research we became well-acquainted with many vulnerable children. One, in particular, offers a vivid illustration of our conception of vulnerability. The most salient features of this case suggest that the child more closely typifies the presenting conditions depicted in field E rather than field A or field I.

> Bub is eight years old, and he is a "vulnerable." We first meet Bub when his social worker brings him and his younger sister to the intake interview. Bub is short and stocky with thick eyeglasses, a round face and a firm stance. He stands close to his sister and behind the interviewers. He and his sister giggle together on the way into the room. When the interviewers approach, he stares straight ahead as if daydreaming. When he is daydreaming, he looks upward without focusing. He smiles and shakes hands.
>
> Bub doesn't talk much at first. When he does speak, however, he talks so softly that it is difficult to understand. He is quite willing to respond to the interviewer's questions but he doesn't make conversation. Bub is only in kindergarten. With much embarrassment he mutters that he "can't read good."

Last month, when he moved into foster care from his parents' home, the social worker discovered that Bub couldn't see very well. He and his sister were moved immediately to a study home for a full evaluation. The social worker explains that they are studying Bub and his sister because they aren't sure how much of their behavior is due to physical problems. Two weeks before the interview, Bub had the first of several operations to correct crossed eyes. He describes the facts of the operation in short two- or three-word sentences. He graphically describes an ointment that he must use and how it makes things blurry. Bub doesn't talk about his feelings. But his voice registers pride in being important enough to receive special treatment. When asked directly about his feelings, Bub shrugs his shoulders, unable to find an answer. He has great difficulty with the portion of the interview which requires reading and writing. He brings the page within three inches of his right eye. That, of course, prevents him from accurately copying shapes or letters.

Bub has lived all of his life with a sister, two brothers, and his mother and father. He has six older half-brothers and sisters, but he has never lived with them. His mother is fifty-two years old. He says that his family, as a whole, has had problems getting along together but that he and his mother have never had any problems. He is very close to his sister, who is one year younger. Throughout the interview Bub and his sister excuse themselves from their respective interviewers in order to huddle together and to compare recollections. Bub tells us about spending all day, every day with his mother and sister. His mom evidently was very affectionate. She wanted to keep the youngest children close to her and frequently made cakes or treats for them. When, after the interview, Bub is asked if anything else has happened to him that we didn't talk about, he tells us about his mother in a matter-of-fact fashion. "She fell asleep, and my Dad burned her hair." Bub's father is a paranoid schizophrenic. Although he functioned well for a number of years, the father has suffered a sudden relapse. "When Mom take a nap, he pour kerosene on her hair and light it. She still in hospital."

Bub loosens up by the end of the interview. He smiles readily and offers information about what he likes to do and what he likes to eat. He begins to talk about the study home and his friends who live there. He stresses several times that he and his sister are there together and that they see each other all the time.

When Bub is offered cookies and is urged to help himself, he rapidly eats one after another. Each time he looks up quickly for permission to take the next cookie. After devouring half a box, the interviewer asks him to wait awhile before eating the next cookie so that he won't get sick. He readily acquiesces. Upon leaving the interview Bub asks for more cookies and chooses two handfuls which are stuffed into his pockets. As he leaves, Bub grabs his sister's hand, skips a few steps and proudly explains to the social worker that he did a good job and that he and his sister will be coming back to join an activity group. He and his sister recite all the things that they will do with their new "friends."

Postscript: Bub and his sister attended our service-research program on a regular basis. After five months they were moved to a permanent children's home but continued to participate in the activity group. Bub learned to read, and he began to close the gap between his age and achievement level.

Victimized Children

Figure 4.1 also clearly illustrates the plight of children who are likely to become victims of behavioral problems. While three different sets of victimizing conditions are postulated in the model, a common feature characterizes all of them: the environmental stressors to which these children are exposed significantly outweigh the coping skills and environmental protectors that can be brought to bear against them. Popular conceptions of the behaviorally-disordered child often exemplify the situation depicted in field G. Here the child with weak coping skills is confronted by a decidedly stressful environment. Because such children are severely disadvantaged in two major respects (namely, weak coping skills and a stressful environment), it is probable that they are victimized to a much greater extent than are the children depicted by either field D or field H. Their status as a victim is likely to be far more stable and irremediable than for other children. To the extent possible, professional interventions should aim to help such children by reducing their environmental stress, strengthening their environmental protectors, and enhancing their personal coping skills.

In fields D and H, the gap between the child's coping skills and net environmental stressors is smaller than in the preceding case. Nevertheless, several key distinctions characterize the two former situations. In field D the child's borderline coping skills are inadequate when he or she is confronted by a decidedly stressful environment. In field H, the child's net environmental stress is merely borderline, but the child is likely to succumb to that stress because of deficient coping skills.

In fields D and H, the child's plight is not as immutable as in field G, and the probability of developing a behavior disorder is lower. Nevertheless, interventions should be directed simultaneously toward the reduction of environmental stressors, strengthening of environmental protectors, and enhancement of personal coping skills. Given the relatively extreme environmental stress depicted in field D, however, somewhat greater attention should be directed toward its diminution than toward enhancement of the child's coping skills. Conversely, perhaps, intervention efforts directed toward the children in field H ought to concentrate more on the enhancement of coping skills than on the reduction of environmental stressors or strengthening of environmental protectors.

Case Illustration: Meeting a Victim. As with the vulnerable children, the characteristics of any particular victim do not always fit neatly and exclusively into one cell or another of the model. Nevertheless, we recall one child who substantially exemplifies the type of victim illustrated by field D.

Tory is thirteen years old and he is a "victim." We first meet Tory for an intake interview at his home. He lives in a downtown area that is newly fashionable among upwardly mobile young families who are rehabilitating older homes. Tory's apartment is on a street with a new brick sidewalk that is lined with green saplings. In seeking his house, we proceed to a narrow garbage-strewn alley between a warehouse and a brick residence. Three broken stairs lead to a center hallway that is mildewed and peeling. Cat excrement and the sharp stench of urine permeate the entrance.

Tory's mother, dressed in a torn robe and slippers, opens the door and allows us to enter without uttering a word. Tory lives with his mother, father, two younger brothers, one younger sister, one cat, and a mangy, scrawny puppy. They reside in a two and one-half room apartment. The living room contains a new super-size color TV. It also has a relatively new set of matched furniture that is covered with dirty torn spreads. A large doorway opens into a small formal dining room that contains a broken dresser, piles of boxes, and two twin beds that are placed foot to foot. Tory and his two brothers sleep in one of these twin beds. His sister sleeps in the other. Tory's parents sleep on a double bed that is placed in a corner of the kitchen.

Tory's brothers and sisters greet us with curiosity and enthusiasm. Their warmth and affection contrasts sharply with their dirty hair, black fingernails, and streaked faces. They speak excitedly about their puppy who is sick "because the cat keeps licking his hair." They giggle at one another, and each child coaxes the others to show us or tell us about something special. Tory's father sits impassively in a corner with a beer can in his hand and stares at the floor. Tory remains in the kitchen until his mother demands that he come out. She introduces him by saying dourly that "this one is my bad one."

Tory is tall for his age and walks awkwardly. His arms and legs seem to move independently of one another and of his body. His sandy hair is uncombed and stands at odd angles. He does not smile or make eye contact and he shuffles awkwardly while being introduced. His brothers and sisters play and talk among themselves.

During the interview we learn that Tory has been placed frequently in study homes and hospitals for testing and then is returned home. His mother is not sure of his diagnosis. "He don't do good in school and he fights a lot." She is concerned that she won't be able to control him.

His mom explains that they just moved into the apartment and that this one is smaller but nicer than the last. She hadn't counted on Tory's return and she states that things are too cramped. The family has moved so many times that neither the mother nor the children can reconstruct their household moves each year. Dad offers no help. He neither attends to nor enters into the general conversation.

Tory's mother and father have remained married throughout a checkered history of separations and reunions. These have been marked by the father's hospitalizations, imprisonments, and periodic disappearances. Dad now is on parole. No one cares to explain any further. However, Tory's referral agent had notified us that his father is an alcoholic. His mother was recently released from her third hospitalization for depression. She is the spokesperson for the family, but only answers direct questions and frequently loses track of her answers. Dad contributes when asked directly about his work. He motions silently toward the window in order to show us a shiny new pick-up truck parked across the street. Tory's brothers and sister jabber enthusiastically about it. In response to our questions, dad mutters that he uses the truck to do "everything people wants." He then stands up without a word and walks casually out of the house. His family had not acknowledged his presence, and it does not acknowledge his absence.

Tory's sisters and brothers quickly answer their interview questions. Each child does well in school, is active in church, and speaks about special friends and interests. With great animation, one brother and the sister offer to take their interviewers on a tour of the neighborhood. The older brother leaves for his part-time job. The two youngest children point out their school and their church and take us into the neighborhood pizza parlor to see how beautiful it is. They confide that some day they will get to eat there. Meanwhile, Tory, who had trouble concentrating on the answers and reading the questions, finishes his interview.

Postscript: Even though all of the children remained in contact with our service-research program throughout the year, Tory's family moved three more times during this period. Tory frequently was not allowed to attend group sessions because he refused to go to church with his family. His grades are failing, he has been suspended twice for fighting, and he has no friends. He has spent one month in a hospital for evaluation. His mother doesn't know what they found or where Tory will be sent. Her voice registers little interest in the topic.

Invincible Children

The model in Figure 4.1 also identifies three different sets of conditions that enable some children to remain invincible to behavioral problems. Such children are at risk only in the sense that they are subject to various environmental stressors that undoubtedly exert an impact on their behavior. In each case, these children are regarded as invincible, or unconquerable, because their personal coping skills substantially exceed the net environmental stress to which they are exposed. As long as the relative balance among environmental stressors, environmental protectors, and personal coping skills remains constant, these children are likely to be affected little, if at all, by the pertinent stresses. Indeed, if their coping skills should improve even marginally they are bound to become even more invincible. In today's world, however, most circumstances which affect a child's behavior usually change over time. Risk factors can either increase or decrease during the course of one's life. Therefore, the pertinent stressors and protectors must be evaluated at periodic intervals to determine a child's vulnerability at any particular moment.

The most stable and desirable conditions exist when children with strong coping skills live in an environment that is decidedly protective (field C). Such youngsters are likely to remain invincible even if their coping skills should deteriorate to a borderline level or, as is more likely, if the net environmental stressors should rise to a borderline level. Policymakers, mental health administrators, and other helping professionals should attempt to stabilize the conditions in field C when they appear and to establish them when they do not. These interventions clearly would represent examples of primary or secondary, rather than tertiary, prevention.

Field B, in contrast, depicts a situation in which a child with strong coping skills lives in a borderline environment. Here, too, the child is relatively invincible, although not as markedly so as in field C. Because the child has strong coping skills, relatively few efforts at preventive intervention need to concentrate on the child. The model in figure 4.1 clearly indicates that fruitful preventive interventions can be directed toward further reductions in the child's environmental stressors and/or gains in environmental protectors. Such interventions would represent a form of primary prevention in which the targets for intervention reside more in the environment than in the individual child. However, if the child's coping skills should deteriorate to a borderline level, or if the environment should become decidedly stressful, the child's status would shift from invincible to vulnerable. Unlike formulations of vulnerability or invulnerability framed essentially in terms of a target child's personal competencies, the current model assumes that one's status as an invincible (or, for that matter, as a victim or a vulnerable) can be altered by a variety of means. Mental health status varies in accord with the relative balance between one's coping skills and net environmental stressors and protectors. If these variables remain relatively constant, the child's vulnerability or invulnerability will be stable. But, if their relationship should change for one reason or another, the child's mental health and corresponding behavior are likely to change accordingly.

A third genre of invincibility is depicted by field F. Here a child with only borderline coping skills encounters easily manageable, low level environmental stress; that is, on balance the environment is protective. In these circumstances, the child's status as an invincible can likely be strengthened only by upgrading his or her coping skills. The net environmental stress already is extremely low and, therefore, unlikely to shift for the better. In contrast, either a deterioration in the child's coping skills, an increment in environmental stressors, or a decrement in environmental protectors could make the child vulnerable. This would occur, for instance, if the net environmental stress shifts from a protective level to a borderline level or, alternatively, if the child's coping skills should deteriorate from a borderline level to a low level. Since environmental changes occur rapidly during childhood, the former likelihood is far more probable than the latter.

Case Illustration: Meeting an Invincible. The present model posits three sets of conditions that enable a child to be invincible. One of the girls who participated in our study clearly exemplifies the situation in field B.

Rosie is fourteen years old, and she is an "invincible." We first meet Rosie and her foster mother when they arrive for the intake interview. They are leaning slightly upon one another and are talking in animated fashion as they approach the door. Rosie is of medium height, very thin, and slightly boyish in build. She carries herself with grace and assurance. Rosie smiles and makes eye contact as the introductions take place. She begins a conversation with the interviewer as they walk toward the office. She is curious about the building and expresses enthusiasm when discussing her visit. Rosie is dressed in somewhat worn knee-length pants and a bright pink blouse. When complimented on her outfit, she explains that she fashioned it herself from an old pair of slacks because the current length is more stylish. She obviously is proud of her ingenuity and delighted that it has been noticed.

Rosie's manner with her foster mother is extremely relaxed and friendly. She neither tries to dominate, nor does she let herself be subjugated. She answers all of the queries addressed to her in complete detail. There is no question that this is *her* interview. Rosie obviously enjoys talking about her life and herself. She is frank about the problems that she has encountered, and she answers the questions briefly and factually. Her eyes brighten and her answers become more detailed and enthusiastic when she discusses her current life and her plans for the future. This is a child who knows what she wants and where she is going. She expresses a deep interest in learning to dance and she signs up for our dance group. She never before has had an opportunity to take any classes, but dancing has been a dream of hers. She likes school and excitedly describes the courses that she will take next year at high school. Her only concern is that her friends won't be in all the same classes with her. Rosie hopes that she will meet new friends, but she does not seem too concerned. She states that she always finds new friends without problems. She just worries "a little ahead of time."

Rosie has not lived with either of her biological parents since she has been two years old. She has no siblings. She has never known her father because he left home before Rosie was a year old. Her mother is a chronic undifferentiated schizophrenic who has been hospitalized and released at regular intervals during the last twelve years. Rosie has not had any contact with her in four years. Rosie expresses little regret at not seeing her mother and no desire to renew the relationship.

Rosie has lived in five different foster homes. One time she had to move because her foster family left town. Once she was removed from a foster family because "they were mean." Twice the family could no longer take foster children. Rosie is content with her current family. They get along "pretty well" and generally like one another. Rosie has a lot of responsibility for cooking and cleaning, in which she takes pride. Her foster mother says that she is no trouble and that she helps with the household. Rosie still writes to the foster family that left town. Some day she hopes to visit them. She lived with them for five years, and they wanted to adopt her. But "it couldn't be done." Rosie tells her story with pride and pleasure rather than with bitter disappointment. The central fact to her is that she was, and is, wanted, not that she can't be with the family.

Rosie quickly finishes her interview and accompanies the interviewer for a tour of the building. She chats comfortably about a variety of subjects. After Rosie's foster mother has completed her own interview, they smile at one another and begin trading anecdotes as they leave the building.

Postscript: Rosie maintained contact with our program throughout the full year. However, when she found that her dance group did not meet her expectations, she called and arranged to join another group. Whenever she has seen the interviewers, she has been sure to stop and chat. As always in the real world, there is some degree of overlap among the various factors that conduce toward classification of Rosie in one diagnostic category or another. All told, however, it is obvious that she thus far deserves to be regarded as an invincible; to date, Rosie seems unconquerable.

SUMMARY AND DISCUSSION

The present chapter sets forth a social interaction model of childhood vulnerability to behavior disorder and mental illness. It is posited that the relative balance between a child's personal coping skills and his or her net environmental stressors and protectors determines whether or not that child will become behaviorally disturbed. In instances when a child's coping skills surpass the net environmental stress, the child is likely to be invincible to a behavior disorder or mental illness. Conversely, when the net environmental stress exceeds his or her coping skills, the child is likely to fall victim to such forces. When the net environmental stress and the child's coping skills are approximately equipotent, however, the child is likely to be vulnerable to a behavior disorder or mental illness. That is, although the child is neither a victim nor an invincible, a slight change in the child's coping skills or in the balance between environmental stressors and protectors could result in a shift toward one status or the other.

The model is not deterministic in either a psychological or a sociological sense, rather, its perspective is social psychological and social psychiatric. Vulnerability is not conceptualized in univariate terms. Instead, three different sets of factors shape one's status. While vulnerability is predicated on differing combinations of environmental stressors, environmental protectors, and personal coping skills, the stability of an individual's vulnerability is virtually the same in all three instances. Similarly, the model posits three different sets of conditions for victim status and three different sets of conditions for invincible status. Some of these are presumed more extreme and less remediable than the others. As a result, risk statuses can be ranked ordinally and, most probably, in interval fashion.

Unlike other formulations of childhood vulnerability, the model suggests that some children who have only borderline coping skills can nevertheless remain invincible to behavioral disturbance. Similarly, some children with weak coping skills need not necessarily be behaviorally disordered. Depending upon their extant environmental stressors and protectors, children may be vulnerable to the adverse effects that often follow from their parents' mental illness, but they need not necessarily fall victim to them. On the other hand, some children with very strong coping skills may be vulnerable to behavior problems in view of the potency of the net environmental stressors to which they are exposed.

Instead of being viewed in simple dichotomous terms, childhood vulnerability and behavioral patterns are presumed to vary along a continuum that encompasses, respectively, the statuses of victim, vulnerable, and invincible. Each status is predicated upon the relative balance between a child's environmental stressors and protectors and his or her personal coping skills. Hence, the model recognizes the fact that any child's vulnerability or invulnerability must be viewed in relative rather than absolute terms. As a result, varying types of intervention strategies can be employed to help a child progress from the status of victim to vulnerable or, more preferably, from vulnerable to invincible. Albeit in rudimentary fashion, the model helps to delineate interventive priorities for the various identified categories of victims, vulnerables, and invincibles.

The model specifies varying combinations of environmental stressors, environmental protectors, and personal coping skills in a relatively discrete fashion, and it identifies their potential influences on childhood behavioral outcomes. Hence, it eliminates much of the conceptual and semantic confusion that has plagued the literature about childhood vulnerability. It suggests furthermore that some children previously deemed superphrenics ought instead be regarded as vulnerables. Even though such children possess strong coping skills, they may be vulnerable to behavior problems because of their exposure to overwhelming environmental stressors that cannot be countervailed by the available environmental protectors. Likewise, some children previously regarded as vulnerables because of their borderline coping skills ought instead be viewed as victims given their inability to withstand overwhelming environmental stressors.

Accordingly, let us now proceed toward a fuller understanding of our subjects' respective attributes and of the unique factors that lead differentially to their designation as either a victim, a vulnerable, or an invincible. Such an analysis should enable us to discover why one child is better able than another to resist the adverse forces that foster behavior problems. Concomitantly, it should permit us to ascertain whether the "web of mental illness" is a unitary construct or whether there are different kinds of "webs" that conduce toward different patterns of behavior disorder.

5 Methods, Measures, and Data Analysis Procedures

THUS FAR, WE HAVE DESCRIBED MANY OF THE KEY FACTORS that determine children's vulnerability to mental illness. In so doing, we have articulated a model of vulnerability that accounts for the relative balance between the at-risk child's net environmental stressors and protectors and his or her personal coping skills. To learn about the complex array of factors that influences whether or not a child will fall prey to behavior problems, the current research examines a sample of 306 high-risk children. These children are deemed to be at high risk for behavior problems because either or both of their parents were diagnosed as mentally ill within six months of the intake interview for the study. As seen in chapter 2, this factor by itself hardly foredooms a child to mental illness. But it does, in fact, mean that a child will be at significantly greater risk for many behavioral difficulties than same-age youngsters who do not have a mentally ill parent. Since there is a strong statistical likelihood that many subjects in such a sample will have significant behavior problems, this particular group of youngsters offers an exceptional opportunity for examining the complex dynamics that determine whether an at-risk child will succumb to behavior problems or whether the child will function well despite being at greater risk than other youngsters.

In essence, our research attempts to refine the conception of risk that is applied to children with mentally ill parents. The vast preponderance of research argues with good reason that such youngsters are at relatively high-risk vis-à-vis other youngsters. Yet, are *all* such youngsters truly at the same high level of risk? Is it possible to identify factors that will cause certain children in this group to be at relatively low-risk while, conversely, causing others to be at extraordinarily high-risk? Only by answering this question can we make sophisticated and discriminating judgments about the true status of putatively high-risk youngsters. By close examination of this sample of children we will be able to analyze in detail the major threads in the web of mental illness and gain insights about ways to help at-risk youngsters avoid significant behavior problems. In later chapters, we will place our findings in bold relief by contrasting them with data acquired from a comparison sample of fifty children who appear to be at relatively low risk because they lack a mentally ill parent. As befits this research, we will refer simply to the former subjects as "Web subjects" and to the latter as "comparison subjects." Likewise, for the sake of convenience we commonly refer to the overall research program as the "Web study."

In this chapter, we explain the methods, measures, and data analysis procedures of the Web study in detail. The main methodological features are the referral, intake, and interview processes. The measures are of three types: those that (1) examine the presence or absence of behavior problems on the part of the at-risk subjects, (2) define environmental stressors and/or protectors to which the at-risk child has been exposed, and (3) indicate the at-risk child's coping strengths and/or weaknesses. Measures devised expressly for the Web study are reproduced in the appendix. Detailed literature citations are set forth for all other measures. Finally, the section on data analysis procedures briefly describes the nature and underlying rationales of the statistical tests and the univariate or multivariate regression analyses employed in the research. The latter are also discussed in detail as they appear in subsequent chapters.

Referred children who participated in the Web study took part in a nine-month program of recreational and learning activities at a community center in suburban St. Louis, Missouri. The basis for referral was the mere fact that one or both of the youngster's parents had been formally diagnosed as mentally ill within the previous six months. Referrals were *not* made on the basis of the at-risk child's own pattern of behavior. Therefore, enrollment in the program did not necessarily mean that the referred child was suffering from a behavior disorder. To the contrary, referral agents were asked to recommend children who were capable of functioning well in an open recreational setting and who did not show evidence of a serious behavior disorder.

As explicated below, all of the referred children and their parents or guardians took part in an extensive intake interview. Data about the referred children pertained to such fundamental aspects of their lives as the presence or absence of behavior problems, environmental stressors and protectors, and personal coping skills. We acquired information about these particular sets of variables from both the children and their parents. In addition, we acquired relevant information about the referred children, their parents, and other family members from such sources as referral agents, therapists, and school teachers. While this chapter explains the referral and intake processes, research instruments, and data analysis procedures of the Web study, the following chapters will describe characteristics of the sample, the subjects' environments, and their behavioral profiles.

REFERRAL PROCESS

The Web study was conducted in conjunction with a program that offered a broad range of recreational activities for the at-risk children of mentally ill parents. Through funds provided by the National Institute of Mental Health, the 306 at-risk children participated in activity groups that met once a week throughout the school year at a suburban community center in St. Louis. Of these youngsters, 176 took part in 1981 and 130 in 1982. Before being admitted to the program, all of the referred subjects and their parents took part in an extensive intake interview, which yielded the basic data employed in the Web study.

To generate referrals to the program, announcements were sent to every psychiatric agency, family service agency, and hospital with a psychiatric ward in the St. Louis metropolitan area as well as private practitioners, pediatricians, and mental health associations. To explain the program and solicit referrals personal visits were made to twenty-five agencies. Referral agents were informed that we sought subjects between the ages of seven and fifteen with at least one parent diagnosed as mentally ill. The DSM-III (American Psychiatric Association 1980) diagnostic system was utilized. The referred child did not necessarily have to reside with his or her mentally ill parents at the time of the study; in fact, the ill parent had often been confined to an institution. To initiate a referral, we requested that the referral agent speak first with the child's parent or guardian, and we asked this individual to describe the activity program to the parent or guardian and acquire verbal consent for an intake interview with a member of our research staff. The referral agent then mailed us a form that listed the names and ages of all children in the family, the name and relationship of the guardian to be contacted, and the name and diagnosis of the mentally ill parent.

INTAKE PROCESS

After receiving a referral form, a member of the research team contacted the parent or guardian by telephone to briefly explain the study and arrange an appointment for an intake interview. Every effort was made to accommodate the family's schedule, and interviews were even conducted on evenings or weekends if more convenient for the family. Participants were encouraged to visit the community center for the interview so that the referred child could become acquainted with the facility and its programs. However, if transportation posed a problem the interview was conducted at the respondent's home. Since the interview required at least one hour, each family received a small payment. To defray the family's transportation costs to the community center, each family received $15 for the interview plus $5 for each additional sibling who took part. If interviewed at home, the family received only $5.

The largest numbers of subjects were referred by family service or child mental health agencies ($n = 96$) and the Missouri Division of Family Services ($n = 82$). Thirty-four subjects were referred by public hospitals and twenty-seven by private hospitals. Twenty-two subjects were referred directly by family members who had learned about the program from news releases or friends. The remaining subjects were referred by psychiatrists in private practice ($n = 18$), friends or neighbors ($n = 9$), juvenile court workers ($n = 7$), psychologists in private practice ($n = 4$), social workers in private practice ($n = 4$), and a local mental health association ($n = 2$). When interviews were conducted, one staff member always spoke with the parent, while another interviewed the child. This reduced the length of the interview and assured privacy for both parent and child. Referral agents and therapists provided corroborative information about the mental health diagnoses of family members, and teachers provided additional information about the child's behavior at school.

Our efforts to arrange interviews for the Web study constitute an interesting commentary both upon the difficulty of research with at-risk children and the dynamics of their families. These issues are highlighted by the procedures we devised to establish contact with the referred families. In numerous instances, these families were highly disorganized, beleaguered by economic crisis, unable to keep appointments, or unstable in terms of composition or place of residence. Many families did not have a telephone. Moreover, the telephones of at least twenty-four referred families had been disconnected in the single week that transpired between their referral and the first effort of the research staff to establish contact. Even when it was possible to initially contact the parent, it sometimes was difficult or impossible to acquire reliable data. For instance, three parents were hospitalized before the interview could take place. Their children were left with neighbors who had little or no information about the family and who were not sufficiently acquainted with them to provide a full and accurate description of the children's behavior. As a result, the interviewers had to make additional appointments and trips in order to acquire necessary information from relatives, neighbors, social workers, or other parties.

The research staff always attempted to interview the most able parent or guardian. Nevertheless, this sometimes was a parent who had been diagnosed as mentally ill. In several instances, a severely depressed parent had received medication following electroconvulsive therapy and, as a result, was unable to remember his or her appointment, too ill to attend, or too disorganized to cancel it. On some occasions, the parent who attended the interview was so heavily medicated that repeated efforts were needed to remain focused on the interview items. Whenever there was reason to doubt the accuracy of a respondent's answers, we crosschecked them with other individuals such as relatives, referral agents, and therapists. These checks confirmed that such respondents' inattentiveness, rather than the accuracy of their responses, was the most problematic aspect of the interviews.

While it is commonly assumed that retrospective data from mentally ill adults are bound to suffer from recall error, the available research indicates that this probably is not the case. Indeed, findings reported by Robins, Schoenberg, Holmes, Ratcliff, Benham, and Works (1985), Finlay-Jones, Scott, Duncan-Jones, Byrne, and Henderson (1981), and Rutter and Brown (1966) suggest that mentally ill respondents may be no more likely than other individuals to suffer from biased recall of prior events. This is particularly the case if the pertinent items are highly factual and do not depend greatly on individual judgments or inferences.

While the Web subjects' recall processes may have been relatively unbiased, it is obvious nevertheless that the prospect of participation in a study proved to be highly problematic for many of them. In several instances, it was evident that the referral agent had not adequately prepared a parent for a telephone inquiry by our staff. Some parents found the prospect of an intake interview so threatening that a crisis reaction was triggered. In one instance, a parent concluded that the interview was a conspiracy by the federal government to take control of his children, and he called the referral agent and a lawyer in order to defend against this "threat." In another case, a family had its telephone disconnected after our initial call and moved secretly to a new address.

Research with these families required considerable tact and organization. After an appointment had been made for the interview, a letter of confirmation, with directions to the interview site and a map, were sent to the referred parents. Families were called twenty-four hours before the interview to introduce the interviewer and to remind the family about the appointment. Even this proved to be upsetting to some parents. One mother, who had already missed two appointments, shouted—perhaps appropriately—over the telephone "My emotions are troubled, not my memory!" Other parents appeared to be highly acquiescent by agreeing to appointments that they had little intention of keeping; it was easier for them to consent than to "disappoint" the referral agent or state directly that they had no desire to participate in the study.

Despite concerted efforts, the referred individuals cancelled 10% of the originally-scheduled interviews, and nearly 33% did not take place because the interviewees did not show up. However, approximately 50% of these persons did, in fact, arrive for a rescheduled interview. Only about 10% of all the families who agreed to an intake interview never kept a scheduled appointment whether at their home or the community center. Seventy-one referred families either never arrived for an interview, declined to participate in the study, or were otherwise unreachable. Altogether, we conducted 86% of the interviews at the community center and 14% at the family's home. Whatever their problems it is plausible to assume that participants in the Web study were less seclusive, disorganized, and resistant than the larger population of referred families from which they had been drawn.

INTERVIEW PROCEDURES

Data from the intake interview and collateral sources refer, for the most part, to the children's behaviors, environments, and coping skills. Several types of data regarding each of these topics were collected either from the parents, children, or other respondents. Here, too, the instability of the children's families posed serious research problems. In the Web study, as in other kinds of field research, it was not possible, for example, to regard the child's "environment" as an unchanging and fully quantifiable construct. In fact, many of the at-risk children had lived in a variety of different environments. Some were relatively enduring while others had been fleeting. In some instances, significant environmental changes occurred at ages purported to be especially crucial for child development. For other subjects this was not the case. In other words, each child's "environmental history" was relatively unique.

To account for such complexities, and to be as comprehensive as possible, we sought multiphasic and multivariate data about the particular family settings in which each child had lived. Through comparable questions information was acquired about three different types of families: (1) the child's current family—the family with whom the child lived at the time of the intake interview; (2) the child's modal family—the family with whom the child had lived for the longest period of time; and (3) the child's biological family—the family to whom the child had been born. For any particular child, these families may or may not be one and the same. A child may currently live with a foster family, for example, even though most of his or her life has been spent with the biological parents. To collect such a broad range of information, the research staff designed a series of parallel interview schedules for the respondents.

We viewed each child's family history from these three perspectives, enabling us to acquire a comprehensive range of information about at-risk children exposed to different kinds of living experiences. Thus, we were able to learn about the environments of children who had lived in a variety of family settings as well as those who had lived with only one family. The resultant data also permitted contrasts among the subjects throughout differing phases of development. Comparable questions were asked about each type of family with whom the subject had lived, that is, the current family, the modal family, and the biological family. The interview schedules, for a subject's current family and modal family were identical in all respects. For instance, each examined whether the at-risk child lived with one biological parent? Two biological parents? One biological parent and one stepparent? Relatives? Foster parents? Adoptive parents? In an institution or a group home? Interview items also examined the socioeconomic status of the family, the social relationships among family members, and a variety of other factors described below.

RESEARCH INSTRUMENTS

We administered all research instruments for the Web study during the intake interview or, in the case of collaborative respondents, during the following two weeks. The instruments provided data about the subjects' behavior problems, environmental stressors and protectors, and personal coping strengths and weaknesses. Copies of the pertinent research instruments appear in the appendix and in the cited references.

Behavior Problems

We employed several measures to examine the behavior problems of the at-risk children. The pertinent data were acquired from parents, school teachers, and the children themselves. The major research instrument for this aspect of the study was the Achenbach Child Behavior Checklist (CBCL).

Achenbach Child Behavior Checklist (CBCL): Parent Report. Parents completed the Achenbach CBCL during the intake interview. This instrument is a normed and standardized 118-item checklist that yields both a Behavior Problem score (described here) and a Social Competence score (discussed later in this chapter) for each subject. The Behavior Problem score (hereafter, simply the CBCL score) has demonstrated high internal consistency (alpha = .98; Achenbach 1978-1979) and high test-retest reliability (r = .93; Achenbach and Edelbrock 1981). It constitutes the primary criterion variable for the Web study. A subject's standardized score on this measure denotes his or her position on the invincible-vulnerable-victim continuum.

This measure can be either self-administered or administered by an interviewer to the child's parent or parental surrogate, who responds to each of the 118 items by checking one of three answer categories. These range, respectively, from zero ("not true of the child") to one ("somewhat or sometimes true of the child") to two ("very true or often true of the child"). Respondents are asked to base their answers on observations of the child's behavior during the six-month period that immediately preceded the interview. Items pertain to such diverse behaviors as psychosomatic illnesses, aggressive behavior, encopresis, and substance abuse. Each child's CBCL score is normalized according to the distribution of such scores within a random sample of the general population.

According to Achenbach and Edelbrock (1981), a normed CBCL score of 63 or above is a useful criterion, or cut-off point, for defining the existence of clinically significant behavior problems on a child's part. This criterion is equivalent to scores at the 90th percentile or above for a normal sample of children who have not been preselected for clinical reasons. Unfortunately, Achenbach's scoring instructions and related publications are limited solely to subjects who register scores at the 55th percentile or above on the CBCL. Although descriptive statistics are not provided for normal population scores that fall below the 55th percentile, the approximate percentage of children who could be expected to attain such scores can be inferred from the normal curve. Children with very low CBCL scores (49 or below) are more likely than others to be positioned in either the invincible or vulnerable—but not the victim—ranges of the behavioral continuum. Achenbach dichotomously categorizes all subjects as either "clinical" or "nonclinical" on the basis of their respective CBCL scores, but we consider such an "either-or" approach to be too global. It takes no cognizance of the fact that very few children are wholly maladjusted or, for that matter, fully well-adjusted; instead, the vast majority of children vary considerably between these polar extremes, especially those who fall into Achenbach's nonclinical category. Many, if not most, of these youngsters can be regarded more properly as vulnerable to mental illness rather than invincible. We proceed beyond Achenbach's application of the CBCL by considering scores at the 10th percentile or lower, corresponding to T-scores of 37 or below, as indicative of invincible status on a child's part. Such scores are the polar opposites of scores that fall at the 90th percentile or above on a normal curve.

Achenbach Child Behavior Checklist (CBCL): Teacher Report. Each referred child's homeroom teacher was also asked to complete the Teacher's Form of the Achenbach CBCL, virtually identical to the one completed by parents. The teachers' responses offer an independent contrast for the parents' assessments of the children's behavior. However, the two measures are not fully comparable since the one refers to behavior observed at school while the other refers to behavior exhibited primarily at home. Since neither Achenbach nor others have reported normed data for this measure we employ raw summary scores for the pertinent analyses.

Behavior Rating Index for Children (BRIC). The subjects also completed the Behavior Rating Index for Children (BRIC), a thirteen-item summated-category partition scale which measures the frequency of problem behavior exhibited by a child (see appendix). The parent version of this brief instrument has demonstrated acceptable levels of test-retest reliability (.83) and internal consistency (.79) (see Stiffman, Orme, Evans, Feldman, and Keeney 1984). Ten items, employed to compute a behavior problem score, refer to such behaviors as hiding one's thoughts from others, saying or doing strange things, quitting a task without finishing it, hitting or hurting others, getting upset, feeling sick, and cheating; the other three items are reverse-worded to inhibit a response set by the respondent. While the latter items are not used to compute a subject's behavior problem score, they indicate selected social competencies. All of the items are rated on a five-point Likert scale that ranges from one ("rarely or never") to five ("most or all of the time"). Parallel versions can be completed by parents (BRIC-P), teachers (BRIC-T), or the children themselves (BRIC-C). Data for the BRIC-C reveal considerably lower test-retest reliability (r = .70) and internal consistency reliability (alpha = .70) than for the BRIC-P.

Environmental Stressors and Protectors

A child's environment encompasses countless stressors and protectors that can affect his or her behavior. Hirsch (1982) suggests that environmental protectors can provide individuals with cognitive guidance, social reinforcement, and emotional support. Moreover, when considered in conjunction with environmental stressors, they significantly enhance one's ability to predict the actual effects of the latter (Marsella and Snyder 1981). An environment rich in protectors should be able to help a child deal more readily with stressors than one relatively devoid of protectors.

Available studies suggest that childhood risk status is directly influenced by a wide variety of environmental stressors including type of parental mental illness, length of a parent's hospitalization, period of time since onset of the parent's illness, socioeconomic status, race, family size, marital discord, out-of-home placement of the child, residential mobility, and community support for the family or at-risk child (cf., for example, Miller, Challas, and Gee 1972; Pearlin and Johnson 1977). The children of mentally ill parents are often exposed to an extremely stressful environment because their parents tend to have high incidences of marital discord, divorce, hospitalization, and unemployment. As a result, the family environments of high-risk children are very unstable (Kreitman 1968; Molholm and Denitz 1972). All these factors can result in sociobehavioral problems on a child's part (Emory, Weintraub, and Neale 1982; Rutter 1981); however, as already indicated, some children are well able to prevail against such circumstances. Again, information about the subjects' environments was obtained from the parents and the children themselves, who responded to research instruments that tapped such diverse variables as social status, life-change events, the mental and physical health of family members, family relationships, and social support.

Demographic Factors. Certain demographic factors are presumed very influential in determining risk status and behavioral outcomes: family composition (Heston 1966; Kety, Rosenthal, Wender, Schulsinger, and Jacobsen 1975), sex of the ill parent (Orvaschell, Mednick, Schulsinger, and Rock 1979), sex of the at-risk child (Gardner 1967a, 1967b; Kokes, Harder, Fisher, and Strauss 1980), and the family's socioeconomic status (Garbarino 1977; Kohn 1969, 1973). The particular impact of any given environmental protector or stressor may depend upon such factors as the child's age and stage of development. Some investigators assume that there are periods of development in which one is particularly vulnerable. To progress through childhood and adolescence, a youngster must experiment with a variety of roles and become increasingly independent. Whereas it had formerly been posited that the first few years of life are especially critical (Clarke and Clarke, 1976), it is now argued that later periods are also critical, especially latency and preadolescence. Certain stressors are presumed to exert long-term developmental effects if they occur at these periods (Clarke and Clarke

1976; Inbar 1976). Hence, demographic data were collected for all developmental phases of the subjects' lives.

Similarly, little consensus exists regarding whether or not the relationship between parental mental illness and childhood behavior disorder is sex-linked. In many instances, the mother appears to be especially influential in the transmission of mental illness (Gardner 1967b; Rutter 1977). However, it is neither absolutely nor consistently clear how mental illness is transmitted on a sex-linked basis from parent to child (Clausen and Huffine 1979; Rutter 1977). Comprehension of this phenomenon tends to be obscured by confounding factors, including serial moves by the child from one parent to another due to separation, remarriage, or other types of relationships among parents and caregivers. To acquire essential demographic information about the children's families, their parents or guardians were asked a broad range of questions, which yielded data about their race, age, religion, occupation, and education. Using Hollingshead's (1974) two-factor schema, the latter two variables were employed to determine the family's socioeconomic status.

Family Mental Health Problems. As shown in chapter 2, children of mentally ill parents are at relatively higher risk than other children for the particular type of disorder manifested by their parents. This is especially true when the parent has schizophrenia or a major affective disorder. Nevertheless, the chronicity and severity of the parent's illness may be better predictors of childhood disorder than the specific diagnostic label (Erlenmeyer-Kimling 1977; Hanson 1974). Furthermore, a child's risk status may increase in accord with the mentally ill significant others who interact with him or her on a protracted basis (Rutter 1977). Risk is greater, for example, when two parents (rather than one) are mentally ill. Regardless of their particular diagnosis, moreover, risk also increases in accord with the number of mentally ill siblings in one's family (Rutter 1977).

We deemed it advisable, therefore, to acquire extensive data about the mental health of all members of the at-risk child's immediate family. During the intake interview, parents gave information about the mental health history of each family member including data about mental health diagnoses, treatment programs, and hospitalizations. We acquired information about the particular type of behavioral or emotional problem manifested, the age of onset, and the family member's current status. DSM-III diagnoses were obtained from the respondent whenever possible and later confirmed by the appropriate treatment or referral agent.

Family Physical Health Problems. It is generally believed that at-risk children have higher incidences of physical illness (Buck and Laughton 1959; Mednick and Schulsinger 1968) and perceptual, visual, or motor problems (Fish and Hagin 1973; MacCrimmon, Cleghorn, Asarnow, and Steffy 1980; Marcus 1974) than other youngsters. This also appears to be the case for mentally ill adults (Mednick 1970). Since these factors may play a role in shaping vulnerability to mental illness, we deemed it essential to gather data about the physical health of the referred children and their families. Therefore, we asked the parent to provide information about the past and present physical health of each person in the family. Data were collected regarding the particular type of physical problem, if any, and the extent to which it limited the individual's ability to function. We employed the four-factor schema devised by the National Center for Health Statistics (Bonham and Corder 1981). Each physical disorder was rated in terms of one of the following categories: (1) the subject encounters no problem or is not limited in any way; (2) the subject can perform major activities but is limited in minor activities; (3) the subject is limited in major activities; or (4) the subject is not able to perform major activities. Typically, major activities refer to housework or employment in the case of adults and to school performance in the case of children. We also obtained related information about the child's allergies and medications.

Life-Change Events. Many studies have linked life-change events to physical illness on the part of children and adults, including coronary heart disease (Rahe and Arthur 1978; Rosenman, Brant, and Jenkins 1976), athletic injuries (Bramwell, Masuda, Wagner, and Holmes 1975), influenza (Imboden, Canter, and Cluff 1963), respiratory illness (Jacobs, Spilken, and Norman 1971), and general ill health (Holmes and Masuda 1974; Mechanic 1976; Wolff 1968). Life-change events and stressful events have also been linked with mental health problems such as depression (Gatchill, McKinney, and Koebernick 1977; Paykel 1978; Paykel, Meyers, Dienelt, Klerman, Lindenthal, and Pepper 1969), psychosomatic illness (Lei and Skinner 1980; Markush and Favero 1974), schizophrenia (Jacobs and Myers 1976), neurosis (Cooper and Sylph 1973), and unspecified psychiatric disorders (Husaini and Neff 1978).

Several studies have explored the specific relationships between stress and illness in children and adolescents. As with adults, these investigations have found consistent associations between life-change events and such problems as cancer (Jacobs and Charles 1980), growth disorders (Coddington 1972), and rheumatoid arthritis (Heisel, Ream, Raitz, Rappaport, and Coddington 1974). Major life-change events are also associated with such problems of adolescence as unemployability (Castillo 1980), delinquency (Gersten,

Langner, Eisenberg, and Orze 1974; Vaux and Ruggiero 1983), unwed pregnancy (Coddington 1979), drug dependence (Duncan 1977), and depression (Friedrich, Ream, and Jacobs 1982). However, the associations between life-change events and such problems have been only in the moderate range (.20 to .40). Furthermore, the findings of these studies have not been easily replicable (Cooley and Keesey 1981).

The multiple respondent interview procedure employed in the Web study afforded an ideal opportunity to explore further the relationships, if any, between major life-change events and children's vulnerability to mental illness. We asked all referred children to provide information about life-change events that had occurred during each year of their life. While it is unlikely that all such events would be recalled accurately by the subjects, we were most interested in learning about the particular life-change events that they deemed most salient and memorable. Accordingly, the interviewer helped the referred children complete a Child Life-Event Timeline that reported the occurrence of major events during each year of their life and the extent to which they had been bothered by such events. Data were collected about each of twenty-six different life-change events that could be viewed as potentially stressful (see appendix). These items were drawn from the earlier stress research of Coddington (1972), Yeaworth, York, Hussey, Ingle, and Goodwin (1980), and others. Each of the cited life-change events usually requires some degree of adaptation or adjustment by an at-risk youngster. We collected retrospective data from each referred child about two major features of his or her life-change events: (1) the age at which the event occurred, and (2) the extent to which the subject felt bothered by the event. The latter was gauged by means of responses to a five-point Likert scale that ranged from one ("did not bother me at all") to five ("bothered me extremely").

This measure yielded two summative scores: (1) the total number of potentially stressful life-change events that have occurred since birth, and (2) the sum of each child's rating of the extent to which he or she has been bothered by the pertinent life-change events. A variety of subscores can also be derived: the average number of events experienced throughout the child's life course, the average extent to which the child was bothered by such events, and the mean number of events, as well as their perceived stressfulness, for any particular year or group of years. Summative scores can also be calculated for subcategories of events or for discrete events such as a move to a new city or a death in the family. Among the key indicators employed in the present research are subscores denoting the number of major life-change events experienced during the year before the interview and the extent to which they bothered the child. These data are not only less subject to errors of recall than those pertaining to more distal events, but they are also comparable to the types of data that appear in the preponderance of research about life-change events. A two-week test-retest assessment of the measure was performed with a subsample of twenty-four at-risk children. We examined these subjects' self-weightings of the "bothersomeness" of each event, and the data yielded a test-retest reliability of .78. Moreover, an analysis of only those weighted items that appear in Coddington's well-validated research reveals a test-retest reliability of .85.

Living Arrangements. As might be expected, many participants in the Web study had lived in a variety of different settings. Because the transition from one type of living arrangement to another may be a major source of stress for the at-risk child, the subjects were asked to review the various living arrangements in which they had resided each year since birth (see appendix). By tracing the child's living arrangements throughout each year of life and from year to year over the life course, we learned whether the child had lived with two biological parents, one biological parent, one biological parent and a stepparent, adoptive parents, foster parents, or in an institution or group home.

Family Social Support. The social supports available to family members may help them avert or cope with adverse environmental forces (Collins and Pancoast 1976). Such supports may be either formal (churches and social service agencies) or informal (friends, relatives, or other individuals). Since these supports may exert an important protective impact for the at-risk child, we deemed it essential to gauge their effects during the course of the Web study. Accordingly, we asked the parents to report the extent to which their family had received formal or informal support for major problems that had occurred in the past year (see appendix). Data were sought about the nature of the problem, the type of support received, the number of supporters, and the extent to which they were considered helpful. The latter was measured by means of responses to a five-point Likert scale in which scores could range from one ("not at all helpful") to five ("extremely helpful").

Family Discord. Available evidence suggests that parents' diagnostic labels are neither the best nor the only predictors of childhood mental illness. Rather, the parent's effect upon the at-risk child may be associated more directly with the way in which the child is involved in the parent's symptomatology (Doane, West, Goldstein, Rodnick, and Jones 1981), the modes of social interaction established between parent and child (Cummings, Zahn-Waxler, and Radke-Yarrow 1981; Fischer 1980), and the nature of the complementary or alternative relationships available to the child and parents

(Sameroff, Seifer, and Zax 1982). Also, the extent of harmony or, conversely, of discord among family members is a crucial modifier of such relationships.

To examine this variable, the parents and children were asked to report the frequency with which discord occurred between mother and child, father and child, mother and father, and within the family as a whole (see appendix). Hence, contrasting perspectives about family discord were taken into account. For each of these relationships, the respondent employed a five-point Likert scale. Scores ranged from one ("rarely or never has problems") to five ("problems most or all the time"). These items are similar to the ones used by Hudson (1982) to validate a twenty-five–item questionnaire about family relationships. He found that responses to each of these questions correlated at a level of .84 or above with the full twenty-five–item measure. While a lengthier version of the questionnaire might have yielded even greater reliability, we opted for the shorter approach because of the amount of time consumed by the intake interview.

Coping Strengths and Weaknesses

As suggested above, contemporary research is progressing toward a comprehensive paradigm that encompasses the mutual interactions between environmental factors and personal competencies. The latter include such variables as problem-solving skills and ego strengths (Jenkins 1979; Pearlin and Schooler 1978), arousal level (Johnson, Sarason, and Siegel 1979; Zuckerman, Kolin, Price, and Zoob 1964), locus of control (Anderson 1977; Rutter, Yule, Quinton, Rowlands, Yule, and Berger 1975; Suls and Mullen 1981), extroversion (Miller and Cooley 1981), and the ability to evaluate an event's effects (Houston, Bloom, Burnish, and Cummings 1978). Certain coping strengths and strategies may enable an individual to modify a stress-provoking event, alter its meaning, or control the symptoms that result. Among other things, one's social competence, self-esteem, and achievement or intelligence may interact with environmental factors to reduce or accentuate the impact of a key life-change event or environmental stressor (Bryant and Trockel 1976; Rutter 1981). Therefore, we also examined these variables in the Web study.

Social Competence. Children who appear invulnerable to environmental stressors or high-risk situations typically have a high level of social competence (Fisher, Kokes, Harder, and Jones 1980; Garmezy 1981; Kauffman, Grunebaum, Cohler, and Gamer 1979; Werner and Smith 1982). Among other things, the ability to communicate one's needs to others and to benefit from their friendship, advice, or resources are considered integral coping skills for children and adults (Anderson 1977; Andrews, Tennant, Hewson, and Vaillant 1978; Hirsch 1982). To measure social competence, the parents responded to the Social Competence scale of the Achenbach CBCL. Items on this scale yield subscores regarding involvement and attainment in three discrete areas: activities, social-interpersonal relationships, and school performance (Achenbach 1978-1979); respectively, we refer to these as activity competence, interpersonal competence, and school competence. Together, they are denoted simply as "social competence." For each construct, the pertinent measures yield data that reflect the extent of the child's involvement and the quality of his or her performance.

Activity competence refers to the child's participation in sports, task-oriented clubs or organizations, jobs, and a variety of chores. Interpersonal competence refers to the child's number of friends, behavior toward others, tendency to be alone, and participation in friendship organizations. School competence refers to the child's performance in academic subjects, placement in regular or special classes, academic promotion or failure, and the presence or absence of school problems. Like the behavior problem scale of the CBCL, this scale has been normed for children from the general population, and responses about a given child yield a normalized T-score on each subscale and an overall T-score for social competence. These scores are arrayed and interpreted in accord with the child's sex and age group. The normed percentiles for social competence scores of boys and girls of a given age are identical. An overall score of 37 or less indicates that the child falls below the 10th percentile of the general population in terms of social competence. Achenbach and Edelbrock (1981) conclude this indicates clinical status on the child's part. They report that the correlation between social competence scores and behavior problem scores on the CBCL is $-.56$.

Self-Esteem. Some types of stressful events produce a threat to any individual's self-esteem, but individuals with low self-esteem may regard many types of external events as threatening (Coyne 1976). Persons with low self-esteem tend to suffer from relatively high rates of stress-induced illness (Kobasa 1979) and to exhibit particularly high incidences of behavior disorder (Langner, Gersten, and Eisenberg 1977). In contrast, high self-esteem is characteristic of children who appear invulnerable to prolonged stress (Garmezy 1981; Werner and Smith 1982). Since the literature suggests that self-esteem is an important coping strength, we considered it desirable to measure this variable, too.

We assessed the children's self-esteem by means of their responses to a brief questionnaire, consisting of four items to indicate how often the re-

spondent feels a given way about himself or herself. Responses can be arrayed along a five-point Likert scale in which scores range from one ("rarely
or never") to five ("most or all of the time"). The selected items were the best
predictors of the four dimensions of the Coopersmith Self-Esteem Inventory
(1975). As revealed by Coopersmith's factor analyses, each item pertains to
a different facet of self-esteem: (1) "How often do you feel there are lots of
things about yourself that you would change if you could?"; (2) "How often
do you feel that your parents expect too much of you?"; (3) "How often do
you feel that kids usually follow your ideas?"; and (4) "How often do you
feel discouraged in school?" The third question, worded positively, is scored
in reverse so that all items can be summed to indicate the extent of the subject's self-esteem. Although the product-moment correlation between the
four-item questionnaire and the lengthier Coopersmith Self-Esteem Inventory is .56, we chose not to employ the latter measure because pretests had
indicated that some of our subjects required as long as an hour to complete it.

Intelligence/Achievement. Numerous investigators have suggested that
the impact of environmental variables is mediated by an individual's intelligence. Thus, while both gifted and ungifted children may be equally sensitive to certain life events (Ferguson 1981), the former may have better problem-solving skills that enable them to cope with environmental stressors
(Haggerty 1980). To measure this variable, all referred children completed
the Wide-Range Achievement Test (WRAT) during the intake interview.
Yielding normed scores in three areas (spelling, mathematics, and reading),
it enabled us to compare the subjects' academic achievement even though
they attended widely differing schools both in terms of geographic location
and academic standards. The WRAT correlates highly with standard measures of intelligence, for example, .75 to .85 with WISC IQ scores and .82
to .87 with WAIS IQ scores.

School Behavior. Poor behavior at school is associated with such factors
as psychosocial maladjustment (El-Guebaly, Offord, Sullivan, and Lynch
1978) and delinquency (Craig and Glick 1968). At-risk children who demonstrate invulnerability have fewer academic and social problems in the school
setting than other youngsters (Garmezy 1974a; Rolf 1972; Rolf and Garmezy
1974). To acquire relevant data regarding school behavior, the subjects'
teachers were asked to rate their performance in the school setting by using
relevant sections of the teacher form of the Achenbach CBCL. These pose
questions about the child's academic achievement and attitudes towards
school. Specifically, the research team obtained information about the average grades received in courses, the subjects' reactions to peers and classroom
assignments, and their rate of learning.

MODES OF DATA ANALYSIS

The analyses that appear in the following chapters are based upon retrospective data. Hence, unlike programs of experimental research, data regarding the subjects are analyzed in terms of a priori characteristics over which the researcher has little or no control. As Robins, Schoenberg, Holmes, Ratcliff, Benham, and Works (1985) note, retrospective studies provide reasonably rapid and inexpensive methods for developing causal hypotheses. They are useful and highly advisable, therefore, as an initial step before proceeding to the more costly methods of prospective studies. If the independent variables selected for measurement at Time 1 in a prospective study are discovered at follow-up to be impotent, the opportunity has been lost to select alternative Time 1 variables. Retrospective analyses do not necessarily bias the selection of statistical tests for the data set, but they do, however, affect the types of inferences that can be drawn from the applied tests. While it is often permissible to generalize the findings of retrospective research to selected populations, care must be taken not to generalize beyond the proper limitations of the data set.

Besides descriptive statistics, two major modes of analysis are employed to evaluate the data collected about at-risk subjects: (1) item-by-item univariate analyses examine how each discrete variable is associated with the subjects' behavior; and (2) the multivariate relationships among key variables are explored. In brief, then, we reviewed the data in terms of descriptive statistics, univariate regression analyses, and multivariate regression analyses.

Descriptive Statistics

Descriptive statistics analyze the data in terms of measures of central tendency (mode, median, and mean), variability (standard deviation and range), and frequency (number of responses for each possible answer to a question, number of subjects who attain a given criterion or score, and number of individuals who fall into a particular category). Such statistics are easily understood and require little explanation. In essence, they provide the basis for the more complex statistical procedures that follow.

Univariate Regressions

With only a single exception, we shall refrain throughout from collapsing continuous data into dichotomous or trichotomous categories. By allowing interval-level data to remain continuous, crucial information is not lost about the major study variables. Likewise, except where clearly justified by empirical evidence or sound conceptual analysis, we do not make causal attributions about the relationships among study variables. We derived most of the results reported in the following chapters from univariate and multivariate regression analyses. Regression methods offer a number of distinct advantages vis-à-vis other modes of analysis. In comparison with simple cross-tabulations or analyses of variance, for instance, they enable the researcher to investigate simultaneously the effects of both continuous and class-level variables. When the latter are included in a regression equation by means of dummy variables, interpretations of the resulting F-values and probability levels are analogous to those for analyses of variance. In effect, the regression equation tests for mean differences between class variables and for the significance of the least-squares linear relationship between continuous variables. Regression analyses yield a significance, or probability, level that enables the reader to ascertain the extent to which the observed results might be attributable to chance variations. They also yield a measure of the variance explained by one predictor (r^2) or multiple predictors (R^2). This measure can indicate, for example, what proportion of the variance in subjects' behavior problem scores is explained by the presence of a mentally ill parent.

Whenever regression analyses or correlation analyses are used to illustrate the relationship between a pair of variables, we pay particular attention to the differences between subjects with especially high and especially low levels of behavior problems. We do so by reporting the results for subjects with CBCL scores in either the highest or the lowest decile of the study sample, based on the actual scores of the referred subjects rather than on normed scores for the general population. To highlight this distinction and to provide conceptual and empirical anchors for each end of the victim-vulnerable-invincible continuum, we refer to the former youngsters as High Prob subjects and to the latter as Lo Prob subjects. These categories vividly demonstrate the findings of the regression analyses. As is appropriate, the significance levels reported for these analyses are based on the overall regression statistic rather than the mean scores for the polar categories.

Multiple Regressions

Multiple regression analyses are used to determine the conjoint and interactive relationships among the key predictor variables and dependent variables of the Web study. This mode of analysis enables one to examine how multiple predictors contribute both separately and jointly to the explanation of variance in the outcome variables. Such a capability is of special importance when examining the effects of multiple determinants such as those investigated in the Web study (compare Cohen and Cohen 1983; Pedhazur 1982).

Each of the following chapters concentrates initially upon the item-by-item univariate relationships between the subjects' CBCL scores and relevant environmental or coping variables. We explore the interactive and cumulative relationships among the predictor variables only after the individual relationships have been analyzed. Subsequent chapters further develop the multivariate predictive model by examining the relationship between parental mental health problems and children's behavior as mediated by environmental stressors or protectors and the children's coping strengths and weaknesses. In each chapter, we follow descriptive analyses of the pertinent variables by univariate regression analyses that examine the relationship between each of the environmental or coping variables and the criterion variable, namely, the subjects' behavior problem scores. In turn, we follow these analyses by multiple regression analyses that elucidate the interrelationships among the larger array of independent variables and the subjects' behavior problems.

SUMMARY AND DISCUSSION

This chapter describes the referral, intake, and interview procedures utilized in the Web study. It also describes the research instruments employed in comprehensive interviews with the at-risk children and their parents or guardians. We acquire relevant data not only from parents but also from teachers, therapists, and referral agents. The central measures focus upon the subjects' behavior problems, environmental stressors or protectors, and personal coping strengths or weaknesses. We measured the subjects' behavior problems by means of the Achenbach Child Behavior Checklist (CBCL), used by parents and school teachers. In addition, parents, teachers, and the children themselves completed a Brief Rating Index for Children (BRIC). We also measured a broad array of environmental stressors and protectors, such as demographic differences among the referred subjects and their families, physical and mental health problems manifested by the subjects and their family members, life-change events to which the at-risk children had been subjected since birth, variations in the subjects' living arrangements and family support systems, and the frequency of discord among various family members. Among the key coping strengths measured are the at-risk children's social competence, self-esteem, intelligence, and social and academic achievement. Finally, the chapter discusses the descriptive statistics and methods of univariate and multivariate regression analysis in the Web study from both conceptual and operational perspectives.

6 The Children

A T THIS JUNCTURE, LET US BECOME BETTER ACQUAINTED
with the subjects who participated in the Web study—the youngsters
who were reared in the web of mental illness. We will examine their demographic characteristics, and, especially, the extent to which they exhibit
significant behavior problems; however, in so doing, it should be recognized
that the presence or absence of behavior problems can be reported by a
variety of different sources including parents, teachers, and the children
themselves. We will not only consider data from all of these parties, but we
will also examine the findings with particular reference to their association
with the subjects' position on the victim-vulnerable-invincible continuum.

BEHAVIOR PROBLEM SCORES

As noted previously, all subjects were referred to the Web study because one
or both of their parents had been in treatment for a mental illness; no child
was referred on the basis of his or her own behavioral or mental health
problems. The subjects' scores on the Achenbach CBCL were employed as
primary indicators of behavior problems. A subject's CBCL score can be
depicted in terms of its position on a continuum that ranges from the complete absence of behavior problems to the presence of extraordinarily severe
problems. In other words, the subject's status can differ from that of victim
(the presence of severe behavior problems) to vulnerable (the presence of
moderate behavior problems) to invincible (the presence of few or no behavior problems). We assume that the child's CBCL score is shaped by the
relative balance between his or her personal coping skills and net environmental stressors and protectors.

In the current study, a subject's behavioral status is indicated by his or her
normalized T-score on the CBCL, ranging from 30 to 90. The normalized
T-score (with a mean of 50 and a standard deviation of 10) yields information
about the relative location of the subject's score within a general population.
In a normal distribution, only 10% of the general population are likely to
have a T-score greater than 63 (Achenbach and Edelbrock 1981); conversely,
only 10% would be expected to have a T-score below 37. However, the

Figure 6.1.

Frequency Distributions of CBCL Scores for a General Population
of Children and for the Web Children

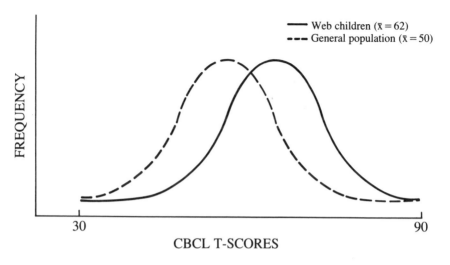

CBCL T-SCORES

T-scores of the Web subjects differ greatly from those in a general population
(see figure 6.1). The majority, or 53% ($n = 162$), of the referred children
have CBCL scores in the highest decile of scores for a normal population. In
a parametric sample of the same size, one would expect to find only 30
children with such extreme scores. Obviously, then, many of the children
referred to the Web study display behavior profiles that identify them as
"victims"; that is, they exhibit severe behavioral problems.

Only five of the children, or fewer than 2%, have CBCL scores within
the lowest decile for a normal population. In a random sample of the same
size, one would expect thirty subjects to have scores within this range. It is
evident, then, that very few of the referred children can be regarded as invincibles. The remaining 45% ($n = 139$) of the Web subjects have CBCL
scores that do not fall into either the victim or the invincible ranges of the
continuum. About 80% of all children in a normal population would be
expected to have CBCL scores within this range. These children, whose
behavior does not clearly identify them as either victims or invincibles, may
be regarded as vulnerables. Their CBCL scores represent a range of behavior that may vary from relatively minor problems to moderately severe
problems. Within the referred sample, the CBCL scores for such subjects
tend to cluster toward the higher, or more problem-ridden, end of the
continuum.

We present the contrasts between the CBCL scores for a normal parametric population and for the Web subjects in figure 6.1. While the latter distribution approximates a normal curve, its mean value is considerably higher than that of the former population. Of a normal distribution 50% ought to have CBCL scores below the midpoint on the victim-vulnerable-invincible continuum, and 50% ought to have scores above the midpoint; however, among the Web subjects only 10% have scores below this point, while 90% have scores above it. Hence, the at-risk children who participated in the Web study clearly have more behavioral problems than other children. It behooves us, then, to discover why such a large proportion of these children have such problems. By the same token, it is important to find out why certain youngsters—even if a distinct minority within the Web sample—are able to avert the severe behavioral problems manifested by the great majority of their at-risk peers.

DEMOGRAPHIC CHARACTERISTICS AND BEHAVIOR PROBLEM SCORES

In many studies demographic factors such as the age, sex, race, or religion of the subjects explain significant variance in criterion behaviors. To begin, let us examine these variables. Because of unequal group sizes, the following analyses of omnibus mean difference tests are based upon the General Linear Model.

Age

Some investigators suggest that at-risk children show evidence of behavior problems from birth onwards (Fish and Hagin 1973; MacCrimmon, Cleghorn, Asarnow, and Steffy 1980; Mednick and Schulsinger 1968). Others assert, however, that significant behavior problems may not show up until early adolescence, particularly if one has schizophrenic parents (Bleuler 1974; Moskalenko 1972). Correspondingly, there is a considerable range of opinion about the effects of significant life events on children's behavior (for instance, Coddington 1979; Sandler and Block 1979; Vincent and Rosenstock 1979). Since many such events occur at patterned intervals throughout the life course, age many be a critical determinant of the behavioral outcomes of at-risk children.

The referred children who took part in the Web study vary in age from 6 1/2 through 15 years (depicted in table 6.1). The mean age is 10.2 years,

Table 6.1.
Age Distribution of Web Subjects

Age	n
6	18
7	35
8	39
9	36
10	44
11	37
12	31
13	27
14	31
15	8

NOTE: $n = 306$.

and the standard deviation is 2.5 years. A linear regression analysis shows that age does not predict the subjects' respective positions on the victim-vulnerable-invincible continuum; that is, a significant relationship does not exist between the subject's age and the presence or absence of behavior problems on his or her part. Bearing in mind that the CBCL is normed for age, the at-risk subjects display the same age-related distribution of scores as children from the general population.

Sex

Many investigators contend that gender predisposes an individual toward risk for certain types of behavior problems. Studies indicate that males are more disposed than females toward physical problems that can heighten their vulnerability to stressful life events and adverse behavioral outcomes (Morris, Williams, Atwater, and Wilmore 1982; Kalverboer and Brouwer 1983). However, some investigators take exception to this conclusion (Miller, Hampe, Barrett, and Noble 1971). Hence, it is pertinent to inquire whether the gender of at-risk children is associated differentially with the presence or absence of behavior problems on their part.

Of the 306 subjects, 58% ($n = 177$) are male, while 42% ($n = 129$) are female. Like age, sex is not associated significantly with the distribution of CBCL scores. Since the CBCL is normed for variations by sex, this finding also indicates that the Web subjects do not differ from a normal population in terms of their gender-based distribution of behavior problems. That is, vis-à-vis other males and females of the same age from a general population, the

referred children exhibit no gender-related variations in the distribution of
CBCL scores.

Race

Some investigators posit that race can influence one's risk status and vulnerability (Scanzoni 1977; Staples 1971; Zegiob and Forehand 1975). Among
the Web subjects, 64% ($n = 196$) are white, and 33% ($n = 101$) are black.
Only four are American Indian, three are Hispanic, and two are categorized
as "other." Since only nine subjects are included in the three latter categories, valid analyses of these categories are not feasible. Hence, two alternative
data analysis strategies were considered: (1) eliminating these subjects from
the analyses or (2) combining them with black subjects in order to create
a category denoted as "nonwhite." In short, both types of analyses yield
similar results. To employ the full sample, therefore, our analyses of the
subjects' race are based upon the white–nonwhite distinction. The latter
category encompasses black, American Indian, Hispanic, and "other" subjects. Again, no significant differences appear between the mean CBCL
scores of the white and nonwhite subjects. Thus, with particular reference to
their CBCL scores, the subject's race contributes little above and beyond the
risk status imposed by his or her parents' mental illness.

Religion

Religious affiliations are sometimes thought linked with value systems that
may influence social behavior (Boshier and Izard 1972) or attitudes towards
mental illness (Erickson 1982). Hence, it was deemed relevant to examine
the relationship between this variable and the subjects' CBCL scores. Since
the children reported their religion directly to the interviewer, the requisite
data pertain to their own religious identification rather than that of their parents or parental surrogates.

Data about religion were not obtained for two of the subjects. Of the
remainder, 44% ($n = 133$) are Protestant, 25% ($n = 76$) are Catholic, 22%
($n = 66$) have no religious affiliation, 9% ($n = 26$) are of "other" religions,
and fewer than 1% ($n = 3$) are Jewish. For purposes of data analysis, therefore, the Jewish subjects were included in the "other" category. No significant religious differences were found in the subjects' CBCL scores.

Thus, major demographic differences among the subjects are not associated with their respective positions on the victim-vulnerable-invincible
continuum. Neither age, sex, race, nor religion are associated differentially

with the CBCL scores of children who already are at-risk for behavior problems in view of their parents' mental illness. These findings suggest that the central sociological and social psychological factors that shape the behavior of at-risk children are more immediate in nature. The key features of the web of mental illness are more likely to be intrafamilial factors influenced in part by the parents' mental illness. These and others factors will be examined in subsequent chapters.

BEHAVIORAL CHARACTERISTICS AND BEHAVIOR PROBLEM SCORES

Besides completing the Achenbach CBCL, the parents of the referred children participated in an extensive interview prior to their child's enrollment in the Web study. During the course of the interview, they indicated whether or not the child had been diagnosed as having a behavioral or mental health problem; if so, they indicated the DSM-III diagnosis that had been applied. They also stated whether or not the child was in treatment for the reported problem. Furthermore, the parents estimated the extent to which the problem interfered with the child's ability to function in normal activities. In conjunction with the CBCL scores, these pieces of information constituted useful checks for the convergent validity of the parents' evaluations of their children's behavior. This is of particular value since the accuracy of parental reports may be open to question when the respondents have been diagnosed as mentally ill. It was essential to employ parental reports because few other persons knew the at-risk child well enough to provide a valid and comprehensive assessment of his or her behavior. Although the best-functioning parent was always selected to report about the child's behavior, this individual had sometimes been deemed mentally ill. Hence, additional measures of the child's behavior problems were obtained from the other parent, teachers, the children themselves, and, in the case of DSM-III diagnoses, from referral and treatment agents. Consistent with the findings of Robins and her colleagues (1985), crosschecks of these assessments revealed no incongruencies associated with parental mental illness.

Mental Health Problems

The parents of the referred subjects were asked whether or not their child had ever been diagnosed as having a major mental health or behavioral disorder. If so, the validity of the reported diagnosis was checked with the mental health professional who had treated the child. The major DSM-III (American Psychiatric Association 1980) categories for childhood disturbance were employed: "behavioral problem," "intellectual problem," "emotional problem," "physical problem," "developmental problem," and "no problem."

Since only thirty-three subjects reportedly had problems other than "behavioral", the foregoing categories were collapsed into "behavioral problems," "other problems," and "no problems." Using this schema, significant differences appear among the subjects' CBCL scores ($p < .0001$, $R^2 = .24$). The three categories predict 24% of the variance in CBCL scores: children with a parent-reported behavior problem ($n = 87$) have a mean CBCL score of 70.2; children with "other" parent-reported problems ($n = 33$) have a mean CBCL score of 68.9; and children with no parent-reported problems ($n = 186$) have a mean CBCL score of only 58.5. Subsequent t-tests reveal no significant differences between the CBCL scores for subjects with behavioral problems and other problems. However, the CBCL scores of these two groups of subjects differ significantly from the CBCL scores of children with no parent-reported behavior problems. This finding tends to validate the accuracy of the parents' CBCL reports.

Treatment Status

The parents also reported whether or not their children were being treated for a major mental health or behavioral problem. Three categories were employed in order to indicate the child's treatment status: "in treatment," had a "problem but was not in treatment," or had "no problem" and therefore was not in treatment. Respectively, the number of subjects in these categories is 97, 39, and 170. The analysis reveals significant differences among the mean CBCL scores of these subjects ($p < .001$, $R^2 = .22$). Thus, the mean CBCL score for children in treatment is 68.4. The mean CBCL score for children not treated despite a mental health or behavioral problem is 70.1. The comparable score for children who have no problem and are not in treatment is only 58.1. Subsequent t-tests reveal that the at-risk children who have a problem and are in treatment have slightly (but not significantly) lower CBCL scores than untreated children who have a problem. In contrast, the no-problem subjects have significantly lower mean CBCL scores than the other two groups.

Child-Reported Behavior Problems

Related data about the subjects' behavior problems obtained from the children themselves offer an additional vantage point from which to examine the subjects' behavior. Although they provide a useful comparison for parental reports, the two data sets cannot be regarded as fully comparable. It is possible that parents and children refer to differing contexts or take cognizance of differing kinds of activities when evaluating behavior. Moreover, because a self-report version of the Achenbach CBCL had not been devised at the time of the study, an alternative self-report measure was employed for the Web study. The subjects were asked to rate their own behavior on the children's form of the Behavioral Rating Index for Children (BRIC-C). Their responses to this measure are correlated significantly ($r = .20$, $p < .001$) with parental responses to the same instrument, the BRIC-P. Importantly, scores on the latter measure also are correlated highly with parent-report scores on the Achenbach CBCL ($r = .76$, $p < .001$; cf. Stiffman, Orme, Evans, Feldman, and Keeney 1984).

The subjects' BRIC-C scores and CBCL scores are significantly correlated ($r = .21$, $p < .0003$), suggesting that the children tend to interpret their own behavioral patterns in much the same way as their parents do. The children and parents tend to agree when the youngster has serious behavior problems and, likewise, when the child does not have such problems. As stated in the preceding chapter, we can provide conceptual and empirical anchors for the victim-vulnerable-invincible continuum by paying special attention to HiProb subjects and LoProb subjects. The HiProb subjects (those who scored within the highest decile of CBCL scores) have mean BRIC-C scores of 35.7. LoProb subjects (those who scored within the lowest decile of CBCL scores) have mean BRIC-C scores of only 25.0. In general, then, it is evident that the at-risk children and their parents agree about the extent of behavior disorder on the child's part.

Teacher-Reported Behavior Problems

The children's teachers were also asked to rate their behavior. Consequently, information was acquired about the children's behavior in two important settings—the home and the school. Scores on the teachers' version of the Behavioral Rating Index for Children (BRIC-T) are associated significantly with the parent-reported CBCL scores ($r = .33$, $p < .001$). HiProb children have mean BRIC-T scores of 39.0, while LoProb children have mean BRIC scores of 23.8.

The teachers also completed the Teacher's Form of the Achenbach CBCL. Although this version of the Checklist has not yet been normed for age or sex, the resultant raw scores agree substantially with the normed results on the parent version of the CBCL ($r = .37$, $p < .0001$). Therefore, the teachers and parents tend to agree substantially in their evaluation of the children's behavior. The mean teacher-reported CBCL raw score for HiProb subjects is 35.2, while the comparable raw score for LoProb subjects is 17.5.

Physical Health Problems

Much of the available literature suggests that children regarded as invincible are physically healthier than their more vulnerable counterparts (Garmezy 1974; Rolf 1972; Rolf and Garmezy 1974; Werner and Smith 1982). They tend to have fewer prenatal and postnatal problems (Rutter 1974) and better general health (Mednick and Schulsinger 1968). To further examine this relationship, we acquired data about the subjects' physical health, allergies, and medications.

Severity of Health Problems. The parents reported the severity of their children's physical health problems by responding to a standard measure employed by the National Center for Health Statistics. Four response categories were provided: (1) no problem/not limited in any activities, (2) not limited in major activities (e.g., school) but otherwise limited (e.g., play, sports, reading), (3) limited in amount or kind of major activity, and (4) unable to carry on major activity. In brief, no significant differences were found between the mean CBCL scores of 22 children with health problems severe enough to limit their daily activities ($M = 67.0$) and 269 children who were not limited by health problems ($M = 62.3$). Although the data suggest that children with poor physical health may have more serious behavioral problems than other youngsters, the trend falls short of statistical significance ($p < .06$). Even the subjects with good physical health have a mean CBCL score that verges on the clinical criterion for significant behavior disorder.

Allergies. Information also was acquired about the subjects' allergies. Significant differences ($p < .008$, $r^2 = .02$) were found between the mean CBCL scores of 227 at-risk children who have no allergies $M = 62.0$) and 77 who have at least one allergy ($M = 66.0$). While providing support for the notion that there may be a relationship between physical health and mental health, the overall trends seem to indicate that the chronicity rather than severity of a child's physical health problems may be a better predictor of behavior problems.

Medications. Similar conclusions tend to emerge when the children's use of medications is examined. A significant difference ($p < .05$, $r^2 = .01$) exists between the mean CBCL scores of children who take medications ($n = 28$, $M = 67.1$) and those who do not ($n = 278$, $M = 62.6$). The primary medications used by the former subjects are stimulants ($n = 7$), anticonvulsants ($n = 4$), minor tranquilizers ($n = 4$), sedatives or hypnotics ($n = 2$), a major tranquilizer ($n = 1$), and other medications ($n = 9$). While medications may diminish the untoward behavior of some at-risk children, it is clear that the subjects who take them have higher CBCL scores than other subjects. Several of the prescribed medications are the type usually employed for the behavioral management of children who have minimal brain damage (Humphries, Kinsbourne, and Swansen 1978). Unfortunately, however, it is not possible to ascertain definitively whether these medications were administered solely for physical problems or, as is more likely, for a variety of behavioral problems. Regardless, in the absence of medication it seems evident that certain of the Web subjects might have had considerably higher CBCL scores than otherwise.

School Performance

Parents and teachers provided relevant information abount the subjects' school performance. The parents reported whether the children had ever repeated a grade and whether or not they had problems at school. The teachers rated the children in terms of actual school performance and observed social behavior.

Parent Reports. The parental report data do not reveal a significant difference between the mean CBCL scores of children who have never failed a class and those who have. The lack of statistical significance suggests that behavior problems and academic performance on the part of at-risk children are discrete phenomena that need not necessarily be associated with one another. This does not appear to be the case for children from the general population; when the latter children have behavioral problems they are more likely to have failed in school (Craig and Glick 1968; El-Guebaly, Offord, Sullivan, and Lynch 1978).

Teacher Reports. Correspondingly, a significant relationship does not exist between the average grades of the at-risk children and the CBCL scores reported by either their teachers or their parents. The teachers provided information about the child's final grade in each academic subject studied during the past year. Using the average grade for all courses, the data from neither teachers nor parents revealed an association between the children's school problems and their behavior problems.

SUMMARY AND DISCUSSION

Altogether, 306 at-risk children participated in the Web study, each referred solely because he or she had a parent diagnosed as mentally ill. Although no child was referred because of personal behavior problems, the available data demonstrate that the Web subjects exhibit significantly more problems than would be found in a random sample of the general population. Using the subjects' scores on the Achenbach CBCL as the criterion variable, more than half of the referred children have behavior problem scores within the clinical range (63 or above). Only 10% of a random sample of children from the general population would be expected to have CBCL scores as high as those registered by 53% of the Web subjects; hence, unusually large numbers of the latter children have serious behavior problems. Likewise, one would expect 10% of children from the general population to have CBCL scores of 37 or lower. Yet, only 2% of the Web subjects have scores within this range. Although the CBCL scores of the Web subjects vary widely, it is clear that they cluster toward the victim end of the victim-vulnerable-invincible continuum. Moreover, the behavior problems of such youngsters do not seem to vary in accord with such factors as their sex, age, race, or religion.

Formal diagnoses of the subjects' mental health problems, reports about their treatment status, and related variables are consistent with these trends. For example, children with a formal DSM-III diagnosis have CBCL scores that average above the clinical cutting point. Reports by the children themselves and by their teachers are consistent with the cited trends. The children's responses to the BRIC-C concur with the parental reports about their behavior problems, and the teachers' responses to the BRIC-T and the CBCL agree significantly with the parental reports. While physical illness is associated with the presence of behavior problems, this appears to be the case primarily for chronic rather than acute health problems. Data regarding the subjects' allergies and use of medications tend to support this conclusion.

Thus, the data in this chapter show that the referred subjects are not only enmeshed in the web of mental illness but also that large numbers of them have already been victimized by it. Scores on the Achenbach CBCL indicate that more than half of the referred at-risk children manifest significant behavior disorders. Yet, aside from the fact of their parent's mental illness, the data provide neither clues about the reasons for the children's behavior problems, nor do they indicate why some youngsters remain problem-free while others develop severe behavior disorders. Accordingly, we must examine the web of mental illness in greater detail, beginning with those threads in the web shaped by the parents of the at-risk children.

7 The Parents

THIS CHAPTER INITIATES OUR EXAMINATION OF THE various strands in the web of mental illness. We begin with the first and foremost components: the parents of the at-risk children. From the outset, our discussion of the parents' role is complicated by the fact that the Web subjects sometimes lived in families with vastly different types of "parents": for example, an at-risk child may live with a biological mother and a biological father; a biological mother and a stepfather; a biological father and a stepmother; a single biological mother or stepmother; a single biological father or stepfather; foster or adoptive parents; or an endless variety of common law parental surrogates. In this chapter we examine the particular living arrangements most common to the Web subjects. Subsequently, we review basic demographic attibutes of the parents—race, religion, age, and mental and physical health.

CURRENT LIVING ARRANGEMENTS AND THE BEHAVIOR OF AT- RISK CHILDREN

As noted above, not every participant in the Web st;udy lives in a conventional family with two biological parents. During the intake interview, we obtained relevant information about the current living arrangement of each subject, including the number and marital status of his or her parents, the total number of individuals living in the household, and the number and behavioral characteristics of siblings in the home. Like many investigators, we assumed initially that children in unstable families and single-parent families might encounter more risk than children in other families.

Examination of the subjects' current living arrangements highlights the instability of their family situations. Only a distinct minority (20%) of the Web subjects still lived with both biological parents at the time of the intake interview. By far the largest proportion (43%) reside with only one biological parent; of these, 127 live with their biological mother, while only 6 live with their biological father. An additional 11% ($n = 34$) live with a biological parent and a stepparent; of these, 32 live with their mother and a stepfather, while only two live with their father and a stepmother. Therefore, 221 of the

Table 7.1.

Associations between Mean CBCL Scores and Current Living Arrangement

Current Living Arrangement	*n*	Mean CBCL Score
Two biological parents	60	63.4
One biological parent	133	65.1
One biological parent and one stepparent	34	62.2
Relatives	28	60.8
Adoptive or foster parents	41	56.4
Group home or institution	10	67.2

NOTE: $n = 306$; $p < .07$, $r^2 = .07$

subjects still resided with their biological mother at the time of the study. Disregarding all other factors, it is evident that the natural families of the at-risk subjects tended to be severely disrupted at some point, after which the child usually resided with the biological mother rather than the biological father.

If the presence of two biological parents is protective, children with both parents should have fewer behavior problems than those who live with single parents or with parental surrogates. However, the available data do not support this hypothesis (see table 7.1). A linear regression analysis reveals significant differences in the mean CBCL scores for children who reside in differing types of situations ($p < .0008$, $r^2 = .07$). Based on subsequent t-tests, children who live with adoptive or foster families tend to have significantly lower CBCL scores ($M = 56.4$) than those who live with one biological parent ($M = 65.1$, $p < .0001$), both biological parents ($M = 63.4$, $p < .002$), one biological parent and one stepparent ($M = 62.2$, $p < .02$), or in a group home ($M = 67.2$, $p < .009$). The fact that one of the at-risk child's biological parents had remarried evidently does little to diminish the child's behavior problems.

Pending more detailed analyses, these findings suggest that fundamental changes in the at-risk child's family, as evidenced by the processes of marital dissolution and remarriage, are more detrimental than beneficial for the youngster. Although we employ several kinds of retrospective data to examine the validity of this supposition, it can be tested fully only by means of rigorous longitudinal investigation. Pending such analyses, the data suggest that the changing social circumstances of the child's family may mediate genetic influences affecting his or her behavior. This may be for the worse, as in the case of a biological parent's remarriage, or for the better, as in the case of placing the child with relatives, foster parents, or adoptive parents.

Web subjects who still live with their biological parents manifest significantly greater behavior problems than those who live with relatives or with foster or adoptive parents. Thus, contrary to popular opinion, overall trends suggest that continuous residence with one's biological parents cannot necessarily be regarded as beneficial for the at-risk child, particularly if the parents are mentally ill. However, removal of a child from his or her biological parents is also not beneficial when the sole alternative is residence in a group home or child care institution.

The behavioral patterns of at-risk children appear to be most positive when they live in a family setting with foster parents, adoptive parents, or relatives. At this early point in our analysis, inferences about the behavioral consequences of shifting at-risk children from one type of living arrangement to another must be tempered by the distinct likelihood that a child's behavior can cause a change in living arrangement as well as result from it, especially in the case of subjects who reside in a group home or institution. Life in such a setting may exert an adverse effect on the child's behavior, but it is also possible that the child's serious behavior problems will lead to placement in such a setting. Similarly, despite considerable controversy about the relative merits of being raised by a single parent or by two parents, the data reveal no significant differences in the mean behavioral outcomes for children who are reared in either circumstance. Indeed, the mean CBCL scores are quite high for *all* Web subjects who live with either or both of their biological parents.

PARENT CHARACTERISTICS AND THE
BEHAVIOR OF AT-RISK CHILDREN

The above data demonstrate that the lives of the Web subjects are sometimes shaped by two different sets of parents, namely, their biological parents and their "current" parents (often not the child's biological parents, but relatives, foster parents, or adoptive parents). In 227 cases, the child's current parents are also his or her biological parents. Given the overlapping categories, we found no significant differences between the current parents and the biological parents in terms of age, race, religion, socioeconomic status, or the relationship of these variables to the children's CBCL scores. Therefore, in this chapter we will limit our discussion to the current parents of the at-risk children, and in chapter 11, we will distinguish more precisely between the biological and nonbiological parents of the at-risk children as we delineate additional strands of the web of mental illness.

Age

At-risk children who have younger mothers tend to have significantly higher CBCL scores than at-risk children who have older mothers ($r = -.21$, $p < .0005$). The mothers ranged in age from 15 through 62 years (clearly suggesting a foster or adoptive parent) at the time of the child's birth. Analogous trends do not appear, however, for the subjects' current fathers. It is quite probable that the observed trends for mothers are attributable to variations in the onset patterns of certain kinds of mental illness. For instance, there is some indication in the literature that adults who are older at the first onset of mental illness may be less seriously affected than those who are younger (Bleuler 1974). The older parents in the Web study do, in fact, exhibit a later onset of mental illness than the younger ones ($p < .001$ for fathers; $p < .001$ for mothers).

Religion

Data regarding religion were acquired only about the subjects' current parents. Compared to some of the other demographic variables, these data are of limited explanatory value. The religion of both the current mother ($p < .001$, $R^2 = .06$) and the current father ($p < .001$, $R^2 = .05$) are significantly associated with children's behavior problems (see table 7.2). Subsequent t-tests reveal that the mean CBCL score of children whose current mothers are Protestant ($M = 60.3$) is significantly lower than those whose mothers are either Catholic ($M = 66.6$), of another religion ($M = 63.8$), or of no particular religious faith ($M = 64.6$). Similar trends are found for the children's current fathers. Children with a Protestant father have CBCL scores ($M = 60.3$) that are significantly lower than children whose fathers are Catholic ($M = 64.8$), of some other religion ($M = 67.4$), or of no religious persuasion ($M = 64.1$).

It is possible that the observed trends are mediated by such factors as socioeconomic status and family size. However, when we entered family size and socioeconomic status as covariates into a hierarchical multiple regression analysis, religion still explains a significant portion of unique variance in the subjects' CBCL scores. Although it might be assumed that Catholic families are larger than Protestant families, this is not the case for the Web sample. Hence, the observed variations by religion cannot be attributed to differences in family size.

Table 7.2.

Associations between Mean CBCL Scores and Selected Parental Characteristics

Parental Characteristic	n	Mean CBCL Score
Religion of Current Mother [a]		
Protestant	129	60.3
Catholic	75	66.6
Other	25	63.8
None	57	64.6
Religion of Current Father [b]		
Protestant	89	60.3
Catholic	72	64.8
Other	27	67.4
None	71	64.1
Physical Health of Current Mother [c]		
No problems or limitations	214	62.1
Some limitations	72	66.1
Type of Mental Health Problem of Current Mother [d]		
Affective	115	67.1
Other	78	62.6
None	90	59.0
Limitations Imposed By Mental Health of Current Mother [e]		
No limitations	87	66.6
Some limitations	68	62.8
Prior Hospitalization of Current Father [f]		
Hospitalized	60	60.1
Never hospitalized	191	64.0

[a] $p < .001$, $r^2 = .06$
[b] $p < .001$, $r^2 = .05$
[c] $p < .008$, $r^2 = .16$
[d] $p < .0001$, $r^2 = .12$
[e] $p < .05$, $r^2 = .03$
[f] $p < .03$, $r^2 = .02$

Race

No significant behavioral differences appear among the at-risk subjects with reference to the race of either of their current parents. Nor do these variables interact with the parents' marital status, socioeconomic status, religion, or age. Unlike some studies in which race is confounded with factors differentially associated with the incidence of parental mental illness, this does not appear to be the case for the Web sample.

Socioeconomic Status

The subjects' CBCL scores do not vary significantly in accord with the SES of their current parents. Hence, this variable does not appear to be a key correlate of behavior problems on the part of at-risk children.

PARENTAL HEALTH AND THE BEHAVIOR OF AT-RISK CHILDREN

As noted in chapter 6, some investigators posit the existence of a correlation between parents' mental illness and physical illness and, moreover, between these factors and the risk status of their children. Accordingly, during the intake interview we took detailed health histories about both the current mother and father and the biological mother and father, including physical health, mental health problems and diagnoses, treatment status, history of hospitalization, and severity of mental health problems.

Physical Health

As discussed in chapter 5, we gathered information about the physical health problems of each parent and the extent to which such problems interfered with the performance of routine activities. The data reveal that the physical health of the mother is significantly associated with the child's behavior problems ($p < .008$, $r^2 = .16$) (see table 7.2). At-risk children whose mothers have no physical problems or only minor problems that do not impede their functioning have a mean CBCL score of 62.1, but children with a mother whose functional abilities are hampered by a physical problem have a mean CBCL score of 66.1. Similar trends are not evident on the part of children who have a father with a physical health problem. Since the mother usually is the primary caregiver, it seems that her physical disability is more detrimental for the at-risk child than is such a disability on the faher's part.

Mental Health

To learn more about the effects of parental mental illness, we need information about specific factors: the type of illness, whether one parent or both are ill, the extent to which the illness limits the parent's ability to function, the treatment status of the parent, and the parent's history of hospitalization. Accordingly, let us examine these factors in detail.

Type of Mental Health Problem. The current parents of the at-risk children exhibit a broad range of mental health problems (see table 7.3). Since many categories have frequencies too small to include in an analysis of mean differences, the data were collapsed into three groups: affective disorders, any other disorder, and no disorder. Given this grouping, the type of mental health problem manifested by the current mother of the at-risk child tends to be associated with the presence or absence of behavior problems on the child's part (p < .0001, R^2 = .12) (see table 7.2). Again, no such relationship appears between the father's particular type of mental illness and the child's behavior. Subsequent t-tests reveal that children whose current mother has an affective problem tend to exhibit significantly higher mean CBCL scores (M = 67.1) than children with a current mother who has "other" mental health problems (M = 62.6, p < .005) or no problem at all (M = 59.0, p < .0001). Furthermore, as might be expected, children with a current mother who manifests an "other" mental health problem have a higher mean CBCL score than children whose current mother has no problem (p < .04). These findings are consonant with the results of prior studies which indicate that mothers who have an affective illness are highly limited with regard to range and type of childrearing skills (see Bastiansen and Kringler 1973; Bleuler 1974; Buck and Laughton 1959; Polansky, Chalmos, Buttenweiser, and Williams 1981; Rice, Ekdale, and Miller, 1971). Even further, they reaffirm the mother's central role in the child's behavior problems because both severity and type of maternal mental health problems are associated significantly with the child's behavioral difficulties. This is not the case for the father. Moreover, the data support the findings of prior studies which suggest that maternal affective illness inhibits important parenting behaviors which influence childhood mental health (Clausen and Huffine 1979; Gardner 1967b).

Severity of Mental Health Problem. During the interview, the parents were asked to indicate the degree to which their mental health problems, if any, limited their ability to perform routine tasks. This question is analogous to the one for physical health problems. It was assumed, of course, that more limited parents would have children with more severe behavior problems. Again there is no relationship between the child's behavior and limitations due to the father's mental health, corresponding to the earlier data regarding the father's physical health. In contrast, a significant relationship exists between the children's behavior and their mother's limitations due to mental health problems (p < .05, r^2 = .03). However, the direction of the relationship is unexpected. To wit, children with mothers who have no limitations because of mental health problems have the highest CBCL scores (M =

Table 7.3.
Frequency Distribution of Parental Diagnoses

Diagnosis	Mother	Father
Affective	115	22
Substance use	10	16
Anxiety	16	4
Schizophrenia	15	7
Antisocial personality	13	5
Psychotic	7	2
Somatoform	2	1
Personality disorder	6	3
Behavioral	4	0
Organic mental disorder	1	0
Psychosexual	0	1
Other	4	1
None	90	76
Total	283	138

66.6). At-risk children whose mothers are limited to some extent have lower CBCL scores ($M = 62.8$) (see table 7.2). This finding may be due to the fact that highly limited mothers are more likely than others to receive assistance from a well-functioning parental "substitute" or surrogate (a homemaker, guardian, relative, or other adult) who can compensate for their limitations and perform essential parenting roles.

Parental Hospitalization. A significant relationship does not exist between prior hospitalization on the mother's part and the CBCL score of her at-risk child; however, such a relationship does exist between the father's prior hospitalization and the child's CBCL score ($p < .03$, $r^2 = .02$). The children of mentally ill fathers who have been hospitalized exhibit relatively low CBCL scores ($M = 60.1$). In contrast, the children of mentally ill fathers who have not been hospitalized display relatively high CBCL scores ($M = 64.0$) (see table 7.2). In the father's case, therefore, temporary removal from the household and/or effective treatment may lead to improved behavior on the part of the at-risk child. In the mother's case, the absence of such a relationship indicates, regardless of maternal mental illness, that, because of the mother-child bond, the child does not benefit as a result of the mother's temporary absence from the household.

Proportion of Mentally Ill Parents. Although the absolute numbers of ill persons may be higher, the relative proportions of mentally ill persons in a family are likely to be lower in large families than in small families. In any given household, it is possible for either one parent or two parents to be men-

Table 7.4.

Distribution of Mental Illness among Parents of At-Risk Children

Parental Mental Health	Daughters	Sons
One-Parent Families[a]		
Mother		
ill	57	66
well	16	14
Father		
ill	4	4
well	0	0
Two-Parent Families[b]		
Mother Ill		
Father ill	16	7
Father well	15	33
Mother Well		
Father ill	10	22
Father well	13	15

NOTE: $n = 292$.
[a] $n = 161$.
[b] $n = 131$.

tally ill. However, any parent—ill or well—is likely to be a particularly potent socializing agent for a child if he or she is the *only* parent in the family. If the mother or father in a single-parent family is mentally ill, 100% of the de facto parents in that family are ill. For better or worse, therefore, the lone parent in a single-parent family is likely to exert an extraordinary amount of influence over a child, especially if the child has no siblings.

By contrast, if one of the spouses in a two-parent family exhibits disordered behavior, only 50% of the extant parents can be regarded as mentally ill. Presumably, the adverse impact of the ill parent will be countervailed somewhat by the adaptive behavior of the well parent. If both spouses in a two-parent family are ill, however, the proportion of ill parents is again 100%. We submit that the greatest likelihood of childhood behavior disorder exists in families where 100% of the parents are ill (that is, either in a single-parent family in which the parent is ill or in a two-parent family where both parents are ill). A substantially lower likelihood exists in families where only 50% of the parents are ill (that is, in a two-parent family with only one ill spouse). The least likelihood of childhood behavior disorder exists in families where none of the parents is mentally ill.

Table 7.4 depicts the distribution of mental illness among the parents of at-risk children in the Web study. More than half of the children live in

Table 7.5.

Associations between Mean CBCL Scores and Proportion of Mentally
Ill Parents

Proportion of Mentally Ill Parents	*n*	Mean CBCL Score
100%	133	65.3
50%	80	61.8
0%	58	59.5

NOTE: $p < .0001$, $r^2 = .04$

single-parent families, 95% of which are headed by a female. In these families, 76% ($n = 123$) of the Web subjects have an ill mother, while only 19% ($n = 30$) have a well mother. In the latter instance, an ill father has usually left the home due to hospitalization; alternatively, a well mother and an ill father have been separated or divorced. Interestingly, 100% ($n = 8$) of the children who live in a male-headed single-parent family do so with an ill father; in effect, then, 100% of their extant parents are mentally ill. None of the subjects lives in a single-parent family headed by a well father. Most of the children in two-parent families have either an ill mother and a well father ($n = 48$) or an ill father and a well mother ($n = 32$). Only twenty-three of the subjects have both an ill mother and an ill father. Moreover, twenty-eight subjects have both a well mother and a well father; these children have been placed with relatives or in foster care after being separated from a biological mentally ill parent. In such instances, the child's current parent is either a stepparent or a duly authorized parental surrogate.

The primary reason for examining the proportionate distribution of mental illness among Web parents is to ascertain whether or not differing concentrations, or densities, of parental mental illness are associated with differing patterns of behavior on the part of at-risk children. A significant relationship, obtained regardless of whether the family is headed by only one parent or two, appears between the proportion of mentally ill parents in a family (treated as a ratio-scaled variable) and the CBCL scores of their children ($r = .21$, $p < .0004$). Table 7.5 presents this relationship graphically where the proportion of mentally ill parents in the family is treated as a categorical variable and entered into a regression equation. The analysis reveals a significant relationship between the proportion of mentally ill parents in the family and the extent of behavior problems on the part of at-risk children ($p < .0001$, $R^2 = .04$). Subsequent t-tests show that children from families where

100% of the parents are mentally ill have significantly higher mean CBCL scores than children from families with either 50% of the parents ill ($p < .02$) or none of the parents ill ($p < .0008$). There are no significant effects attributable to either the sex of the child or to the interaction between sex of the child and the proportion of mentally ill parents in the family.

The importance of these findings is vividly illustrated when they are examined from a slightly different standpoint—the respective proportions of mentally ill parents in the families of HiProb children and LoProb children. In the former families, the mean proportion of mentally ill parents is 0.9; in the latter it is only 0.6. In other words, HiProb children live in families that consist overwhelmingly of mentally ill parents. Yet, LoProb children, too, live in families where the mean proportion of mentally ill parents is relatively high. As will be seen in the following chapters, the families of LoProb children are characterized by certain attributes that help protect the at-risk youngster from the effects of the parental mental illness.

SUMMARY AND DISCUSSION

As might be expected, the parents of the Web subjects play an integral role in their children's behavior. Moreover, the quantitative and qualitative features of the children's family are related to the presence or absence of significant behavior problems. Children who have moved away from a mentally ill parent, or whose mentally ill parent has left the home, exhibit significantly better behavior than children who continue to reside with a mentally ill parent. The sole exceptions are children placed in group homes or institutions; typically, these youngsters require special care because their behavior is too disturbed to be managed by foster families.

The parent's age, among other factors, is associated with the behavior of the at-risk child. Children whose parents were older when they were born are better behaved than children whose parents were younger. The data indicate that the mental health problems of these parents tended to emerge later in life. Likewise, the parent's religion is associated with the child's behavior problems. Whether one refers to the father or the mother, children with a Protestant parent have significantly lower CBCL scores than children of parents from any other religious background. This finding is of interest since the children's self-reported religion bears no relationship to their behavior problems.

Both the physical and mental health of the at-risk child's mother are significantly related to the child's behavior. When the mother's physical health limits her ability to perform normal roles, her child tends to behave significantly worse than when her problems are nonlimiting; the reverse is true when the mother's functioning is limited by a mental health problem. Mothers who report no limitations in their ability to function have children with more severe behavior problems than mothers who contend their functioning is affected adversely by mental health problems. Perhaps mothers with self-admitted problems turn to other sources of support for childrearing assistance, but parents who feel competent—whether warranted or not—may fail to seek assistance that could help their at-risk child avoid behavior problems.

The particular type of mental health problem exhibited by the mother is also associated with her child's behavior. If the mother manifests an affective illness her child is likely to have significantly more behavior problems than if she has any other type of mental health problem or no problem at all. This trend obtains for both the current and the biological mother of the at-risk child but not for the current or biological father. Hence, certain types of mental health problems may hinder the mother's constructive influence on childrearing more seriously than the father's. An affective illness, in particular, may deter her ability to respond to the at-risk child with sensitivity and emotional warmth.

The nature of the father's mental health problems seems much less determinate for the at-risk child than the nature of the mother's problems. Thus, the type or the severity of the father's mental health problems or the nature of his treatment status are not significantly associated with the behavior of the at-risk child. However, prior hospitalization on the father's part is significantly associated with the at-risk child's behavior problems. Children with a mentally ill father who has been hospitalized exhibit significantly fewer problems than children with a mentally ill father who has never been hospitalized; apparently a father's hospitalization may remove, even temporarily, a key source of strain for the at-risk child. Even more, the father's hospitalization may lead to greater self-awareness and/or control of his childrearing functions. Finally, the at-risk child is likely to have the most severe behavior problems when 100% of his or her current parents—either the sole parent in a single-parent family or both parents in a two-parent family—are mentally ill. The child's problems are likely to be less severe, respectively, when only one parent is ill in a two-parent family or when none of the parents are ill.

Thus, the behavior of at-risk children is associated integrally with the social status and behavioral patterns of their parents and other family members. Significant predictive factors include the proportion of mentally ill parents in the family, the age and religion of the mother and the father, the mother's physical and mental health, and the treatment status of both the mother and the father. Although each of these variables constitutes a major univariate thread in the web of mental illness, subsequent chapters will examine these and other variables from a multivariate and interactive perspective. In so doing, we will further elucidate how the strands of the web are interwoven to influence the fate of the at-risk child.

8 Family Relationships and Children's Behavior Problems

POPULAR WISDOM ASSERTS THAT "THE APPLE DOES NOT fall far from the tree." When applied to the mental health realm, this metaphor suggests that the behavior problems of children are likely to reflect the behavior problems of their parents. After all, most observers consider the family—more than any other sociological unit—the predominant factor that shapes children's behavior. Indeed, as seen in chapter 2, countless studies have documented the close relationship between parental mental illness and the behavioral problems of children.

Some clear trends are evident in the available literature: inadequate parenting, for example, is likely to result in a variety of childhood behavior problems (Patterson 1982); parental discord is likely to cause stress and subsequent behavior disorders on the part of young children (Rutter 1980); antisocial parents are more likely than other parents to rear antisocial children (McCord and McCord 1957). Yet, even these well-documented findings must be couched in cautious terms. The preponderance of research about these variables is based on univariate analyses which assume that "all other relevant variables are held equal." But it is all too evident that the relevant variables which shape a child's behavior are rarely, if ever, held constant outside the experimental laboratory. To the contrary, relevant variables usually interact with one another in a complex fashion. One variable (for example, spousal discord) may shape another (such as inadequate parenting), or two variables may be related reciprocally (ineffective parenting may produce spousal discord which, in turn, further diminishes the quality of parenting). Moreover, any pair of variables that affects childhood behavior may be influenced concurrently by a common antecedent. Thus, spousal discord and ineffective parenting may both be influenced by parental unemployment. Even further, pertinent family variables sometimes covary in an inverse fashion and may thereby neutralize one another. It is conceivable, for instance, that the effects of parental unemployment on childhood behavior may be countervailed by the effects of welfare assistance or personal counseling.

Although welcome changes are taking place, only a small portion of the extant research about childhood mental health examines the interactive and causal relationships among relevant variables. And few studies investigate the differential amounts of variance in children's behavior problems explained by given sets of predictors. The available studies seldom distinguish between two interrelated but clearly separable variables—parents and family. All too often it is presumed that the "family" of an at-risk child is tantamount to his or her "parents," and vice versa. But the family is a far more complex and inclusive social unit than is the parental dyad. As a result, researchers usually opt to study the relatively straightforward relationships that exist between parents and children while neglecting the more intricate ones that obtain in the larger family unit; this distinction is important. Families are of extraordinary social complexity when one accounts for the many siblings and relatives who may live together under the same roof, whereas the parental dyad shrinks to a mere monad when it is struck by death or divorce. Parents' relationships with one another are usually considered additive, while the relationships among the many members of a large family tend to be exponential in their permutations and combinations. Family relationships change more frequently than parental relationships. And, most perplexing from a conceptual and methodological standpoint, children must necessarily be viewed as part of the family unit while, on the other hand, clearly distinguished from the parental dyad. Small wonder that researchers prefer to concentrate upon parental, rather than familial, determinants of childhood behavior disorders.

In this chapter we adopt several strategies to avoid some problems that have plagued prior research. First, our conception of family functioning, although attending to the parental dyad, extends far beyond that unit of analysis. We examine family discord as manifested not only in the affectional and social relationships between spouses but also in the relationship between each parent and the at-risk child. Furthermore, we study discord in the family unit as a whole and examine the role siblings play in family mental illness. Second, we investigate mental illness from an ecological perspective. We examine the extent to which maladaptive behavior is manifested in the entire family system and, in turn, how characteristics of the latter shape the behavior of at-risk children. To perform such analyses with rigor it is necessary to distinguish carefully among the various attributes of one-parent families and two-parent families, families with a single child and families with many children, and families with only a single mentally ill member and families with two or more persons who are mentally ill. Third, we investigate both the univariate and multivariate effects of the crucial variables that influence children's behavior.

FAMILY DEMOGRAPHY AND CHILDREN'S BEHAVIOR PROBLEMS

One of the most salient demographic features of any family is its size. While the size of a family is highly correlated with the number of siblings in it, the correspondence between these two variables is obviously not perfect. In any nuclear family this correlation depends upon the specific number of parents in the family, the number of siblings, and the number of relatives or relevant other individuals who share a given household. Accordingly, our analyses will constantly strive to distinguish these variables from one another. The major variables studied include the mental health of siblings, the proportion (density or concentration) of mentally ill persons in the family, and the extent of discord between various family members and within the family as a whole.

Family Size

Some studies have found little relationship between family size and children's behavior disorders (Marjoribanks 1981; Touliatos and Lindholm 1980). Nevertheless, the available literature about single-child families clearly suggests that family size may exert a number of important effects on at-risk children. Singletons or those reared in very small families tend to have high IQs and relatively high levels of achievement (Clausen 1966), but they also have more symptoms of psychopathology than other children (DeAlmeida-Filho 1984). In contrast, children from large families are considered more cooperative and more conforming but less happy (Clausen 1966; Dreikurs and Soltz 1964). However, few studies have yielded useful information about the operational relationships between family size and specific childhood behavior problems. Because family size is a correlate, but not a direct cause, of such problems, its effects are mediated by other variables more directly responsible for children's behavior. These variables include the amount of individual attention accorded to each child, the extent of intrafamily competition for resources, and the amount of parental tolerance for deviant or nonconforming behavior. Each of these variables—as well as many others—is likely to have a distinct impact on children's behavior; yet each is also likely to be affected in part by family size.

Table 8.1.

Correlations between Children's CBCL Scores and Selected
Family Variables

Family Variable	r	p	PROBLEM STATUS	
			Hi Prob	Lo Prob
Number of persons in household	−.19	<.001	4.4	5.8
Number of siblings with behavior problems	.15	<.01	0.7	0.3
Number of siblings without behavior problems	−.20	<.001	0.2	0.9
Proportion of siblings with behavior problems	.14	<.02	0.4	0.1
Number of parents and siblings with behavior problems	.20	<.0007	1.7	1.2
Proportion of parents and siblings with behavior problems	.27	<.0001	0.6	0.3

NOTE: *n* = 291.

In this chapter, the associations between many of the pertinent variables are examined by means of product-moment correlations and multiple regression analyses. The association between family size and children's CBCL scores is a significant and inverse one (r = − .19, p < .001) (see table 8.1). Contrary to the findings of most other studies, at-risk children in large families tend to exhibit fewer behavior problems than their counterparts in small families. As with previous analyses in this book, end points are employed as descriptive anchors. The end points in table 8.1 consist, respectively, of the mean scores for HiProb subjects, those children in the Web study who had CBCL scores within the highest decile, and LoProb subjects, those children who had CBCL scores in the lowest decile. The average size of Web families with a HiProb child is 4.4 persons, while the average size of families with a LoProb child is 5.8 persons. Hence, the HiProb children in the Web study were usually reared in families with significantly fewer members than LoProb children. This finding alone dramatizes some of the difficulties encountered in research using family size as a predictive variable; it is consistent with prior research findings that regard single children as less happy than children from larger families, but it also challenges the veracity of findings that regard such youngsters as conforming and high-achieving. Clearly, family size alone does oittle to explain children's behavior. Instead, it is more useful to ascertain how family size is linked with more direct behavioral determinants.

It is probable, of course, that the inverse association between family size and children's behavior problems is linked in part with the tendency of severely ill parents to give birth to fewer children than less ill parents, particularly if childbearing patterns are interrupted by early onset of mental illness, late marriage, or prolonged separation from a spouse due to hospitalization or other reasons. However, the putative childrearing advantages of large families can also be attributed to other factors. Such families are likely to provide many role models for young children. They encourage and demand a wide range of social competencies and adaptive behaviors on the part of family members. Autonomy and individual initiative are likely to be promoted and reinforced at a relatively young age. Moreover, the influence of an ill parent is likely to be relatively weak because many other individuals are available to socialize the at-risk child. This is especially important if the mentally ill parent serves as a poor role model. In addition, other family members can serve as "functional substitutes" for the mentally ill parent (Freeman and Simmons 1958) by performing key roles—housekeeping, child care, and wage-earning—formerly the responsibility of the ill parent. Under such circumstances a family with an ill parent ought to be able to sustain its functioning in a relatively well-equilibrated manner. The other members of the family can substantially offset the potentially damaging effects of the ill parent's dysfunctional behavior.

Number of Siblings

As might be expected from the above findings about family size, LoProb children in the Web study tend to have more siblings ($M = 2.3$) than HiProb children ($M = 1.5$). However, the relationship between number of siblings in a family and child behavior problems is not statistically significant. Since the number of siblings in a family is correlated at only a modest level with family size ($r = .44$, $p < .0001$), it appears that much of the variance in the latter variable is attributable to individuals other than children in the household, such as grandparents, aunts, and uncles. In some instances, this variable also refers to infants who are the offspring of siblings of the Web parents. The total number of siblings per family ranges from 0 to 7. Less than one-quarter of the Web subjects ($n = 70$) are singletons. The modal number of siblings is

Table 8.2.

Hierarchical Multiple Regression Analysis Assessing the Effects of
Sex of Mentally Ill Parents and Sex of Child on CBCL Scores[a]

Source	df	SS	F	p	R^2
Model	3	1,778.28	4.76	.003	.06
Error	206	25,649.99			
Total	209	27,428.27			
Source			F	p	
Sex of child			0.47	NS	
Sex of ill parent			12.93	.0004	
Sex of child x sex of ill parent			0.87	NS	

NOTE: $n = 210$
[a] Families with only one ill parent.

one ($n = 99$) while seventy-eight subjects have two siblings, forty-two have
three, and fourteen have four. Two of the subjects have five siblings, and one
has seven. Regardless, it is not so much the absolute number of siblings in a
family that determines a child's behavior pattern as it is the nature and
quality of the relationship with siblings.

Sex of the Mentally Ill Parent

One of the most thoroughly explored relationships in the mental health literature is the association between children's behavior and the sex of the mentally ill parent. As seen in chapter 2, some investigators contend that behavior disorders are sex-linked, while others argue to the contrary. The former
assert, for instance, that a young girl is more likely to emulate her mother's
behavior disorders than her father's. Analogously, a young boy is more
likely to imitate the maladaptive behavior of his father. In other words, these
investigators hypothesize the existence of a sex-of-child by sex-of-parent
interaction in the prediction of childhood behavior problems. However, our
data suggest that the mother's influence is prepotent with children of *either*
sex. It seems unlikely, therefore, that behavior problems are based merely on
the child's modeling of the same-sex parent or upon sex-based linkages
between the parent and child.

A multiple regression analysis for families with one ill parent reveals a
significant association between the sex of the mentally ill parent and behavior
disorders on the part of the at-risk child ($p < .003$; $R^2 = .06$) (see table 8.2).

Children who live with a mentally ill father have significantly fewer behavior problems ($M = 58.2$, $n = 40$) than children who live with a mentally ill mother ($M = 65.2$, $n = 170$). The sex of the at-risk child and the sex-of-child by sex-of-parent interaction do not explain significant variance in the subjects' CBCL scores. Hence, it is clear that the mental illness of a mother is associated more closely with behavior disorder on the part of her child—whether male or female—than is the mental illness of a father. It is probable, then, that maternal nurturance is not only crucial for normal child development but also that other persons in the family cannot readily substitute for the mother in this regard. In contrast, it appears that parental surrogates may be able to substitute rather adequately for the father when he is beset by mental illness.

FAMILY MENTAL HEALTH AND CHILDREN'S BEHAVIOR PROBLEMS

The above findings suggest that factors such as family size, number of siblings, and sex of the mentally ill parent are important predictors of children's behavior problems. However, the behavioral impact of these variables is probably indirect. They are likely to shape dynamic factors that exert a more direct and immediate impact upon children's behavior. The dynamic factors are likely to be reflected in the patterns of social behavior prevalent in the family as a whole.

One approach toward measuring family mental health is based upon assessment of the *proportion* of all persons in a family who exhibit behavior disorders. In the preceding chapter we examined the proportions of mentally ill parents in the participating families. By extending our conception to include siblings and others who reside in the household, this approach offers a comprehensive but concise measure of the concentration, or density, of mental health problems in any given family. As the proportion of mentally ill persons in a family increases, it can be assumed that important changes take place in its internal dynamics. Dysfunctional role models are likely to proliferate in number and potency, and social reinforcement is more likely to be preferred for maladaptive than adaptive behavior. Important family functions are likely to be performed with less efficiency and effectiveness. Furthermore, the members of the family are more likely to be labeled pejoratively by relevant others. This may result in stigmatization or premature foreclosure of valuable social opportunities that might otherwise be available. To be of maximum value, such a measure must account for not only the particular proportions of ill and well persons in a family but also the related factors that determine their respective influence as role models or agents of socialization.

Many subjects in the Web study have siblings who exhibit behavior problems. In fact, seventy-one of the subjects have one such sibling. Seventeen of the subjects have two siblings with a behavior problem, and one has three such siblings. As reported in table 8.1, a significant association exists between children's CBCL scores and the number of siblings who have behavior problems ($r = .15$, $p < .01$). HiProb children have an average of 0.7 siblings with a behavior problem, while LoProb children have only 0.3 such siblings. It is likely that these siblings model and reinforce maladaptive behavior for the at-risk child. In addition, of course, both groups of children may be subjected to common stimuli or to shared environmental demands that exert an adverse impact on their behavior. In all likelihood, these factors and others operate interactively.

As might be expected, data (see table 8.1) also reveal that LoProb children have more siblings who are free of behavior disorder ($M = 0.9$) than do HiProb children ($M = 0.2$). More important, the proportion of siblings with a behavior disorder is four times greater for HiProb children ($M = 0.4$) than for LoProb children ($M = 0.1$). Hence, the at-risk children in the Web study are quite likely to exhibit behavior problems if they already have siblings with such problems. Consistent with earlier findings, these data suggest that children from larger families fare better because their families are *proportionately* less likely to consist of persons with behavior disorders, whereas such disorders are likely to be most concentrated in relatively small families.

Finally, in this regard, it is germane to report that children's CBCL scores vary in accord with the total proportion of mentally ill persons (namely, parents *and* siblings) in the family ($r = .27$, $p < .0001$). The mean proportion of mentally ill persons in families with LoProb subjects is 0.3, while the comparable proportion for HiProb subjects is twice as large ($M = 0.6$). In other words, nearly two out of every three persons in the latter families suffer from a behavior disorder; to be symptom-free in such a family may represent a special form of deviance. Both conceptually and empirically, it is evident that this variable reflects key aspects of family functioning that influence the behavior of at-risk children. Accordingly, it will be scrutinized closely in this chapter and throughout the remainder of the volume.

DISCORD IN FAMILY RELATIONSHIPS

The above findings about the concentration of mental illness in families suggest that the primary determinants of children's behavior may inhere in genetic predispositions, the social and behavioral relationships that exist among family members, or both. Because we are interested primarily in the relationship between children and their environment, however, we pay special attention to the types of social relationships within the family. Both clinicians and researchers have asserted that such relationships are critical determinants of child development. Some clinicians contend that disturbed parental relationships are the root of virtually all forms of childhood disorder (cf. Emory, Weintraub, and Neale 1982; Klein and Shulman 1980; Satir 1972). A substantial body of research indicates that behaviorally disturbed children have more frequent relationship problems not only with their mothers and fathers but also with their siblings and other persons in the family (Fowler, Tsuang, and Cadoret 1977; Lewis, Beavers, Gossett, and Phillips 1976). However, since most relevant studies are merely correlational, it is difficult to assess causal relationships among the key variables.

Although correlational data can inform one's suppositions about causal relationships, throughout this volume we emphasize the need to view such data from a conservative perspective. We can infer cause-effect relationships on occasion, but in no way can we prove their existence on the basis of the available correlational data. Hence, all the correlational relationships cited here should be regarded strictly and solely as evidence of covariation among the correlated variables. For instance, we cannot necessarily conclude that problematic family relationships cause a child to become disturbed or, conversely, that disturbed children stimulate problematic family relationships. Since these variables probably interact in a reciprocal fashion, intervention programs would do well to concentrate upon both the at-risk child and the child's family.

The available research demonstrates that a positive relationship between parent and child heightens the prospects of successful behavioral modeling by the latter (Bandura 1969). In contrast, if the parent-child relationship is distant or hostile, the parents' behavior is less likely to be modeled. Moreover, if a poor relationship develops between the parent and child, the child is less likely to accept the values of the former (Becker 1964), more likely to experiment with drugs and alcohol (Newcomb, Huba, and Bentler 1983), and less likely to resist peer pressures that conduce toward antisocial or delinquent behavior (Friday and Hage 1976; Lee 1983; Linden and Hackler 1973). The various interactions among parental mental health, parent-child

128   FAMILY RELATIONSHIPS

Table 8.3.

Product-Moment Correlations among Seven Measures of
Discord in Family Relationships

	Parent Reports		
	Mother-father	Mother-child	Father-child
Parent Reports			
Mother-father	—		
Mother-child	.25†		
	(*n* = 115)	—	
Father-child	.34‡	.32‡	
	(*n* = 115)	(*n* = 150)	—
Family	.45‡	.29§	.35‡
	(*n* = 115)	(*n* = 288)	(*n* = 153)
Child Reports			
Child-mother	NS	NS	.18*
			(*n* = 142)
Child-father	NS	NS	.18*
			(*n* = 144)
Family	NS	NS	.20†
			(*n* = 151)

* p = < .05   ‡ p = < .001
† p = < .01   § p = < .0001

relationships, role modeling, and childhood behavioral outcomes are far more complex than might be imagined. In some instances, the quality of a child's relationship with the parent may remain relatively unaffected by a parent's mental illness, but in others—particularly if the parent suffers from an affective disorder—the quality of the parent-child relationship may change dramatically.

When the at-risk child has a close relationship with a mentally ill parent, some studies suggest that the latter's maladaptive behaviors or thought processes are likely to be emulated by the child (Anthony 1972). On the other hand, if the child has a poor relationship with a mentally ill parent the consequent rejection and hostility may cause the child to develop deviant behavior patterns (Bell and Vogel 1960). Such disparate views do little to explain why some children remain invincible in the face of their parents' mental illness and others do not. Accordingly, a major objective of the present research is to ascertain more clearly the interrelationships among parental mental illness, functional and dysfunctional family relationships, and children's behavioral outcomes by scrutinizing the particular social relationships that exist among parents, siblings, and at-risk children. Discordant or problem-

| | Child Reports | | |
Family	Child-mother	Child-father	Family
—			
NS	—		
NS	.16* ($n = 214$)	—	
.14* ($n = 288$)	.41‡ ($n = 256$)	.30‡ ($n = 246$)	—

atic relationships within a family can be manifested in countless ways. They may exist between husband and wife, parent and child, or within the family as a whole. Moreover, the pertinent actors may view such discord from differing perspectives or may interpret it in different ways.

Data about family relationships were obtained from all the Web children and from one of their parents. We asked the respondents to report how frequently problems occur in the mother-child relationship, the father-child relationship, and the family as a whole. In addition, we asked parents to evaluate the frequency of problems in their own relationship with one another, using a five-point scale that ranged from "seldom or never has problems" to "has problems most or all of the time." These measures succinctly describe the frequency of discord within the family. If a respondent no longer lived with the individual who was being rated, a sixth response alternative was permissible, "never see or hear from one another."

Table 8.3 presents product-moment correlations for the parents' and children's assessments of varying types of discord in their respective families. Parents evaluated the frequency of mother-father discord, mother-child discord, father-child discord, and discord in the family as a whole. Children evaluated the frequency of child-mother discord, child-father discord, and discord in the family. Significant correlations are evident for thirteen of twenty-one pairs of the relevant variables. As might be expected, there is substantial agreement about the frequencies of the various types of discord within each group of respondents but much less agreement between the two groups. The greatest consensus is evident in the respondents' evaluations of discord in the father-child relationship.

Parental Assessments of Discord in Family Relationships

The parents were highly consistent in their evaluations of different types of problems within the family. Their ratings indicate that family discord is associated most closely with problems in the mother-father relationship ($r = .45$, $p < .001$). When problems occur frequently between spouses, the family as a whole is likely to be characterized by frequent discord. Similarly, if family discord occurs often, the spouses are likely to have frequent problems in their own relationship. The frequency of family discord is also associated with the frequency of discord in the relationship between father and child ($r = .35$, $p < .001$) and between mother and child ($r = .29$, $p < .0001$). Hence, the father-child relationship is more closely linked with family discord than is the mother-child relationship.

Likewise, both the father-child relationship and the mother-child relationship are associated with spousal discord. The parental evaluations reveal that frequent problems between the father and child are more likely to be associated with spousal discord ($r = .34$, $p < .001$) than are frequent problems between the mother and child ($r = .25$, $p < .001$). If the father and child have a warm relationship, the two spouses are more likely to get along well with one another, and vice versa. Conversely, if the father-child relationship is discordant, the husband-wife relationship is also likely to be discordant. As might be expected, a strong association exists between father-child discord and mother-child discord ($r = .32$, $p < .001$). Hence, when the child's relationship with one parent is characterized by frequent problems a distinct likelihood exists that the relationship with the other parent will also be problem-ridden.

Children's Assessments of Discord in Family Relationships

Parents and their children obviously view the world from very different perspectives. Therefore, these parties express only a modest degree of consensus about problems in the family as a whole ($r = .14$, $p < .01$) (see table 8.3). Yet, given the disparity in the respondents' ages, mental health, and social needs, even this extent of consensus is noteworthy. While the parents and at-risk children also express a modest degree of consensus about the frequency of discord between father and child (r = .18, p < .05), they do not concur in their judgments about discord between mother and child.

When one reviews the various relationships, a relatively high degree of consensus appears about the father's role, regardless of whether one refers to the father's relationship with the at-risk child or with the family as a whole. The possible reasons for this finding are manifold. As suggested by Hammer (1963–1964), in many families the father's various functions and roles may be more salient than the mother's. Consequently, family members' judgments about his role performance may be based upon relatively clear and consensually-validated criteria. Alternatively, it is also possible that young children are prone to deny or distort problems in family relationships, particularly if they are attributable to the mother's maladaptive behavior. Because acknowledging the mother's role in family problems may jeopardize her nurturance, parents' and children's judgments about maternal behavior may sometimes disagree with one another. Support for this supposition emerges from the data provided by the at-risk children. Specifically, a stronger association exists between their assessments of child-mother discord and family discord (r = .41, p < .001) than between child-father discord and family discord (r = .30, p < .001).

The parental reports differ from the children's reports since the parents do not deem the mother-child relationship as closely linked with family discord as the father-child relationship. This suggests that at-risk children view the father-child relationship as more important for family functioning than do the parents themselves. A related datum supports this interpretation: the parents' assessments about father-child discord tend to concur with the children's assessments (r = .18, p < .05). However, the parents and children do not agree to any significant extent about the frequency of problems in the mother-child relationship. The primary reasons for this finding again seem to inhere in the differential salience of paternal and maternal roles in the family and in possible distortions of the children's judgments about the mother-child relationship.

The extent of parent-reported discord between the father and child tends to be associated with the children's assessments of problems in the mother-child relationship (r = .18, p < .05) and in the family as a whole (r = .20, p < .01). Consequently, a rather uniform pattern emerges in the web of mental illness. From several different perspectives, problematic relationships between the father and the at-risk child are linked consistently with the children's reports of problems elsewhere in the family system. While mother-child problems are linked with such difficulties, it seems that they are less often recognized or acknowledged by the at-risk child.

Table 8.4.

Associations between Proportion of Mentally Ill Parents in Family and
Selected Types of Parent-Reported Discord in Two Parent Families

| | TYPE OF DISCORD | | |
Proportion of Mentally Ill Parents	Family Discord[a]	Mother-Child Discord[b]	Father-Child Discord[c]
100%	4.0 (*n* = 23)	2.4 (*n* = 23)	3.2 (*n* = 22)
50%	3.4 (*n* = 80)	2.7 (*n* = 80)	2.7 (*n* = 79)
0%	2.6 (*n* = 27)	2.7 (*n* = 28)	2.0 (*n* = 26)

[a]$p < .001$, $R^2 = .11$ [c]$p < .0001$, $R^2 = .21$
[b] NS

MENTAL ILLNESS AND DISCORD IN FAMILY RELATIONSHIPS

The child's relationship with either or both parents is associated closely with
discord in social relationships throughout the entire family system. The
father-child relationship, in particular, seems to be highly salient to family
members. Paradoxically, this may be due to the fact that the mother's nurturance is of such paramount importance that the at-risk child distorts or de-
nies its true nature in order to protect that relationship or achieve a certain degree of psychological comfort. Perhaps the best way to learn more about this
question is by examining how various patterns of mental illness are associated with differing patterns of discord in the family.

Parental Mental Illness and Discord in Family Relationships

Table 8.4 presents parent-reported data for two-parent families in which
none of the parents, one of the parents, or both of the parents are mentally ill.
As noted previously, the former are typically foster families or families in
which a well parent left an ill spouse. As might be expected from the previous analyses, family discord varies directly with the proportion of mentally
ill parents in the family ($p < .001$, $R^2 = .11$). Subsequent t-tests show that
families without mentally ill parents have significantly less discord than
families with either one mentally ill parent ($p < .001$) or two mentally ill parents ($p < .0001$). Likewise, families in which only one parent is mentally ill

have significantly less discord than families with both parents mentally ill ($p < .002$).

The effects of the proportion of mentally ill parents on father-child discord follow a similar pattern ($p < .0001$, $R^2 = .21$). Subsequent t-tests show that families with no mentally ill parents have significantly less discord between the father and child than families with either one mentally ill parent ($p < .008$) or both parents mentally ill ($p < .0002$). Furthermore, father-child discord occurs less frequently in families with only one mentally ill parent than in families with both parents mentally ill ($p < .04$). By contrast, the proportion of mentally ill parents in the family has no effect on the frequency of mother-child discord.

It is conceivable, of course, that mentally ill mothers distort or deny threats to the mother-child relationship. However, many at-risk children are able to sustain a constructive relationship with their mother despite the latter's mental illness; this is especially important in the case of two-parent families in which the father is also mentally ill. These findings suggest that maternal mental illness may be less dysfunctional than paternal mental illness with respect to its effects on the parent-child relationship. More important, they seem to indicate that the bond between mother and child is less vulnerable to disruption by mental illness than the bond between father and child. The quality of the mother-child relationship appears relatively immune to the major forces usually presumed to influence it, such as whether or not mental illness exists on the mother's part, whether the family is single-parent or two-parent, whether only one parent or both parents are mentally ill, and whether the at-risk child is male or female. In short, mentally ill mothers seem as capable as well mothers of maintaining a positive relationship with their at-risk sons and daughters. Moreover, they are able to do so regardless of whether they have the additional burden of a mentally ill husband or, even, no husband at all. Thus, the relationship between the mentally ill mother and the at-risk child appears to be highly resilient, actively nurtured, and protected by all concerned. Yet, when this crucial relationship does in fact become disrupted, especially deleterious consequences may ensue for the at-risk child. Later in this chapter we will complement the data about discord in family relationships with information concerning the children's actual behavior.

Finally, the linkage between parental mental illness and family discord is also affirmed by the correlations reported in table 8.5. A positive association exists between family discord and the proportion of mentally ill parents in the family ($r = .28$, $p < .0001$). Unlike data in table 8.4, however, these data pertain both to one- and two-parent families.

Sibling Mental Illness and Discord in Family Relationships

A positive association exists between family discord and the number of siblings in the family ($r = .33$, $p < .0001$). The greater the number of siblings,
the more likely that discord will occur (see table 8.5). However, the relatively frequent discord in large families does not necessarily result in maladaptive behavior on the part of the at-risk child (cf. table 8.1). To the
contrary, as posited by some conflict theorists (cf. Coser 1954), discord ac-
commodated in a healthy manner may enhance one's social skills.

The data regarding sibling mental illness are consistent with the earlier-
cited trends. Family discord is directly associated with both the absolute
number of mentally ill siblings ($r = .37$, $p < .0001$) and the proportion of
mentally ill siblings in the family ($r = .27$, $p < .0001$) (see table 8.5). It is evident that high absolute or proportionate numbers of mentally ill siblings may
lead to frequent family discord and, conversely, that frequent family discord
may generate a high incidence of mental illness among siblings. Together
these findings lay the groundwork for examining the most central question
of the present chapter: are the effects of discord in various types of family
relationships associated with the differential behavior patterns of at-risk
children?

CHILDREN'S BEHAVIOR AND DISCORD IN FAMILY
RELATIONSHIPS

Thus far we have identified several key strands of the web of mental illness.
It is now evident, for instance, that the proportions of mentally ill siblings
and mentally ill parents in a family are associated with the frequency of
family discord. Likewise, it is clear that the respective proportions of mentally ill siblings and mentally ill parents are associated with the CBCL scores
of at-risk children. It seems plausible, then, for discordant family relationships to be associated with children's CBCL scores.

Family Discord and Children's Behavior

The data in table 8.6 provide support for the foregoing supposition. Moreover, both the Web parents and their at-risk children tend to concur about the
pertinent associations. A positive association exists between the frequency of
family discord and the severity of children's behavior problems ($r = .26$,
$p < .0001$). According to the parents, the mean frequency of discord in fam-

Table 8.5.

Correlations between Parent-Reported Family Discord and Selected
Family Variables

Family Variables	r	p
Number of siblings	.33	<.0001
Number of siblings with mental health problems	.37	<.0001
Proportion of siblings with mental health problems	.27	<.0001
Proportion of parents with mental health problems	.28	<.0001
Proportion of parents and siblings with mental health problems	.23	<.0001

NOTE: *n* = 291.

Table 8.6.

Correlations between CBCL Scores and Selected Measures of Discord
in Family Relationships

Type of Discord	r	p	Hi Prob	Lo Prob
Family discord[a]	.26	.0001	4.0	3.1
Mother-child discord[a]	.42	.0001	3.9	2.1
Father-child discord[a]	.26	.001	3.5	2.9
Family discord[b]	.14	.02	3.6	2.7
Child-mother discord[b]	.17	.006	2.5	1.9
Child-father discord[b]	—	NS	2.2	2.0

[a] = reported by parent
[b] = reported by child

ilies with a HiProb child is 4.0; this indicates that such families have problems "a good part of the time." The mean frequency of discord in families with a LoProb child is 3.1; hence, such families experience discord only "some of the time." One feature of the lattermost datum should not go unnoticed: even LoProb children experience some family discord. But the fact that they are relatively unaffected by it may be attributable to two factors.

First, of course, such children encounter family discord less often than HiProb children. Second, their personal coping skills and unique environmental protectors may be able to neutralize the adverse effects of frequent family discord. We will examine the latter possibility later in this volume.

Table 8.6 provides additional data about the children's assessments of discord in the family. In short, the observed trends are quite similar to the ones reported by parents. Again, a direct association exists between family discord and children's behavior problems (r = .14, p < .02). On the average, HiProb children report substantially higher frequencies of family discord (*M* = 3.6) than LoProb children (*M* = 2.7). Nonetheless, both groups of children report somewhat lower frequencies of family discord than their parents, but it is not possible to determine whether this is due to the parents' tendency to exaggerate the extent of family discord, the children's ability to tolerate it, or the children's possible predilection to deny it or otherwise remain oblivious to it.

These findings pertain only to families with whom the children lived when we conducted the intake interview. In addition, we acquired evaluations of family discord about the children's previous families (those families in which some of them had lived before acquiring stepparents or being transferred to foster homes). Here, too, the association between family discord and children's behavior problems is positive and significant. Although the relationship is somewhat weaker than for the child's current family, it is evident that discord in a previous family setting can be associated with maladaptive behavior on a child's part long after he or she has left that family.

Mother-Child Discord and Children's Behavior

Virtually identical trends appear when comparable data about the mother-child relationship are examined. A direct association exists between mother-child discord and children's behavior problems, regardless of whether the data are reported by the parents (r = .42, p < .0001) or their children (r = .17, p < .006) (see table 8.6). Again, the parents and children tend to corroborate each other's reports. Three findings are especially noteworthy.

First, as we have found for previous associations, the at-risk children tend to report less frequent mother-child discord than their parents. Unlike their assessments about family discord, however, the children's evaluations of mother-child discord are markedly lower than the ones provided by parents. Again, the HiProb children report significantly higher frequencies of mother-child discord than do the LoProb children.

Second, the parents report that HiProb children, on the average, are subjected to frequent discord in the family ($M = 4.0$) and in the mother-child relationship ($M = 3.9$). They report that LoProb children also are subjected to rather frequent family discord ($M = 3.1$); however, they clearly are able to cope with it. In contrast, LoProb children, on the average, encounter very low frequencies of mother-child discord ($M = 2.1$), even lower than father-child discord frequencies ($M = 2.9$).

Third, mother-child discord explains far more of the variance in children's behavior problems than does any other variable in table 8.6. The parents' reports explain 19% of the variance, nearly three times the variance explained by either father-child discord ($r^2 = .07$) or discord in the family as a whole ($r^2 = .07$). In part, this finding may be due to the fact that mothers were usually the only respondents to perform both assessments—mother-child discord and children's behavior problems. Nonetheless, when mother-child discord occurs, it seems strongly associated with behavior problems on the child's part, and vice versa. Similar trends also emerge in the children's reports, showing that child-mother discord ($r^2 = .05$) explains more than twice the variance explained by family discord ($r^2 = .02$). In the children's judgment, discord in the child-father relationship explains none of the variance in behavior problems.

Thus, it seems that at-risk children may often be unable or unwilling to recognize the extent of discord that exists in the relationship with their ill mother. But, if and when such discord is evident, it is strongly associated with the severity of their behavior problems. Moreover, similar findings appear when one examines the child's former relationship with a mother from whom a separation has occurred ($p < .001$). Even if an at-risk child has moved to a foster family or acquired a stepmother, it is evident that the previous problems with his or her former mother may continue to exert an adverse impact on the child's behavior.

Father-Child Discord and Children's Behavior

As noted above, parents reported a high mean frequency of father-child discord ($M = 3.5$) in families with HiProb children but only a moderate frequency in families with LoProb children ($M = 2.9$). A positive relationship exists between father-child discord and children's behavior problems ($r = .26$, $p < .001$) (see table 8.6). But, interestingly, the children themselves do not report the existence of such a relationship. As with the mother-child relationship, HiProb children may be especially prone to distort or deny the extent of discord that exists in the relationship with their father. Also, akin to the mother-child relationship, frequent problems with one's former father are related significantly and positively to subsequent behavior problems on the child's part.

Mother-Child Discord versus Father-Child Discord

The above data lead inexorably to a fundamental question: is the relationship with the mother more influential at shaping the behavior of the at-risk child than the relationship with the father? To answer this question, a simultaneous multiple regression analysis examined whether or not mother-child discord and father-child discord together predict more of the variance in CBCL scores than either variable alone. While father-child discord is significantly associated with children's CBCL scores on a univariate basis, it explains little variance above and beyond that which is explained by mother-child discord (see table 8.7). Hence, a problematic relationship with one's father produces little additional risk for the child. Moreover, a positive relationship with the father does not appear to mitigate the adverse consequences of a poor mother-child relationship. Conversely, however, a positive relationship between the mother and the at-risk child *does* appear to mitigate the deleterious effects of a poor father-child relationship. Moreover, as noted previously, a poor mother-child relationship is less likely to occur than a poor father-child relationship in families where both parents are mentally ill. It is possible, then, that mentally ill mothers are somewhat better able than mentally ill fathers to exert constructive controls over the relationship with their at-risk child. In many respects, therefore, the mother-child relationship appears to be the linchpin for the child's behavioral outcomes.

Husband-Wife Discord and Children's Behavior

Because a significant association does not exist between husband-wife discord and children's behavior problems, it appears that discord between spouses need not necessarily be associated with behavior problems on the part of an at-risk child. This is especially the case as long as the parents are able to prevent their problems from spilling over into their respective relationships with the at-risk child. Mentally ill parents, like well-adjusted parents, are often able to exert this form of protective self-control for the at-risk child. Nevertheless, large numbers of parents in the Web study were not able to offer such protection: spousal discord is associated with discord between the child and the parents or with discord in the family as a whole (see table 8.3). When parents are unable to insulate the at-risk child from spousal

Table 8.7.
Simultaneous Multiple Regression Analysis Assessing the Effects of
Mother-Child Discord and Father-Child Discord on CBCL Scores[a]

Source	df	SS	F	p	R^2
Model	2	3392.36	16.59	.0001	.18
Error	147	15030.47			
Total	149	18422.83			

Source			t	p	
Father-Child Discord			1.93	.06	
Mother-Child Discord			4.53	.0001	

NOTE: $n = 150$
[a] In two-parent families.

discord, the behavioral consequences for the child may be especially deleterious.

Family Mental Health, Discord in Family Relationships,
and Children's Behavior

Much of the mental health literature concentrates solely upon the putative consequences of the relationship between the ill parent and the at-risk child. Some observers refer to this relationship as a form of *folie à deux* (Anthony 1972; Rutter 1966). Others emphasize the mentally ill parent's presumed inability to nurture (Lidz 1970). And still other investigators focus upon the detrimental effects of maladaptive role modeling by the deviant parent (McCord and McCord 1957). In various respects, the data from the Web study either modify, affirm, or refine these conceptions. Regardless of one's standpoint, most investigators assume that the sex of the child, the sex of the ill parent, and the nature of the parent-child relationship all contribute integrally to the child's behavioral outcomes (Orvaschel, Mednick, Schulsinger, and Rocke 1979; Walters and Stinnett 1971). However, the preponderance of studies examine these variables only from a univariate perspective. In our judgment, the practical significance of such variables can be best understood by examining their multivariate relationships.

Thus far our analyses indicate that certain patterns of mental illness and/or discord in the families of at-risk children are associated with behavioral outcomes. In many instances, however, univariate analyses can be misleading due to intercorrelations among the predictor variables. For example, it was shown earlier in this chapter that both mother-child discord and father-child discord are related to children's behavior problems on a univariate basis (see table 8.6). By accounting for the intercorrelations among the pertinent predictors, however, the results of a multiple regression analysis (see table 8.7) demonstrate that father-child discord explains very little unique variance in behavior problems above and beyond that which is explained by mother-child discord; hence, it will be eliminated from subsequent analyses. This finding highlights the efficacy of examining in detail the multivariate relationships among the major threads in the web of mental illness thus far identified: family discord, mother-child discord, and the proportion of mentally ill persons in the family.

On both a conceptual and an empirical basis, proportionate measures of family mental illness appear to be superior to absolute numerical measures because they take account of the diffusing and eufunctional effects of healthy family members on the at-risk child. Of the family mental illness measures reported in table 8.1, it is not surprising, therefore, to discover that children's behavior problems are linked most closely with the one that best describes the family's actual composition (that is, that includes both parents *and* siblings) and, moreover, that takes account of the *relative* proportions of ill and well persons within the family.

From the many variables examined in this chapter, mother-child discord, family discord, and the proportion of mentally ill family members appear to be the best predictors of children's behavior problems. Therefore we entered these variables simultaneously into a multiple regression analysis to assess their individual contributions toward the prediction of the children's CBCL scores (see table 8.8). Both mother-child discord and the proportion of mentally ill family members contribute significantly to the behavior problems of at-risk children. In contrast, the frequency of family discord explains no additional variance in CBCL scores above and beyond the two other variables. Moreover, no significant multiplicative relationships appear.

At this juncture, then, it is evident that the two most potent predictors of children's behavior problems are the extent of mother-child discord and the proportion of mentally ill persons in the immediate family. As with numerous other studies, the mother's relationship with the at-risk child seems to be of greater importance than the father's relationship, and such discord is substantially associated with the child's behavior regardless of whether or not the mother is mentally ill. However, if mental illness on the mother's part disrupts the quality of her relationship with the at-risk child, the child is especially prone to maladaptive behavior. The frequency of mother-child discord

Table 8.8.

Simultaneous Multiple Regression Analysis Assessing the Effects of
Mother-Child Discord, Family Discord, and Proportion of Mentally Ill
Family Members on CBCL Scores

Source	df	SS	F	p	R^2
Model	3	9035.53	32.04	.0001	.25
Error	283	26,602.81			
Total	286	35,638.34			

Source			t	p	
Family Discord			1.81	NS	
Mother-Child Discord			7.24	.0001	
Proportion of Mentally Ill Family Members			4.29	.0001	

NOTE: $n = 287$

is a crucial predictor of the at-risk child's behavior regardless of how mental
illness is distributed in the family. In other words, its effects are independent
of the relative proportions of mentally ill persons in the family.

   In similar fashion, regardless of the extent of mother-child discord, the
concentration of mental illness in the family is a potent predictor of children's behavior problems, suggesting the existence of genetically-linked
behavioral predispositions within the family. At the same time, however, this
indicates that the patterns of behavioral modeling and social reinforcement
within the family become more pervasive, potent, and dysfunctional for the
at-risk child as increasing proportions of family members become mentally
ill. Such adverse social circumstances are far less likely to be amenable to
professional intervention than is the mother-child relationship. Nevertheless,
these are but two critical strands in the web of mental illness. We must
delineate others to better comprehend the range and influence of the various
factors that determine childhood behavior disorders.

SUMMARY AND DISCUSSION

The data in this chapter shed considerable light on the web of mental illness.
Here the families of at-risk children are treated as multifaceted social systems. We employed several different perspectives to examine various patterns of mental illness among parents and siblings, the frequency of discord

among particular members of the family, and the independent and interactive contributions of these variables and others to the prediction of behavior disorder on the part of at-risk children.

The *social relationships* among family members are by far the best predictors of children's behavioral outcomes: the severity of behavior problems on the part of at-risk children increases in accord with the number of siblings exhibiting such problems and decreases with the number of siblings free of behavioral problems. If, as is often the case, a child has several siblings who manifest a behavior problem and several who do not, it is the relative *proportion* of such siblings that best predicts disorder on the part of the at-risk child. This finding is highly consistent with the model of childhood mental illness that appears in chapter 4. In particular, it supports the hypothesis that the relative balance between environmental protectors and environmental stressors is a crucial determinant of susceptibility to mental illness. It implicitly recognizes such factors as the overt and covert conformity pressures within a family and the particular patterns of social and material reinforcement employed by parents and siblings.

On a univariate basis, discord between mother and child, father and child, and within the family as a whole are significantly associated with adverse behavioral outcomes. At-risk children who experience the greatest discord manifest the most severe behavior problems. However, multiple regression analysis reveals that only mother-child discord, as opposed to father-child discord, predicts unique variance in the maladaptive behavior of at-risk children. Hence, when the mentally ill mother proves incapable of sustaining a positive mother-child relationship, the consequences for the child tend to be especially deleterious. In general, both healthy mothers and mentally ill mothers seem able to maintain a positive relationship with their children. Discord occurs much more frequently in the father-child relationship than in the mother-child relationship, but father-child discord does not seem as harmful as mother-child discord. Finally, although multiple regression analysis reveals that mother-child discord and the proportion of mentally ill family members predict the behavior problems of at-risk children in a relatively independent fashion, when considered together, these variables further enhance our ability to identify crucial features of the web of mental illness.

9 Family Support Networks

TO PARAPHRASE JOHN DONNE, "NO FAMILY IS AN ISLAND entire unto itself." When mental illness strikes a parent, most families are able to draw upon relatives, friends, or social service agencies to help them cope with the problems either directly or indirectly associated with the illness. Nevertheless, some families have greater access to such sources of support than others. Moreover, some draw very readily upon the available resources, while others choose not to do so. And, of course, when sources of social support are utilized it does not necessarily follow that their impact upon the family will be beneficial; some families may benefit greatly from the available sources of support, while others may not. In accord with the model set forth in chapter 4, social support networks, if effective, must be regarded as important environmental protectors for high-risk children and their families. Supports can reduce the likelihood of mental illness in a family and help the family cope more readily with a member's mental illness. However, the crucial research question is not whether social support networks can help high-risk children and their families but, rather, which sources of support can help *most* for *which* types of high-risk children and families? In other words, how can social support systems help to disengage high-risk children from the web of mental illness or, more accurately, to avert harm from being entangled in it?

Many researchers assert that social support is one of the most critical variables enabling individuals and families to cope with the stress caused by mental illness (Antonovsky 1979; Caplan and Killilea 1976; Wolfe and Huessy 1981). Indeed, a burgeoning literature documents the importance of social support networks for family well-being and the promotion of community mental health. Most writers posit that networks which effectively integrate family members into the surrounding community are likely to promote mental health on their part (Bott 1971; Caplan 1974; Collins and Pancoast 1976; Pancoast 1980; Phillips 1981).

A considerable body of research indicates that a parent's physical and mental illness tends to be associated with a lack of social support during periods of high stress. In effect, social supports mediate important life stresses so as to attenuate their impact upon illness (Andrews, Tennant, Hewson, and Vaillant 1978; Haggarty 1980; Jenkins 1979; Myers, Lindenthal, and Pepper 1972). Some studies demonstrate, for instance, that a lack of social support contributes to schizophrenic pathology and expedites the removal of ill or isolated individuals from the open community (Marsella and Snyder 1981).

Knowledge about a family's support systems greatly increases the ability to predict the behavioral effects of life-event stressors, whether alone or in combination with a myriad of socioeconomic factors (Marsella and Snyder 1981; Myers, Lindenthal, and Pepper 1972). As Hirsh (1982) asserts, social support networks can provide individuals with much-needed cognitive guidance, social reinforcement, and emotional support to help one cope more effectively with stress. Clearly, however, not all social support networks are equally helpful in mediating the relationship between life stresses and physical or mental health (Caplan and Killilea 1976). All stressful life events are not equally amenable to amelioration, nor are all individuals equally engaged in effective support networks. Rather than those which try to control the difficulty itself, the most useful support networks seem to be those which help an individual cope with the meaning of his or her difficulty, reinforcing the individual's sense of control and expanding his or her repertoire of potential responses (Andrews, Tennant, Hewson, and Vaillant 1978; Barnes 1975; Mitchell 1969).

Social support networks are particularly important for child and adolescent development (Gottlieb 1975). However, the respective contributions of such networks may vary by the sex of the youth; females seem to utilize social supports more effectively than males (Burke and Weir 1978). Such supports may influence the child directly, or, alternatively, they can influence the child's parents so that a more positive childrearing environment is established. Research indicates that the particular impact of social support on children is shaped by the family's ability to utilize it (Gottlieb 1980).

Studies about the effectiveness of social support networks have been deterred, for the most part, by difficulties in conceptualization and measurement. The literature reveals considerable controversy about these topics. Indeed, there is virtually no consensus about the preferred ways to measure the presence of social support. Little consensus exists about such fundamental measurement questions as "who helps," "how much help is received," and "how does one measure the relationship between help received and its effects upon a family's particular types of problems." Some problems seem relatively amenable to help from certain sources of support, while others appear less so. Methods of measurement commonly entail techniques of network mapping (Sokolsky and Cohen 1981) or conceptual definition (Lin, Dean, and Ensel 1981; McFarlane, Neale, Norman, Roy, and Streiner 1981). However, neither of these approaches is particularly useful for the Web study. Therefore, we deemed it necessary to develop our own research instruments to study the effects of social networks on the child's ability to withstand parental mental illness. These measures examine the prevalence of a given family problem, the type of problem, its perceived severity at two points in time, and the formal or informal support networks that may have helped the family cope with the problem. The measures also enable us to study the interrelationships among selected family problems and the effects of a broad range of social support networks. Our analyses focus solely upon support networks used by the entire family rather than by the particular high-risk child. Hence, this chapter examines the various types and severities of family problems, the help or support received from relevant agencies and individuals, and the interrelationships among these sets of variables.

FAMILY PROBLEMS AND SOCIAL SUPPORT

While many Web families must face problems that arise directly from a parent's mental illness, they must also cope with problems due to a variety of other causes. Accordingly, the parents were asked about the foremost problem their family had encountered in the year immediately prior to the intake interview.

Types of Family Problems

Of the 306 Web children, 19.5% ($n = 57$) are from families that have not encountered a noteworthy problem during the year (see table 9.1). In contrast, the remaining children—nearly 80% of the Web sample—live in families that have faced one or more significant problems. Importantly, parental mental illness is regarded as the most significant family problem for only 10% of the Web subjects. Other problems are much more common.

The most frequent problem reported by the parents pertains to childrearing. In fact, 24.3% ($n = 71$) of the Web subjects live in families where the parents report serious problems with their children, not all of whom participated in our study. In many instances they are either biological or foster siblings of the Web subjects. Initially, it appears that the most common problem faced by Web families is not a parent's mental illness but the inability of parents to exercise effective control over their children. An

Table 9.1.

Family Problems During the Past Year

Type of Family Problem	Number of Children with Problem	Percent of Children with Problem	Mean Severity of Problem
Problem with children	71	24.3	3.3
Financial problem	49	16.8	3.4
Parental mental illness or hospitalization	30	10.3	2.1
Severe illness or death	22	7.5	2.5
Separation or divorce	20	6.8	3.1
Marital problem	9	3.1	3.0
Children placed outside of home	8	2.7	2.2
Other problem	26	8.9	2.8
No problem	57	19.5	NA
Missing data	14	0.0	NA
Total	306	99.9	

additional 2.7% ($n = 8$) of the subjects are from families concerned about problems related to the placement of one or more children outside the home. Clearly, the most prevalent problems in Web families—of greater concern than the actual mental illness of a parent—are associated with the care and rearing of children.

Finances are another major problem for many Web families. Whether financial problems contribute to or are exacerbated by the parent's mental illness remains unknown. It is probable that many mentally ill parents are unable to maintain a job. Moreover, the cost of their care may impose a major financial burden on the family. Altogether, 16.8% ($n = 49$) of the Web children reside in families where financial problems were considered of paramount importance during the preceding year. Death and severe physical illness had also struck a substantial number of Web families during the year. Thus 7.5% ($n = 22$) of the Web children live in families affected by one of these setbacks. In addition, the turbulent state of husband-wife relationships in the Web families is illustrated by the fact that nearly 10% of the children live in families in which the parents encountered severe difficulties with one another. Specifically, 3.1% ($n = 9$) are from families in which marital problems are paramount, while another 6.8% ($n = 20$) were subjected to their parents' separation or divorce during the year. Finally, 8.9% ($n = 26$) of the children are from families in which the parents encountered serious problems not revealed to the interviewer.

Thus, the vast majority of Web subjects live in families afflicted by severe problems. In the parents' opinion, parental mental illness is seldom the worst of the family's many problems, largely because its adverse effects appear to be indirect. Although the parent's illness seems to interfere with such important matters as childrearing, spousal relationships, and the family's financial well-being, it is neither the most crucial nor the most informative variable for understanding the dynamics of childhood vulnerability. Rather, one must comprehend how this variable exerts an impact upon fundamental social relationships within the family and how these, in turn, shape the behavior of the at-risk child.

Severity of Family Problems

While the above enumeration of family problems may be informative, it is more germane to inquire about the severity of these problems. Do they transcend the family's ability to cope, or are they regarded as readily manageable? To shed light upon these questions, parents were asked to rate the severity of the main problems that had confronted their family during the previous year. A five-point Likert scale was employed in which responses could range from "not at all severe" to "extremely severe." On the average, Web parents rated their main family problems as "somewhat severe" ($M = 3.0$) at the time of the interview. In addition, the respondents were asked to report the severity of the cited problem at its "worst point" during the year. The mean for this datum was 4.2—between "very severe" and "extremely severe." On the average, therefore, the Web families had faced very difficult times during the preceding year but had somewhat "weathered the storm." The severity of their self-reported problems had diminished, on the average, to a moderate level by the time of the interview.

The most severe problems for the Web families are also the very ones that occur most frequently. Even at the time of the interview (by which point their foremost problem had generally subsided) the financial problems of Web families ranged, on the average, from moderately severe to very severe ($M = 3.4$). Problems with their children were also deemed severe ($M = 3.3$) by the Web parents. Respectively, these problems affect 16.8% and 24.3% of the Web subjects. Moderately severe to very severe problems regarding finances or childrearing were found in the families of nearly two out of every five Web children.

Whereas problems such as separation or divorce ($M = 3.1$) and marital difficulties ($M = 3.0$) were deemed moderately severe at the time of the interview, other problems such as death or physical illness ($M = 2.5$), placement of a child outside of the home ($M = 2.2$), and, even, a parent's mental illness or hospitalization ($M = 2.1$) were deemed of little severity. These problems tended to be acute when they first occurred, but their adverse impact was apparently short-lived. Financial and childrearing problems, in contrast, tend to be debilitating to a family because of their chronic nature. Parents sometimes regard hospitalization or placement of a child as beneficial for the family even though it may be a temporarily wrenching experience. The latter supposition is affirmed by the fact that the parents rated foster placement of their child as an "extremely severe" problem ($M = 4.8$) at its worst, but of only minor severity ($M = 2.2$) by the time of the interview. In this regard, it is pertinent to note that state-sanctioned out-of-home placement in Missouri cannot be accomplished simply on the basis of a parent's request. Typically, public authorities initiate such placements because of parental negligence, abuse, or incompetence.

To a somewhat lesser extent, the same pattern also appears for the sometimes mysterious "other" problems reported by Web parents. At their worst point during the preceding year, these problems were regarded as quite severe ($M = 4.7$), but by the time of the interview their severity had diminished considerably ($M = 2.8$). Although the respondents steadfastly refused to describe the nature of these problems, we learned subsequently in two instances that they referred to incest and child abuse. Several other instances were associated with a parent's arrest for a criminal offense. In any event, it is clear that the vast majority of Web children live in families afflicted by rather severe problems. Moreover, because of mental illness on the part of one or both parents, their families seem less prepared than others to cope with the potentially debilitating effects of such problems. If so, how are these families able to survive their travails? Even more importantly, how are so many of the children who reside in them able to maintain their mental health? At least in part, the answers to these questions can be found in the social environs of the Web families. Specifically, certain of the families receive timely assistance from individuals and/or human service agencies.

FORMAL AND INFORMAL SUPPORT SYSTEMS

A variety of sources, either formal or informal, potentially can assist families beset by problems (see table 9.2). Formal sources include organizations such as social service agencies, hospitals or clinics, schools, financial aid agencies, and employment agencies. Informal sources include relatives, friends, or neighbors. To ascertain which sources of support are employed most frequently and successfully we asked the Web parents to provide several

Table 9.2.
Sources of Family Support

Source of Support	Number of Children Whose Family Received Support	Percent of Children Whose Family Received Support
Agency		
Social service agency	114	48.5
Hospital	33	14.0
School	15	6.4
Financial assistance agency	3	1.3
Employment agency	0	0.0
Other agency	6	2.6
No agency support	64	27.2
Total	235	100.0
Individual		
Relative	40	14.6
Friend	76	27.7
Neighbor	11	4.0
Other individual	32	11.7
No individual support	115	42.0
Total	274	100.0

items of information about relevant agencies and individuals. We asked parents not only to cite which categories of agencies or individuals were helpful to them but also to report the total number of agencies and individuals who provided assistance.

Formal Support Systems

The families of 235 Web children reported major problems of varying severity during the year before their interview. Strikingly, 27.2% received no help from an organization or agency. Formal support systems were either unavailable to such families or, more likely, the family was reluctant or unable to draw upon the available agencies or organizations. Hence, large numbers of Web children and their families received no formal assistance even though they had a variety of severe problems.

By far the most frequent assistance came from social service agencies. Nearly half (48.5%) of the Web children whose families reported a problem had been assisted by a social service agency; however, this is to be expected since such agencies were a prime source of referrals to the Web study. Hospitals (14%) and schools (6.4%) also provided meaningful assistance to problem-ridden families in the Web study. In contrast, formal assistance for financial problems was virtually nil. None of the Web families received help from an employment agency, and only 1.3% had received assistance from a financial aid agency. This is especially distressing since financial problems were frequent and severe for the Web families.

Informal Support Systems

Since many Web families did not receive formal assistance of any kind, one might speculate that they acquired considerable help from informal sources such as relatives, friends, or neighbors. Indeed, perhaps the need for formal support is vitiated if informal support systems are readily available. Contrary to such speculation, however, an extremely large number of families who needed help for a major problem did *not* receive assistance from a relative, friend, neighbor, or any other individual. Altogether, 42% of the Web children lived in such families. Hence, many families had both a mentally ill parent and one or more other problems they regarded as significant; yet, they received neither formal nor informal help. Whether due to the parent's mental illness or not, numerous families and at-risk children were isolated from important sources of potential assistance.

The nature of this isolation becomes evident when one examines the specific sources of informal help for families who faced significant problems. Friends provided assistance nearly twice as often (27.7%) as relatives (14.6%), and neighbors provided much less assistance (4%) than either friends or relatives. The fact that Web families are somewhat isolated from relatives and neighbors—at least with reference to receiving assistance for important problems—may help to account for their difficulties in coping with parental mental illness. Finally, 11.7% ($n = 32$) of the Web children lived in families that received informal help from a variety of other individuals such as ministers, physicians, and storekeepers.

Helpfulness of Support Networks

Assistance from agencies and individuals is of little significance unless it actually helps a family cope with its problems. Regardless of variations in helping patterns, therefore, it is germane to inquire whether any given source of support is more or less useful than others. Hence, parents were asked to rate the helpfulness of each of the agencies or individuals from whom they received assistance. Again, we arrayed the possible responses along a five-point Likert scale that ranged from "not at all helpful" to "extremely helpful." An analysis of informal sources of support demonstrates that no single group of individuals is regarded as more or less helpful than the others; for example, relatives are no more helpful than neighbors. Likewise, despite the relatively great frequency with which they provide assistance, friends are not judged more helpful than either neighbors or relatives.

When formal sources of support are considered, a significant relationship exists between the total amount of help received by families and the type of formal support provided ($p < .001$; $r^2 = .06$). A comparison between social service agencies and all other agencies shows that the former provided twice as much assistance as the latter, despite the fiscal cutbacks imposed upon social service agencies of all kinds. On the average, social service agencies are regarded as moderately to very helpful. Schools and hospitals are regarded as even somewhat more helpful, while financial aid agencies are not considered very helpful.

FAMILY PROBLEMS AND CHILDREN'S BEHAVIOR

The prime focus of the present study is the behavior of at-risk children. Our examination of family problems must aim, therefore, to illuminate the relationship between these problems and children's behavior. Accordingly, we will investigate how the behavior of high-risk children is associated with the particular types of problems confronting their families. As noted above, the preponderance of Web families had suffered in the past year from a significant problem above and beyond a parent's mental illness. Yet, many of the children in these families were able to avoid behavioral difficulties, suggesting that some types of family problems are more closely linked than others with maladaptive childhood behavior. Our data tend to corroborate this supposition.

A significant association exists between the CBCL scores of the Web children and the particular types of family problems they have encountered ($p < .009$; $r^2 = .06$). As might be expected, the lowest CBCL scores ($M = 58.9$) are found for Web children whose families had no problems during the preceding year. Nearly all such families have at least one mentally ill parent, but they do not regard this as a significant problem. In fact, the at-risk children in such families have mean CBCL scores well within normal limits. Contrary to popular opinion, perhaps, children whose parents were separated or divorced during the year also have comparatively low CBCL scores ($M = 60.2$). Their parents' separation or divorce was evidently not traumatic enough to result in clinically disordered behavior. Indeed, the CBCL scores of such children differ hardly, if at all, from the ones of children who live in problem-free families. Above and beyond the parental mental illness that may exist, separation or divorce does not seem to promote significant behavior problems on the part of Web children. Indeed, one wonders whether divorce or separation might alleviate the stress experienced by spouses and, in turn, by the at-risk child? Children from families that have encountered a death or a serious physical illness during the year have relatively low CBCL scores ($M = 61.3$). Hence, at-risk children whose families are problem-free or who have experienced a separation, divorce, death, or severe physical illness do not differ significantly from one another in terms of CBCL scores. Children from these families have mean CBCL scores within normal limits. While the family problems of these children may be acute, they also are rather time-limited; hence, their adverse effects on the at-risk children appear relatively limited.

The highest CBCL scores are associated with "other" problems ($M = 66.1$), parental mental illness or hospitalization ($M = 65.4$), and problems with children ($M = 65.3$). Financial problems are associated with slightly lower CBCL scores ($M = 63.0$). The mean CBCL scores for these types of problems differ significantly from the ones for the previously cited problems and range above the clinical criterion. Naturally, problems with children are likely to be associated with high CBCL scores. As has been evident throughout, parental mental illness or hospitalization bode ill for the behavior of at-risk children. Most important, all the problems linked with high CBCL scores seem to be chronic. Unlike the effects of death or divorce, anguishing as they may be, the stresses that follow from inadequate finances, childrearing problems, and parental mental illness are likely to remain with the family for a sustained period of time. The family, as well as the at-risk child, must try to cope daily with these problems. Yet, as the data suggest, these are precisely the types of problems that seem most closely linked with severe behavior disorders on the part of at-risk children.

SOCIAL SUPPORT AND CHILDREN'S BEHAVIOR

When confronted with a major problem, as we have noted, families can seek assistance from formal or informal sources or both. Also, of course, they can choose not to seek assistance. In general, our data show that the mean CBCL scores for Web children are higher in families that seek help for problems, especially those seeking formal assistance, than in families that do not seek help. A family may seek help for a variety of reasons: it may request assistance when confronted by a single, especially severe problem, or it may alternatively seek aid because of accumulated unmanageable problems. Chronic problems may be more burdensome for a family than short-lived acute problems and, therefore, more likely to promote help-seeking behavior. To learn more about help-seeking, we examined the total number of individuals and agencies from whom each family received assistance. Consistent with the above findings, families that have children with high CBCL scores tend to receive help from more agencies and organizations than families that have children with low CBCL scores ($p < .01$; $r^2 = .03$). On the average, Web families with HiProb children were helped by 1.5 agencies, while families with LoProb children were helped by 1.2 agencies. However, both types of families are equally likely to seek assistance from informal sources.

Additional analyses of the Web families' help-seeking behavior were performed by controlling for the differential severity of the major problem cited. Controls were introduced for problem severity at both the time of the interview and the point in the preceding year at which the problem was deemed worst. In both instances, the findings are consistent with the trends cited above. Again, a significant relationship exists between children's CBCL scores and the number of agencies or organizations from whom help was received ($p < .02$; $r^2 = .03$). Likewise, no relationship is found for the number of individuals from whom help is received. Thus, regardless of whether a family faces a severe or minor problem, it is likely to receive help from more agencies if it has a child with a high CBCL score. Though the evidence is far from definitive, this suggests that serious problems concerning a child's behavior are more likely to engage a family with formal sources of social support than are other types of family problems. Moreover, the extent of engagement seems to vary in accord with the severity of the child's behavior problems. Yet, these trends evidently do not occur with reference to informal sources of support.

To further examine the utility of social support networks we asked the parents to identify the individuals or agencies who assisted them with the family's problem and evaluate their helpfulness, utilizing a five-point Likert scale that ranges from "not at all helpful" to "extremely helpful." Rather than calculate the mean helpfulness of each source of support, however, we attempted to ascertain the *total* amount of help each family received by summing the assessments of helpfulness for all the agencies and individuals who reportedly assisted a given family. Although some families received help from only a single agency, others received help from two, three, four, or even more agencies. Again, a significant relationship was found between the total amount of help received from agencies and the children's CBCL scores

$(p < .003; r^2 = .04)$; families with HiProb children received 50% more help than families with LoProb children. Again, too, no such relationship was found for the amount of help received from individuals. Evidently, relatives, neighbors, and friends were not deemed particularly helpful with regard to the families' childrearing problems. Furthermore, controls for the severity of the family's major problem—whether at the time of the interview or at its worst point during the preceding year—indicate that this variable exerts no impact on the observed relationships. Regardless of problem severity, a highly significant relationship exists between the amount of help received from formal sources and the CBCL scores of the Web children $(p < .005; r^2 = .05)$. The amount of assistance received from such sources is linked most closely with the extent of the children's maladaptive behavior.

PARENTAL MENTAL ILLNESS, SOCIAL SUPPORT, AND CHILDREN'S BEHAVIOR

In essence, this chapter examines three different threads of the web of mental illness: the first pertains to the types of problems encountered by the Web families, their severity, and their relation to the at-risk children's behavior; the second concerns the help-seeking activities of the families and their association with the children's behavior; and the third considers the amount of help the families received and its relationship to various types of family problems, formal and informal support systems, and the children's behavior. An overview of the relationships among these variables helps clarify the role of support systems in the lives of the Web families. The utilization of such systems appears linked with both the nature of the foremost problem confronting the family and the behavior of its at-risk children. In effect, key threads of the web of mental illness are integrally related to one another.

The data reveal that 80% of the Web children's families encountered a major problem in the year preceding their interview for the study. Childrearing and financial problems, far more prevalent than other types, represent 40% of those reported. In contrast, the mental illness of a parent was deemed the foremost family problem for only 10% of the subjects. Other significant family problems were death or severe physical illness, separation or divorce, marital problems, out-of-home placement for a child, and, to a much lesser extent, incest, child abuse, and arrest for a criminal offense.

It is evident that one-third of the families that experienced a major problem in the last year had no contact with a formal support system, perhaps indicating that many Web families were sufficiently resilient to cope with problems on their own. The severity of acute, but transient, problems quickly diminishes in the respondents' view. Examples include death and severe physical illness, separation or divorce, and out-of-home placement for a child. In contrast, some chronic family problems were regarded as key family concerns throughout the year. Foremost among these are childrearing and financial problems. While most of the Web families have a mentally ill parent, few regard this as the family's foremost problem. Evidently the impact of a parent's mental illness is felt most profoundly as a result of its indirect effects on marital relations, childrearing, and the family's finances.

In almost half the instances where a major family problem exists, the family receives no support from individuals such as friends, neighbors, relatives, ministers, or physicians. If friendships are regarded as mutual aid systems, many Web families are bereft of this form of support. Perhaps their difficulties militate against reciprocal and mutually beneficial friendships. Certainly, it is difficult for beleaguered families to offer much to a social relationship. It is virtually impossible to develop long-lasting extrafamilial ties if one is always on the "receiving end" of a relationship since lasting friendships must be based on the reciprocal ability to give and take. The unstable lives of many of the Web families make it extremely difficult for them to generate or sustain this sort of relationship.

The coping skills of the Web families frequently seem exhausted by the demands of day-to-day living. Few resources are left for reaching out to others. Unlike the case with formal support networks, where reciprocal exchange is not always expected, it is virtually impossible to sustain informal support systems for long without some degree of reciprocity. Ironically, those families in greatest need of informal support may be precisely the ones least able to acquire or sustain it. As a result, the Web families are in double jeopardy. Not only must they deal with the demands imposed by the mental illness of a parent, but they are also severely hampered by their inability to cultivate key environmental protectors—informal systems of social support —that could potentially help them to deal with major problems. This dual burden seems to be imposed on many families with a mentally ill parent. From an intervention perspective, it would seem advisable not only to help such families develop social skills that can foster reciprocal relationships but also to systematically establish social support groups that consist of families with similar problems and needs. Paradoxically, these capabilities must be imparted by the formal sources of support, such as social service agencies, to which these families have access.

We observed several interesting trends among the families that did, in fact, acquire social support. When assistance was received from informal sources, no particular group of individuals seemed to offer greater help than the others. Friends provided help much more frequently than relatives who, in turn, provided help much more frequently than neighbors. However, the respondents did not consider relatives or friends more helpful than, say, neighbors or store clerks. In contrast, there is a distinct association between the various agencies that lend assistance and their reported helpfulness. Schools, hospitals, and social service agencies—especially those offering mental health services—are deemed more helpful than other types of agencies. Even though the subjects had been referred to the Web study because of a mentally ill parent, relatively few of their parents mentioned that mental illness was a major family problem during the year. It seems, then, that many of the social service agencies provided useful programs enabling them to serve as key environmental protectors for the at-risk families. Their missions and service-delivery programs extended beyond mere casework treatment by offering services that addressed such issues as family relationships, child-rearing, and unemployment. In contrast, even though many parents considered finances to be a major problem, agencies that concentrated on financial aid were not deemed very helpful.

The data also revealed clear relationships between the particular types of problems encountered by the Web families and the behavior of at-risk children. The children's behavior disorders were less severe in families that had experienced problems requiring adjustment to an acute but time-limited difficulty—a major physical illness or the death of a family member, separation or divorce of the parents, or other relatively insignificant family problems. These usually entail either a temporary or a permanent loss of a family member and the subsequent need to redistribute the various roles and functions that had been performed by that individual. Children's behavior problems were most severe in families that encountered chronic stress or continuous friction among its members—relationship problems between a child and others in the family, spousal discord, financial problems, parental mental illness, and long-term hospitalization. In most such instances, the family's chronic problem affects its full range of activities and social relationships. Consistent with our original model, such problems seem to create a highly stressful environment which, because of its continuous pressures, is associated with severe behavior disturbance on the part of at-risk children. In turn, the child's behavior disturbance plays an integral role in sustaining the severity, chronicity, and intransigence of the family's other problems.

Web families that experience a major problem and seek help from an agency or formal organization tend to have children with more severe behavior disorders than families that do not seek help. This finding—along with the fact that the severity of family problems plays no role in the acquisition of formal support—clearly suggests that difficulty with childrearing is one of the key factors which impels Web families to seek formal assistance. Regardless of whether they do so for the good of the child, the well-being of the family, or both, this finding indicates that parental mental illness does not necessarily blind a family to the needs of its own children. Families whose children have severe behavior problems are more inclined to seek help and be offered help than families whose children do not.

Some Web families that had a major problem sought help from only a single agency or individual, and others sought help from many agencies and individuals. The latter families presumably had more extensive support neworks than the former. Nevertheless, we did not find a significant relationship between the extent of a family's informal support network and the behavior of its at-risk children. Rather, there is a significant association between the extent of formal support and children's behavior. Families with children who have a serious behavior problem have a much larger formal support network than families whose children are comparatively well-behaved. Families with multiple problems may require help from a multitude of agencies. Statistical analyses that control for differences in the severity of family problems, both currently and at their worst point in the past year, reveal that families with severely disturbed children receive help from more agencies than families with relatively well-adjusted children. Thus, regardless of other family problems, it seems that the extent of disturbed behavior on the part of an at-risk child is what impels the family to reach out to formal agencies or to be sought out by them.

Just as there is a relationship between the extent of formal support and children's behavior, there also is a significant association between the reported helpfulness of formal systems and the children's behavior. Families with children who have more severe behavior problems acquire a greater amount of help. However, since these findings are based on reports from parents, it is conceivable that concerns about their children's misbehavior could have skewed the respondents' perceptions and assessments. The parents' perceptions of an agency's helpfulness might be shaped by their feelings of concern or desperation about their children's behavior. Yet, this is obviously not the case for other problems of great import such as divorce, death, or financial difficulties. Hence, despite their many difficulties, Web parents either are extremely sensitive to the needs of their children, or, more likely, they evaluate agency helpfulness according to the actual utility of the services provided.

Together, these findings reveal clear patterns of association between various types of family problems and the behavior of at-risk children. Problems that contribute to intense and prolonged stress within a family are associated with greater behavioral difficulties on the part of at-risk children. Consistent with our model, children who live in highly stress-ridden families seem more vulnerable to behavior problems. Although most families may have access to formal or informal sources of support that can potentially alleviate their stress, many seem unable or unwilling to seek such assistance. For the most part, Web families are satisfied with the social support provided by formal organizations. In contrast, informal support systems are neither considered to be particularly helpful, nor are they frequently called upon for assistance.

SUMMARY

The findings in this chapter reveal many consistencies, as well as several unresolved questions, about the social interaction model of childhood vulnerability. First, families with chronic problems are more likely than others to have children victimized by a behavior disorder. Second, the presence of a behavior disorder on the part of a child is more likely than other problems to engage a family with formal sources of assistance. Third, extrafamilial social support systems do not necessarily reduce the victimization of at-risk children even though they are considered helpful for addressing other family problems. Fourth, a child's behavior disorders and other family problems may interact with one another in a particularly deleterious manner, even to the point of hindering the family's ability to acquire potentially helpful social support. Family stress may stimulate or exacerbate the child's problematic behavior; in turn, the child's maladaptive behavior may generate stress in the family that hinders its ability to cope with key problems.

Many children not only become enmeshed in the web of mental illness but, far worse, become threads of the web itself. In doing so, they inadvertently strengthen the web, victimizing not only the other family members who are already enmeshed but also themselves. The findings in this chapter do not necessarily refute the cherished belief that social support networks can assist families victimized by mental illness, but they do show that many at-risk families are isolated from social support, sometimes due to the nature of their mental health problems or related difficulties. As a result, those enmeshed within the web—parents and children alike—are often unable or unwilling to respond to their own dire plight.

10 Life Events of At-Risk Children

WHEN PARENTS ARE BESET BY MENTAL HEALTH PROB-
lems their children are likely to encounter a variety of stressors:
family members may be separated from one another time and again; the
family may move frequently; and crucial parental roles may be performed
inadequately or not at all. Since at-risk children can be greatly affected by
these life events, it is pertinent to determine their prevalence and to ascertain
their relationships to the Web subjects' behavior. However, as we explore
these questions, it is important to remember that the effects of stressful life
events on children's behavior can be mediated by a number of factors. These
factors include not only the frequency with which such events occur but also
the children's awareness of them, the extent to which they are recalled, and
whether the subjects regarded them as stressful.

EFFECTS OF STRESSFUL LIFE EVENTS

Life-change events—the death of a sibling, failure of a school grade, divorce or remarriage of one's parents, and a move to a new city—result in
significant alterations of an individual's status from one time to another.
Frequently such events and the accompanying transitions result in significant
physical and emotional stresses. When this is clearly the case, they sometimes are denoted as life-stress events. Among adults, certain life-change
events have been linked with coronary heart disease (Rahe and Arthur 1978;
Rosenman, Brant, and Jenkins 1976), athletic injuries (Bramwell, Masuda,
Wagner, and Holmes 1975), general ill health (Holmes and Masuda 1974;
Mechanic 1976; Wolff 1968), influenza (Imboden, Canter, and Cluff 1963),
and respiratory illnesses (Jacobs, Spilkin, and Norman 1971).

Life-change events have also been associated with mental health problems
such as depression (Gatchill, McKinney, and Koebernick 1977; Paykel
1978; Paykel, Myers, Dienelt, Klerman, Lindenthal, and Pepper 1969),
psychosomatic illness (Lei and Skinner 1980; Markush and Favero 1974),
schizophrenia (Jacobs and Myers 1976), neurosis (Cooper and Sylph 1973),

and unspecified psychiatric disorders (Husaini and Neff 1978). However, many observers are wary about inferring causal links between stressful life events and psychiatric illness merely on the basis of retrospective studies. They contend, in particular, that ill individuals tend to inflate the number of stressful events recalled retrospectively (cf. Hudgens, Robins, and Delong 1970).

Several studies have explored the relationship between stress and illness among adolescents and young children. As with adults, they report consistent associations between life-stress variables and children's physical health, including cancer (Jacobs and Charles 1980), delayed growth (Coddington 1972), and rheumatoid arthritis (Heisel, Ream, Raitz, Rappaport, and Coddington 1974). Life-stress variables are also associated with such problems as delinquency (Gersten, Langner, Eisenberg, and Orze 1974; Vaux and Ruggiero 1983), unemployment (Castillo 1980), drug dependence (Duncan 1977), depression (Friedrich, Ream, and Jacobs 1982), and teen pregnancy (Coddington 1979).

Typically, the association between life-change events and physical or mental illness has been moderate (r = .20 to .40, cf. Cooley and Keesey 1981). Consequently, researchers have expressed concern about the relatively poor predictive potency of life-event measures and have sought to derive more useful research tactics. One approach entails expanding research designs about the relationship between stressful life events and illness from simple bivariate to multivariate designs. Like other investigations, the analysis in this chapter concentrates essentially on first-order relationships between these two sets of variables. Nevertheless, we believe that the effects of stressful life events upon individuals are usually mediated by significant personal and interpersonal factors. Hence, later chapters will explore the relationships among these variables from a multivariate perspective.

PREVIOUS RESEARCH ABOUT STRESSFUL LIFE EVENTS

Most studies conclude that stress occurs in conjunction with life-change events that require major adaptations by an individual. These investigations typically ask respondents to recall whether or not a particular event occurred within a given time period. Some studies also require the respondent to interpret and report the extent of stress caused by a particular event, while others assign a predetermined value to the stress presumably generated. However, recall of life events and interpretation of their stressfulness is bound to be influenced by various factors, including the subject's intellectual ability, self-esteem, and mood, as well as time elapsed since the event.

Instruments that focus upon stressful life events typically present a list of occurrences quantified by the degree of emotional or behavioral disruption that "usually" ensues for individuals subjected to them (Chandler 1981; Coddington 1972; Ferguson 1981; Sandler and Ramsey 1980; Yeaworth, York, Hussey, Ingle, and Goodwin 1980). There are two major ways of performing this quantification: (1) assign an automatic weight of one, or unity, to each event simply by summing the events that have transpired, and (2) use expert judges to assign differential weights to each event. Most instruments measure only recent life events (those that have occurred within six months to one year of testing).

When examining children's stress, it is usually necessary to pose different kinds of questions than those asked of adults. The particular developmental period in which a stressful life event occurs and the cumulation of such events over the child's life course may critically influence the child's responses to an interview item. Furthermore, different children may interpret a given event in differing ways. A child's unique interpretation of a life event may shape his or her reaction to it as much as the event itself. Hence, it is essential to measure not only the frequencies and incidences of particular life events but also the extent to which respondents regard them as stressful or not.

Weighting Life Events

To acquire self-report data about the stressful life events of children, Coddington (1972) modified the social readjustment rating questionnaire devised by Holmes and Rahe (1967). He created a separate scale for each of three age groups: elementary, junior high, and senior high school children. Parents, pediatricians, and other adults supplied the weightings for the items. However, it is doubtful that adults can make valid inferences about the social and psychological adjustments required of adolescents or young children who encounter stressful life events. Studies of adults invariably employ expert judges of adult age to assign weightings for particular life events. Yet, research with children and youths seldom employs same-age subjects in order to derive "expert" weightings. This is especially unfortunate since the particular competencies and developmental demands imposed by their age may lead adult respondents to perceive a given event differently or to experience more or less stress from it than younger respondents.

Time Period Measured

To compute stress scores, many investigators examine only life events that have occurred within six months or one year of the subject's interview (Dohrenwend, Krasnoff, Askenazy, and Dohrenwend 1978; Holmes and Rahe 1967). Although our data can be used to derive such a time-specific measure, we are able to proceed beyond this approach by employing self-report information about all the major life events remembered about each year of the subjects' lives. As a result, one can examine not only age-specific differences but also the effects of cumulative life-change events. Some investigators restrict their focus to events that occur within a recent time frame because they presume that the recall of distal life events is faulty. However, we contend that the true meaning or stressfulness of a life-change event is based not on an absolute amount attributed to a given event but, more properly, on the extent to which the individual perceives the event as stressful. In large part, of course, this is associated with the extent to which the event is recalled.

STRESSFUL LIFE EVENTS OF AT-RISK CHILDREN

We collected extensive data about the life events of all Web children by employing a Child Life-Change Timeline that measures the frequency and degree of stress produced by twenty-six major changes or transitions experienced throughout a child's life. Thirteen of these appear on Coddington's measure. We collected retrospective data from each child about two major factors: (1) the age at which each event transpired and (2) the degree to which the child was bothered by the event (indicated by the subject's response to a five-point Likert scale that ranged from "not at all" to "completely").

The resultant information accounts for key changes that require a significant transition or adaptation on the child's part and that can, therefore, be regarded as potentially stressful. Concurrently, it offers data about the child's subjective interpretation of each event's stressfulness. The instrument yields three summative scores: (1) the total number of life-change events that have occurred since birth, (2) the sum of the child's estimates of their stressfulness, and (3) the sum of all the items used by Coddington, weighted in accord with his protocol. Analyses reveal a test-retest reliability of .86 for scores based on Coddington's (1972) weighted items and .79 for scores based on the children's subjective estimates of the stress caused by the listed events.

The instrument can also be used to derive a variety of subscores. For example, it yields scores regarding the average number of life-change events experienced throughout the child's life course, the average amount of stress experienced throughout the life course, the total number of events experienced during any year or any particular age period, and the average stressfulness of the events for that period. It also yields summative scores for specific events or categories of events. Although the subjects vary in age from only six and one-half through fifteen years, they have encountered many potentially stressful life events which can be grouped into the following discrete categories: moves from one living arrangement or place of residence to another; family composition events, such as death, divorce, or the birth of a sibling; health problems such as a severe illness or injury; school failure; delinquent behavior; and other unspecified events.

Moves to a New Setting

We asked the subjects if they had ever moved from one city to another, one home to another, or one school to another. The vast majority ($n = 253$) had never moved from the St. Louis metropolitan area. In fact, only 17.3% ($n = 53$) had ever experienced such a move. Of these, twenty-nine had moved only once. However, two children had moved to a different city as many as five times.

In contrast, many subjects had moved from one home to another. In fact, only ninety-three had never engaged in such a move. Nearly 70% ($n = 213$) had moved at least once; of these, eighty-two moved only a single time. One nine-year-old child had moved as many as nine times. Furthermore, almost all of the children had at one time or another experienced a move to a different school; only fourteen had never done so. Six children had changed schools as many as eight times. The average number of moves per child was 4.8, while the range varied from no moves to a total of thirteen moves. The subjects indicated, on the average, that each move had bothered them only "a little" ($M = 2.1$). Hence, they apparently accept with some degree of equanimity the disjunctures caused by a move from one setting to another.

Family Changes

We also queried the subjects about important changes in their family, including the death of a sibling or parent, parental divorce, parental remarriage, acquisition of a stepparent, birth of a sibling or step-sibling, and foster placement. Seven children had experienced the death of a sibling, while eight had experienced a mother's death. Nearly 8% ($n = 24$) had been confronted by the death of a father, and almost 44% ($n = 133$) of the children had experienced the death of a grandparent. Hence, given their relatively young age, the subjects had a high incidence of death-related losses.

The children's families are also in flux due to other reasons. For instance, 28 children had acquired a stepmother or a surrogate mother at some time, 59 had acquired a stepfather or surrogate father, and 151 had gained one or more siblings through birth or adoption. Moreover, relatives or friends moved into the home of 74 subjects at some point.

Perhaps more important, 115 children (slightly more than one-third of the sample) had experienced the divorce of their parents. Since some of the at-risk children had been born to unwed mothers, the occurrence of two-parent families that were divorced was well above 50%. In addition, many of the subjects had experienced some kind of temporary or partial loss of an important family member. For example, 60 of the children had a sibling who had left home. Moreover, 27.1% ($n = 83$) of the subjects had spent some time in a foster home or group home. This means that more than a fourth of the children had been removed from their biological family at least once. In the state of Missouri laws do not allow a parent to voluntarily place a child in public foster care because of personal problems; instead, the family must be declared incompetent prior to the child's removal to a foster home. With the exception of expensive private placements, the process is not an elective one. Hence, only the children of the most severely disturbed parents would be likely to qualify for out-of-home placement.

Although the range varied from 0 to 11, each at-risk child experienced an average of 3.6 major changes in his or her family. On the average, the subjects reported that they had been "somewhat bothered" ($M = 2.8$) by such changes. In general, they experienced three times as many losses of family members as gains, and they regarded these losses as 25% more bothersome than the gains.

Health Problems

Many of the children also had a serious illness or injury that had kept them in a hospital or bed-ridden for at least two weeks. In fact, 24.1% ($n = 74$) had suffered a serious illness, and 16.3% ($n = 50$) had a serious injury. The children viewed such incidents as quite stressful ($M = 3.1$). Hence, they rated personal health problems as more stressful than major family changes, including the death of an immediate relative.

School Failure

In general, the at-risk children fared poorly in school. Five children had failed two grades, and 30.1% ($n = 92$) had failed one grade. Hence, the subjects' adjustment problems were frequently reflected in a very important performance area—academic achievement. In general, the subjects regarded their failures as moderately stressful ($M = 2.8$).

Delinquent Behavior

About 12.1% ($n = 38$) of the children had been reported to the authorities or other individuals as a result of delinquent activity. Given their young age, this is a relatively high incidence. The subjects regarded such events as relatively stressful ($M = 2.7$).

Other Life Events

"Other" life events refer to unspecified occurrences that the subjects mentioned on their answer sheets. Some of these undoubtedly pertained to instances of child or sexual abuse. The mean number of unspecified events per child was only 1.4. On the average, however, the subjects regarded these events as quite bothersome ($M = 3.2$).

STRESSFUL LIFE EVENTS AND THE BEHAVIOR OF AT-RISK CHILDREN

Among other things, the data permit examination of the relationship between life events and the children's current physical and mental health. As noted previously, the measures used to evaluate the latter include the children's reports of their own behavior on the Behavior Rating Index for Children (BRIC-C), the parents' reports of the children's behavior on the Child Behavior Checklist (CBCL), the severity of physical health problems from which the children suffered, the number of allergies that afflicted the children, and the medications taken by the children.

Number of Life Events

There are no consistently significant correlations between any of the measures of life events and the children's physical or mental health. This is true whether one examines the average number of life events as weighted by Coddington, the number of life events in the past year, or the extent to which the children were bothered by the events that occurred in the past year. The average number of life events, as weighted by Coddington, is correlated with the children's ratings of their own behavior ($r = .12$, $p < .04$). However, this may be a chance finding since it is the only significant one of the kind.

Types of Life Events

An examination of the various types of life events that occur with sufficient frequency to permit statistical analysis (number of moves, number of family losses or separations from family members, and number of additions to the family) reveals no association with any of the subjects' physical or mental health measures. While some events were more stressful than others, there are no discernible relationships between this factor and the subjects' physical or behavioral patterns.

Age at Occurrence

Some studies of childhood vulnerability suggest that a critical relationship emerges between children's behavior and the life events that occur during certain developmental periods. Consequently, we examined several of these periods: birth through three years of age, birth through six years of age, and four through six years of age. For these particular age periods there are no significant correlations between stressful life events and the subjects' physical or mental health. Tentatively, then, the data suggest that a continued search for "critical" age periods is likely to be conducted in vain. Typically, such quests concentrate solely on the personal strengths or weaknesses of the at-risk child. However, in terms of the model set forth in chapter 4, critical periods are likely to occur only to the extent that concomitant variations take place in the net balance between the at-risk child's environmental protectors and stressors. It is not particularly probable that such variations will have a strong and consistent relationship with age-related developmental phases.

Changes in Stress Levels

Some investigators believe that individuals eventually become inured to a given level of stress. If so, Web subjects who have experienced frequent stress might come to regard it as relatively "normal" or acceptable. Regardless of the number of stressful life events to which at-risk children are accustomed, however, are they likely to suffer adverse effects from a sudden surge in their frequency? To examine this question, we grouped the subjects into two categories: (1) those who experienced a greater number of life events in the last year than they had encountered, on a yearly average, throughout the rest of their life, and (2) those who experienced fewer life events in the last year than they had encountered, on a yearly average, throughout their life. In short, there are no significant associations between the children's physical and mental health and either of these categories of subjects. This finding raises the question of whether or not acute stresses are as deleterious for at-risk children as chronic ones, even though the latter may tend to be less severe.

In sum, examination of the data from several different perspectives reveals no association between stressful life events and the physical or mental health of the at-risk children. This is the case whether one looks simply at the life events that occur within a brief period, such as the year that preceded the study, or at the events that occur throughout the subjects' lifetime. Similarly, the findings are the same whether life events are weighted for stressfulness by either the individual subject or by the Coddington method. The lack of association may be due to a variety of factors. For example, because many of the subjects were only six or seven years old, they needed a considerable amount of help to articulate their responses to the Child Life-Change Timeline. Moreover, the timeline requires subjects to recall events that have occurred since birth. Subjects who have encountered a multitude of events may have forgotten some of the earlier ones. Likewise, there are no significant differences either for recent events (ones that have occurred within the past year) or for more distal events (ones that have occurred since birth). While the instrument may be of questionable utility for subjects with such a wide range of ages, test-retest analyses of reliability do not reveal significant differences between the older and younger subjects.

Measurement and Interpretation

Since the Child Life-Change Timeline appears to be quite reliable on a test-retest basis, and since there are no differences in the correlations between the stress scores of either older or younger children and their physical or mental health, it can be assumed that other factors account for the lack of significant trends. Yet, clear trends may be absent merely because some high-risk children are vulnerable during *all* phases of their life. Similarly, it is conceivable that some high-risk subjects experience an extreme degree of chronic stress throughout the life course and subsequently become desensitized to it. They may simply accept stressful life events as normal features of their daily life.

Moreover, it is possible that our sample of subjects is skewed in terms of its distribution of stressful life events; it may consist essentially of children who have experienced extremely large numbers of stressful life events. The at-risk subjects' CBCL scores indicate, for example, that they have more behavior problems than children in the general population. Hence, the sample's capacity to reveal a clear association between life events and children's behavior may be somewhat truncated. In effect, the apparent lack of association may be due to the fact that there are not enough at-risk subjects with low CBCL scores and only a modest number of life changes. We will examine these issues in detail when we review the differences between the at-risk subjects and a comparison sample of children who do not have mentally ill parents.

Furthermore, the lack of association between stressful events and the children's behavior may perhaps be due to either environmental factors that mitigate their relationship or to the existence of a threshold effect. The latter can obtain if there is a discernible point at which further increments in a child's stressors make no difference in his or her behavior. Indeed, it is conceivable that parental mental illness itself generates enough stress to approach such a threshold. Additional life changes might then be of little meaning to the at-risk child. In contrast, such changes might be regarded as highly significant by youngsters with healthy parents who have encountered only a few life events. Nevertheless, the analysis of comparable data for the latter type of children does not support this supposition (see chapter 14).

Last, but certainly not least, the data raise the distinct possibility that major life events are not by themselves the most direct and prepotent causes of children's behavior disorders. Rather, to the extent that such events generate stress, if at all, their effects appear to be mediated by other factors that shape the child's ultimate behavioral outcomes. Indeed, this conclusion follows from the model set forth in chapter 4. Some children may encounter extremely stressful life events yet, on balance, remain unaffected by them as long as they are protected by potent environmental supports. In contrast, other children may suffer debilitating consequences from rather modest stressors simply because they are unable to draw upon adequate environmental protectors. Even if only in preliminary fashion, then, the data suggest the efficacy of the model proposed in chapter 4.

STRESSFUL LIFE EVENTS AND THE CHILDREN'S FAMILIES

To complete the present discussion, it is pertinent to ascertain how, if at all, family mental illness is associated with stressful life events. Hence, we now will examine how the life events of at-risk children are related to selected attributes of their families.

Extent of Mental Illness in the Family

No significant associations were found between the proportion of mentally ill parents or family members and any of the measures of stressful life events —average number of life events, average number weighted by the children, average number weighted by the Coddington method, or the amount of stress within the last year. Therefore, families do not necessarily experience large numbers of stressful life events merely because they are populated by large numbers of mentally ill persons. Again, it is possible that a threshold effect may obscure the actual trends. That is, families with only a single mentally ill member may experience so many life-change events that additional ones are unlikely to occur even if more members are mentally ill. We will explore this hypothesis when we examine a comparison sample of children from the general population. The lack of association between life-change events and the proportion of mentally ill family members raises a relevant point; a strong association exists between the children's CBCL scores and the proportion of mentally ill persons in their family. When considered together, these findings suggest that it is not the extent of change or stress in families that generates childhood mental illness but, more probably, the maladaptive role models, reinforcement systems, and parent-child relationships that exist within them.

Socioeconomic Status

A significant negative association exists between the parents' socioeconomic status and the number of stressful life events that their at-risk children experienced during the past year ($r = -.23$, $p < .001$). Likewise, there is an inverse association between SES and the extent of stressfulness that the children attribute to such events ($r = -.19$, $p < .002$). At-risk children from lower socioeconomic strata seem to experience more life-change events during a given year than do children from higher strata, but this alone does not conduce toward behavior problems on their part.

Race and Religion

No significant associations were found between the family's race or religion and any measure of stress on the part of the at-risk children. Thus, at-risk children of a given race or religion do not experience either more or less stress than any other children.

Family Size

Likewise, there are no significant associations between family size and any of the life-stress variables. Larger families, for example, do not experience more stressful events than smaller ones.

Physical Health of Parents

Although parents in the Web study have physical health problems, there are no significant associations between the mother's or father's physical health and the stressful life events reported by their children. In other words, children with physically handicapped mothers or fathers are not subjected to more stressful life events than children with nonhandicapped parents. Whatever the parents' physical disabilities, they are not unduly hampered in their ability to protect the at-risk children from stressful life events.

Mental Health of Parents

The data reveal a significant positive association between fathers' mental health problems and the mean number of stressful life-events experienced by their at-risk children ($p < .04$). Likewise, there is a significant positive association between fathers' mental health problems and the mean number of life events weighted by the Coddington method ($p < .03$). However, no significant associations are found between the mothers' mental health problems and the children's stressful life events.

These findings suggest that the father's inability to perform key roles, typically in the financial realm, is associated with the occurrence of stressful life events for the family and the at-risk child. The mother's inability to perform key roles, in contrast, is not especially associated with stressful life events. Hence, mothers may be more resilient and better able than fathers to perform their basic roles, even when suffering from a mental health problem. Alternatively, however, the nature of maternal roles may allow a greater degree of flexibility in the quality and timing of performance. The findings of earlier studies (cf. Freeman and Simmons 1958) suggest that "functional substitutes" (such as older children in the family) may be better able to perform traditional maternal roles than paternal roles. As a result, the family's functioning is more likely to be sustained when the mother is ill than when the father is ill. The association between socioeconomic status and stressful life events lends additional credence to this view of maladaptive parental functioning and family stress.

Finally, the findings in this chapter require a methodological comment. Since the at-risk children are the primary informants about life-change events, one might speculate that subjects with superior intelligence are better able than other children to remember such events. Similarly, it could be hypothesized that children who encounter many stressful life events might achieve at a lower level than other subjects. Although we did not administer a direct measure of children's intelligence, scores on one instrument, namely, the Wide-Range Achievement Test (WRAT), correlate highly with scores on standardized intelligence tests. Yet, we found no consistent associations between the children's WRAT scores and their recall of either proximal or distal life events that might be associated with stress. Moreover, since recent life events, as well as distal ones, are not associated with the children's behavior, it is unlikely that the findings can be attributed to the subjects' differential ability, if any, to recall significant life events.

SUMMARY AND DISCUSSION

The findings in this chapter suggest that stressful life events do not necessarily generate severe behavior problems on the part of at-risk children. Rather, the effects of such events seem to be mediated by several variables. This finding is consistent with the model of childhood vulnerability set forth in chapter 4: the absolute number of stressors to which a child is exposed does not appear as crucial as the net balance between the stressors and environmental protectors that influence his or her behavior. The data suggest, also, that the most deleterious effects upon children's behavior may be due to chronic rather than acute stressors. Few clear associations are found between stressful life events and children's behavior; furthermore, the most consistent link is between stressful life events and the father's physical or mental health. These data raise the possibility that it may be somewhat more difficult to find functional substitutes to perform the father's familial roles than the mother's roles. Nevertheless, while maladaptive paternal functioning may produce a wide range of problems for a family, it seems to have relatively little bearing on the behavioral outcomes of the at-risk children.

11 Living Arrangements of At-Risk Children

THUS FAR IT IS EVIDENT THAT THE FAMILIES OF THE Web children play an integral role in shaping their mental health. However, the exact nature of the familial influence remains somewhat obscure partially because these families are in a constant state of flux with reference to not only the number of persons who reside in them but also, more importantly, the nature of the members' social and interpersonal relationships with one another. Changes occur in terms of communication, affection, mutual help, respect, and countless other variables. Furthermore, many of the Web children have resided in several different settings or with several different "families" during the course of their lives. Their parents may have divorced and remarried. They have often been placed with relatives, friends, foster parents, or adoptive parents. Some have been remanded to group homes or child care institutions. In such instances, a variety of biological parents, stepparents, parental surrogates, biological or step siblings, or other individuals may play a role in shaping the child's behavior. Although it is virtually impossible to discern the exact contribution of each person to the at-risk child's behavior, we can identify some general patterns that shed further light on the web of mental illness.

FAMILY CHANGE AND CHILDREN'S LIVING ARRANGEMENTS

Unlike two or three generations ago, very little consensus now exists about the proper definition of "family." The American family has become increasingly amorphous and ephemeral. For decades the nuclear family was regarded as the ideal family type and was deemed to consist merely of two biological or natural parents plus their children (Parsons 1965; Skolnick and Skolnick 1977). This model clearly specified the key family members who could influence a child's behavioral development. Moreover, it was thought that parents would be influential for a prolonged period of time because of increased life expectancy and a steadily declining incidence of family dissolution due to death. Nevertheless, there have been significant, if not startling, increases in family dissolution for a variety of reasons, foremost among these are divorce, desertion, and court action as a result of parental neglect or abuse. For example, there has been a rise in divorce from 2.5 per thousand in 1965, peaking at 5.3 per thousand in 1981 (United States National Center for Health Statistics 1985). In 1985 the number of divorces was 1,187,000, or 5.0 per thousand (United States National Center for Health Statistics, 1986). Of even greater significance is the fact that children are involved in divorces much more frequently than before. The number of children who were involved in a divorce reached over 1,000,000 per year by 1975 (United States National Center for Health Statistics 1985).

Separations and desertions affect almost as many children as divorce. While it is difficult to acquire accurate data, it seems that these forms of marital dissolution occur most frequently among urban families, low-income groups, nonwhites, and families with mentally ill parents. Desertion may run as high as 400,000 to 500,000 per year (Freed and Foster 1969). As a consequence of high rates of marital dissolution because of divorce, separation, desertion, death, or illegitimacy, it is estimated that in the near future only a bare majority (55%–60%) of American children will grow up in a traditional two-parent family in continuous, permanent, and undisrupted contact with both biological parents (Bane 1976).

Although these trends are of great significance, it is relevant to note that lowered incidences of parental death in the past century have offset increases in family dissolution due to divorce, desertion, and illegitimacy. Consequently, today's child has a better chance of being reared in a two-parent family than a century ago. However, childrearing in this context now is more likely than before to occur in serial fashion. That is, the child is more likely to reside for a period of time with stepparents, foster parents, or parental surrogates. The chance that the child will remain with his or her biological parents until adulthood is much slimmer than one hundred years ago. While nearly 80% of all children lived in a two-parent family in 1976, only 67% were residing with both of their biological parents; 13% were living with a stepparent in a reconstituted family following the divorce or death of one parent or after the marriage of an unwed mother to a man who was not the father of her child (Carter and Glick 1976). In 1970, 15.1% of all children under age 18 were living with only one parent, and currently 45.8% of all children live with only one biological parent. Moreover, 11.4% of all children live with neither biological parent (*Statistical Abstracts* 1982–1983). At some point in their childhood, then, four out of every ten children will live in a single-parent family (Glick 1979).

The nature of family life has changed profoundly in recent decades. Hence, it has been essential both to revise traditional conceptions of the family and to devise more adequate ways of measuring key differences among the various family settings and residential environments in which a child can be reared. Today, many youngsters have lived, at least for a while, in a variety of family or residential settings. They sometimes reside in one setting (such as a stepfamily or a foster home) while, at the same time, maintaining a meaningful relationship with other persons who formerly comprised their immediate family (such as their siblings, biological parents, stepparents, or foster parents). In the Web study, many children were able to maintain contact with their biological parents even after a court or social service agency had placed them with relatives, foster parents, or a child care agency. Similarly, some children maintained a viable relationship with the latter individuals or organizations after they had returned to their natural homes. Unfortunately, however, the pace of conceptualization in research has lagged behind the actual rate of change in family structure. Hence, it has been difficult to account for such changes in field studies of at-risk children and their families.

Only a handful of research instruments utilize the child's perspective to examine changes in family life and in the living arrangements of at-risk children (cf. Coddington 1972; Yeaworth, York, Hussey, Ingle, and Goodwin 1980). These instruments typically attempt to measure general life events or life changes that affect the whole family, and they rarely account for the extent to which a child moves from one family to another. Their measures usually treat such transitions merely as one facet of more broad ranging life-change events or life stresses that may affect the child (cf. Coddington 1972; Goldberg and Comstock 1976; Rahe 1981). Therefore, as noted previously, we devised measures that specifically examine this phenomenon. They are especially apropos for the present research because children with mentally ill parents are more prone than other youngsters to move from one family or living arrangement to another, whether at their own volition or due to a court order.

CHANGES IN THE LIVING ARRANGEMENTS
OF AT-RISK CHILDREN

The life histories of the Web children reveal an extraordinary amount of instability and change. Large numbers of subjects have moved frequently from one type of living arrangement to another. We have identified four distinct patterns of change in the subjects' living arrangements or residential settings and, therefore, four discrete categories of subjects: No-Change, Change-Biological Parent, Change-Alternative Family, and Change-Institutional.

No-Change subjects are children who have spent their entire life with the parent(s) present at their birth. In nearly all instances this refers to the child's biological mother and biological father. However, also included in this category are several subjects born to an unwed mother who have lived solely with her since birth. Although these children have resided in a single-parent family, their basic living arrangement has not been altered since birth. In three instances, a Web subject lived with one biological parent and one stepparent who was present at the time of his or her birth. Although the child did not reside with two biological parents, this living arrangement, too, had not changed since birth. The common characteristic of all the No-Change subjects, then, is continuous habitation with the parents or parental surrogates who were present since their birth. Altogether, only 19.9% ($n = 61$) of the Web children can be regarded as No-Change subjects, an incidence substantially lower than for the general population.

Change-Biological Parent subjects are children who have expeienced at least one significant change in their living arrangement since birth but nevertheless have always resided with at least one biological parent. In most instances, this type of change pattern emerges when the at-risk child lives with a biological parent who has been divorced and remarried one or more times. Even though a significant disruption has occurred in the child's living arrangement, the youngster has resided continuously with one of his or her biological parents. In contrast with the following two patterns, this form of change seems to represent the least radical departure from the traditional family model in which a child lives until adulthood with both of his or her biological parents. However, the inherent stability of this pattern is associated more with the child's continuous link with one of his or her biological parents than in being reared by a full complement of two parents or parental surrogates. If a child must be subjected to a major change of parents or living arrangements at some point in life, presumably this pattern is less traumatic than the other alternatives. In all, 39.2% ($n = 120$) of the Web children can be regarded as Change-Biological Parent subjects.

Change-Alternative Family subjects are children who have lived at some point in an alternative family setting. Although they have been separated from their biological parent(s) for some period of time, they nevertheless have always resided in a familial type of environment. After being removed from their biological parents, for instance, such children may have lived either temporarily or permanently with relatives (grandparents, aunts, uncles, or older siblings), friends, foster parents, or adoptive parents. In all, 32% ($n = 98$) of the Web children can be regarded as Change-Alternative Family subjects.

Change-Institutional subjects are children who have experienced the most radical departure from the traditional family model. These youngsters have lived for some period of time in an institution or a group home. Thus, not only have they been separated from their biological parents, but they have also been reared for a period of time in a nonfamily, or institutional, setting. These settings differ from the foregoing ones in view of the absence of full-time parental surrogates, biological siblings, and stepsiblings. Only 8.8% ($n = 27$) of the Web children can be regarded as Change-Institutional subjects.

It is presumed that variations in the patterns of children's living arrangements will exert a major impact on their behavior. Moreover, these variations may be associated with key life events that sometimes shape the residential arrangements of children and, in turn, are shaped by them. We discuss these relationships between children's living arrangements and certain life events in the following sections.

Change Patterns and Moves to a New Setting

Most observers posit that a change of residence from one family or institutional setting to another represents a major life transition for a child. No-Change subjects have resided in only one family setting during their lifetime. Children who exemplify any of the other three change patterns have resided in multiple settings. Change-Biological Parent subjects lived, on the average, in 2.8 different family settings. In the overwhelming majority (92.2%) of cases, Change-Biological Parent subjects shifted from residence with two biological parents to a situation in which they then lived with only one of their biological parents or with a biological parent and a stepparent. Typically, the change was due to their parents' divorce, and the at-risk child usually lived with his or her divorced mother and a stepfather. In some instances, the child's mother was married and divorced several times, resulting in further transitions for the at-risk child.

Change-Alternative Family subjects moved from one living situation to another an average of 3.7 times. These are children who lived for some period with neither biological parent but who resided nevertheless in a family setting. Three-quarters of the subjects in this group had resided with both biological parents in early childhood. Following their departure from the traditional setting, 45% lived with relatives, foster parents, or adoptive parents. About one-third resided initially with a single parent or with a stepparent after having left both biological parents; thereafter, they usually gravitated from one alternative family setting to another.

Change-Institutional subjects experienced the greatest number of transitions in their living arrangements. On the average, they were involved in 5.2 moves to a new residential setting. After placement in a group home or child care institution, 37.5% of the Change-Institutional subjects remained in that setting until the time of the Web study. However, 32.1% subsequently left the institution to join relatives, friends, foster parents, or adoptive parents. Moreover, 26.8% rejoined a single biological parent or a biological parent and a stepparent. Only 3.6% ever returned to both biological parents. Change-Institutional subjects frequently moved back and forth among foster homes, group homes, treatment institutions, biological families, and other settings. Once in the "placement cycle," then, it is evident that at-risk children are prone to numerous residential transitions. While most Change-Institutional subjects have lived at one time with both biological parents, more children from this category than from any other began life with only a single parent. All of the Change-Institutional subjects lived in at least three different settings. One eleven-year old subject from this category had lived in fourteen different settings. The significance of these transition patterns can be gauged, in part, by examining their associations with major life-change events and life stresses.

Change Patterns and Stressful Life Events

Analyses of the pertinent data reveal, in short, that the mean stressfulness of moves to a new living arrangement, the total number of life-change events experienced over a lifetime, the stressfulness of these events, and the number and stressfulness of events in the last year tend to vary significantly in accord with the at-risk child's change pattern. Thus, stressful life events of all kinds occur least frequently for No-Change subjects and with progressively greater frequency for Change-Biological Parent, Change-Alternative Family, and Change-Institutional subjects. This trend obtains whether one considers the total number of stressful events that occur in a child's life and their mean stressfulness or alternatively the total number of stressful events during the past year and their mean stressfulness. Hence, both the total number of stressful events and their mean stressfulness are linked with the particular types of changes that occur in a child's living arrangements. Generally, stressors are manifested with greater frequency or severity as the at-risk child

Table 11.1.

Current Living Arrangements, Residential Change Patterns, and Mean
CBCL Scores

Current Living Arrangement	*n*	CBCL	Change Pattern	*n*	CBCL
Two biological parents	60	63.4	No-Change	61	63.6
One biological parent and one stepparent	34	62.2	Change-Biological Parent	120	64.6
One biological parent	133	65.2	Change-Biological Parent	120	64.6
Alternative family	69	58.2	Change-Alternative Family	98	59.3
Group home or institution	10	67.2	Change-Institutional	27	67.7

takes part in increasingly disruptive transitions, more removed from the
traditional family model. Analogous trends also appear for the year that
preceded the subjects' participation in the Web study. Clearly, then, life
stresses and major changes in children's living arrangements are integrally
linked with one another. Consequently, it is germane to ask whether or not
variations in the change patterns of at-risk children are associated with behavior problems.

Change Patterns and Children's Behavior

A significant association exists between the subjects' change patterns and the
extent of their behavior problems ($p < .0006$, $R^2 = .06$) (see table 11.1).
However, the nature of this relationship differs from the progressions
observed for the life-change events cited above. At-risk children who
have moved more frequently or who have experienced greater stress do not
necessarily have higher CBCL scores than other children. As might be expected, subsequent t-tests show that the Change-Institutional subjects exhibit the highest CBCL scores ($M = 67.7$) vis-à-vis the Change-Alternative
Family subjects ($M = 59.3$, $p < .0007$), Change-Biological Parent subjects
($M = 64.6$, $p < .0005$), and, even, the No-Change subjects ($M = 63.6$,
$p < .02$).

These data clearly indicate that placement away from one or both biological parents is not necessarily associated with severe behavior problems on the
child's part, especially if either or both parents are mentally ill. The findings
are particularly significant when one considers that stressful life events are
associated differentially with the four types of change patterns but, nevertheless, that the behavior outcomes for children who live in alternative family

settings are *not* particularly deleterious. Recall from chapter 10 that stressful life events are not associated directly with children's CBCL scores. The meaning of this seeming anomaly is now evident since it appears that the effects of such events are mediated by the child's pattern of living arrangements. In the case of children with mentally ill parents, habitation with one or both biological parents or in an institution is associated with relatively severe behavior problems. By comparison, habitation in an alternative family setting is associated with fewer children's behavior problems. Hence, the data suggest that neither a completely stable living arrangement nor continuous residence with one's biological parents are *sine qua nons* for proper behavior adjustment on the part of an at-risk child. Instead, the potentially adverse consequences of stressful life events and disjunctive living arrangements appear offset by the benefits that accrue from residing in a healthier family setting (with foster parents, adoptive parents, friends or relatives).

CURRENT LIVING ARRANGEMENTS OF AT-RISK CHILDREN

The above data suggest that at-risk children may benefit significantly from placement in an alternative family setting. However, fully reliable information is not available about the qualitative features of the settings in which the subjects lived during their early years. Nor have we yet established whether there are important links between these settings and the subjects' living arrangements at the time of the Web study (i.e., the subjects' "current" living arrangement).

Current Living Arrangements and Past Living Arrangements

About 75% of the subjects who resided with both biological parents at the time of the Web study have never experienced a change in living arrangement; they have resided with the same family throughout their entire life. However, one-quarter of the subjects who resided with both biological parents at the time of the study had, in fact, experienced another living arrangement at some time in the past. They may have lived with relatives, stepparents, a single parent, or even in an institution before returning to both biological parents. In contrast, 44% of the subjects who reside currently with one biological parent and one stepparent have lived previously in a more disjunctive setting (an alternative family setting or in a group home or institution). Of the subjects who reside currently with a single biological parent 30% have lived for some period of time in an alternative family setting or an institution. Only 9% of the subjects who reside currently in an alternative family setting had once lived in an institution.

At the time of the Web study, then, the vast majority of subjects were residing in the most disjunctive of the various settings in which they had ever lived; Web subjects seldom returned to a previous living arrangement that had been a less radical departure from the traditional family model than the one in which they resided at the time of the study. Importantly, the subjects' CBCL scores vary consistently in accord with their current living arrangement. Thus, as seen in table 11.1, the lowest CBCL scores are manifested by subjects who reside currently in an alternative family setting ($M = 58.2$) or whose most disruptive past living arrangement had been in such a setting ($M = 59.3$). Conversely, the highest CBCL scores are manifested by subjects who reside currently in a group home or institution ($M = 67.2$) or whose most disruptive living arrangement had been in such a setting ($M = 67.7$). Subjects whose current living arrangement or most disruptive past arrangement was with one or both biological parents exhibit CBCL scores that cluster between these extremes. It appears, then, that alternative family settings exert a relatively positive effect on the behavior of at-risk children. Therefore, it is pertinent to inquire what makes one type of setting more or less beneficial than another for an at-risk child.

Current Living Arrangements and Children's Behavior

In previous chapters we isolated several variables characteristic of the living arrangements of at-risk children and also associated with the extent of their problem behavior. The two most pertinent from both a theoretical and a predictive standpoint are the extent of mental illness in the child's family and the frequency of discord in family relationships. At-risk children with a greater proportion of mentally ill persons in their family tend to have higher CBCL scores than other youngsters. Likewise, the frequency of mother-child discord is associated directly with the CBCL scores of the at-risk children. Although family discord, father-child discord, mother-child discord, and the proportion of mentally ill persons in the family are all associated significantly with the subjects' CBCL scores, only the latter two variables contribute unique variance when all four are entered simultaneously into a multiple regression analysis.

It is likely that the differing CBCL scores of subjects who reside in different living arrangements are in fact due to the unique features of their respective settings rather than to variations in such factors as socioeconomic status, race, religion, or family size. If so, when the differences in pertinent predic-

Table 11.2.

Hierarchical Multiple Regression for the Association between Current
Living Arrangements and CBCL Scores, Controlling for Proportion of
Mentally Ill Persons in Family and Frequency of Mother-Child Discord

Source	Degrees of Freedom	Sum of Squares	F value	Probability	R^2
Model	5	8915.6	18.31	.0001	.25
Error	282	27463.7			
Total	287	36379.3			
Contribution of each variable			F value		p level
Proportion of mentally ill persons in family			29.29		.0001
Frequency of mother-child discord			61.98		.0001
Current living arrangement			0.09		.96

NOTE: $n = 288$

tors are controlled, the type of living arrangement should explain no additional variance in the subjects' CBCL scores. As shown in table 11.2, a hierarchical multiple regression analysis shows this to be the case. When considered alone, the children's living arrangements significantly predict their CBCL scores ($p < .0007$, $R^2 = .06$). But, after the proportion of mentally ill family members and the frequency of mother-child discord are entered into the equation, the unique contribution of the subjects' current living arrangements becomes insignificant. Thus, virtually all the variation in subjects' CBCL scores that initially seemed due to their respective living arrangements is, in fact, attributable to two specific features of those living arrangements—the proportion of mentally ill persons in the household and the frequency of mother-child discord. This finding highlights the fact that it is essential for investigators to look beyond mere descriptive typologies of families or living arrangements. Rather, they must examine the specific features that make one setting more or less pathogenic than another. Often the typological labels used to identify particular environments do little else than obscure the real forces within them, those most influential at shaping the behavior of their inhabitants.

The differences in the subjects' CBCL scores before and after the two covariates are entered into the linear regression further demonstrates this point (see table 11.3). In each instance, the lowest CBCL scores appear for subjects who live in an alternative family setting. This living arrangement, characterized by less frequent mother-child discord than any other living ar-

Table 11.3.

Mean Proportion of Mentally Ill Persons in the Family, Mean Frequency of Mother-Child Discord, and Mean CBCL Score, by Current Living Arrangement

Current Living Arrangement	Proportion of Mentally Ill Persons in Family	Frequency of Mother-Child Discord	Mean CBCL	Least Squares Mean CBCL
Two biological parents	.42	2.8	63.4	63.7
One biological parent and one stepparent	.49	2.4	62.2	63.1
One biological parent	.57	3.0	65.2	63.2
Alternative family	.17	2.5	58.2	62.7
Group home or institution	NA	NA	67.2	NA

rangement except possibly those with a biological parent and a stepparent, also has the lowest concentration of mentally ill persons in the household. Furthermore, the reported differences between the subjects' mean CBCL score and least square mean CBCL demonstrate that the initial variations between groups disappear once controls are introduced for the two key variables (i.e., proportion of mentally ill family members and frequency of mother-child discord). These data attest further to the validity of the assumption that the observed slopes are homogeneous. No interaction appears between these two factors and the subjects' current living arrangement.

Mother-Child Discord. As noted previously, mother-child discord is an exceptionally strong predictor of at-risk children's behavior. Moreover, it varies significantly from one setting to another ($p < .01$, $R^2 = .04$). Such discord occurs least frequently when the child lives in an alternative family setting ($M = 2.5$) or with a biological parent and a stepparent ($M = 2.4$). In terms of statistical significance, as indicated by subsequent t-tests, the key variation is between these two settings (respectively, $p < .006$ and $p < .009$) and settings with a single biological mother ($M = 3.0$). The comparable mean for settings with two biological parents is 2.8. It is evident, then, that a discordant mother-child relationship occurs most frequently when a single parent must cope with the demands of rearing an at-risk child.

Proportion of Mentally Ill Persons in the Family Setting. The mean proportion of mentally ill persons varies significantly by the particular type of family setting ($p < .0001$, $R^2 = .25$). Indeed, one of the most salient findings in the present chapter pertains to the fact that the mean proportion of mentally ill persons in alternative family settings is exceptionally low ($M = .17$)

vis-à-vis all other family settings (p < .00001). In contrast with settings in which a biological parent is present, the low concentration of mental health problems in alternative family settings is especially pronounced. This further explains why at-risk children are relatively free of behavior problems when they are reared in alternative family settings. Besides their other strengths, such settings are relatively devoid of deviant role models and dysfunctional socializing forces on the part of parents or siblings. By comparison, there are extremely high concentrations of mentally ill persons in families where the at-risk child is reared either by a single biological parent ($M = .57$), both biological parents ($M = .42$), or a biological parent and a stepparent ($M = .49$).

It is especially germane to note that the marriage of one biological parent to a stepparent is *not* associated with a reduced concentration of mental health problems in the at-risk child's family—at least in comparison with families where two biological parents are present. In fact, remarriage may produce the opposite effect, lending credence to the notion that parents' assortative mating plays a major and continuing role in the lives of at-risk children and clearly dramatizing the potential benefits of placement in an alternative family setting. Taken together, the practical implications of these findings cannot be dismissed lightly. They raise serious doubt about the hallowed principle that at-risk children should seldom be placed away from their biological family. In fact, the data suggest that this principle may clash directly with the competing principle of maximum "normalization" of the child's environment. Resolution of this conflict depends upon the answer to a fundamental question: is it more normal or beneficial for an at-risk child to live with nonbiological parents or parental surrogates who are mentally healthy than with one or more biological parents who are mentally ill? The data clearly indicate that mental health professionals must give serious attention to this and related questions.

SUMMARY AND DISCUSSION

This chapter examines the various types of living arrangements of the Web children through two different perspectives. First, the at-risk child's life history is examined to ascertain the extent to which he or she has moved from one residential setting or living arrangement to another. This analysis reveals four patterns of change in the living arrangements of at-risk children: No-Change, Change-Biological Parent, Change-Alternative Family, and Change-Institutional. The denotations refer, respectively, to subjects who have lived with either or both biological parents since birth and have not resided with any other parents or parental surrogates; with one biological parent since birth but with changes in the presence or absence of another parent or parental surrogate (e.g., a stepparent); with friends, relatives, foster parents, or adoptive parents at some point in their life; and in a group home or institution at some point in their life. Each pattern represents a progressively more radical departure from the traditional family model in which a child resides continuously with both biological parents. Second, the child's living arrangement at the time of the Web study is examined. This form of analysis examines five discrete types of current living arrangements in which an at-risk child can reside: (1) with two biological parents, (2) with one biological parent and one stepparent, (3) with a single biological parent, (4) with non-biological parents (friends, relatives, foster parents or adoptive parents), (5) in a group home or child care institution.

As our analysis of at-risk children proceeded from No-Change subjects to Change-Biological Parent, Change-Alternative Family, and Change-Institutional subjects, corresponding progressions occurred on a number of dimensions. These include the total number of times that the subjects moved to a new setting, the mean stressfulness of such moves, the total number of stressful events to which the subjects had been exposed in their lifetime and in the year that preceded the Web study, and the mean stressfulness of the major events that occurred during these periods. However, the subjects' behavior problems are not characterized by the same type of progression. Change-Alternative Family children exhibit significantly fewer behavior problems than other subjects, including those who have lived continuously with one or both biological parents.

In concert with the data from preceding chapters, these findings demonstrate that the effects of stressful life events are mediated by the particular types of settings in which an at-risk child resides. Alternative family settings seem particularly able to reduce the likelihood of a child's behavior problems. In effect, they help the at-risk child to successfully elude the web of mental illness in which he or she otherwise might become entrapped. While alternative family setttings may not be as affluent as the child's biological family, they are characterized by significantly lower concentrations of mental health problems. In fact, the adults in alternative family settings have disproportionately fewer problems of *either* a physical or a mental health nature. Furthermore, mother-child discord, father-child discord, and discord within the family as a whole occur much less frequently in alternative family settings than in the other types of living arrangements. Since these factors are strongly associated with behavior problems on the part of at-risk children, it seems evident that alternative family setings offer important environmental protectors for such children. In short, they provide an important mechanism for disengaging the at-risk child from the web of mental illness. The quality of a child's living arrangements appears to be substantially more important than the particular transitions and stressful life events to which the child has been exposed. Indeed, competent parental surrogates may enable a child to transform stressful life events into constructive learning experiences.

To our knowledge, no other studies have examined the particular interrelationships among living arrangements, stressful life events, mediating factors, and the behavior of children who have mentally ill parents. Unlike previous investigations, our data indicate that neither the total number nor the mean stressfulness of major life events are the most critical factors in a child's development. Rather, the effects of these variables are mediated by the quality of the child's living arrangement. Stressful life events and major life changes need not be inevitable correlates of behavior disorder. If a child who experiences many stressors is aided by healthy and supportive adults— even if foster or adoptive parents—the consequences are likely to be less adverse than for a child who encounters such stressors in a family where one or both parents are mentally ill. In terms of the model set forth in chapter 4, habitation in an alternative family setting affords important environmental protectors that readily offset the environmental stressors to which an at-risk child is exposed. In effect, risk status diminishes as the child successfully eludes the web of mental illness formed by his or her biological parents.

12 Coping Skills of At-Risk Children

F OR THE MOST PART, THE LITERATURE ABOUT CHILDHOOD vulnerability presumes that the main—and often sole—determinants of vulnerability or invulnerability are the child's unique coping skills. Children who fare well in a given environment are deemed to have adequate coping skills, while those who fare poorly are presumed to have inadequate skills. We now know, however, that the child's coping skills are not the only determinants of vulnerability or invulnerability. Environmental stressors and protectors are also of critical importance. Nevertheless, we have not yet established whether the Web subjects who exhibit behavior problems are truly deficient in coping skills or, instead, if their coping skills are at normal levels but hopelessly inadequate in the face of potent environmental stressors. In this chapter, therefore, we attempt to learn more about the coping skills of the at-risk subjects and the relationship between these skills and their behavior. This analysis will serve as a prelude to our subsequent examination of the multivariate associations among coping skills, environmental factors, and children's behavior.

CHILDREN'S COPING SKILLS

The available literature indicates that the key coping skills of at-risk children include problem-solving ability and ego strength (Jenkins 1979; Pearlin and Schooler 1978), arousal level (Johnson, Sarason, and Siegal 1979; Zuckerman, Kolin, Price, and Zoob 1964), internal locus of control (Anderson 1977; Rotter 1975; Suls and Mullin 1981), extroversion (Miller and Cooley 1981), and the ability to properly assess an event's stressfulness (Houston, Bloom, Burnish, and Cummings 1978). The univariate predictive potential of environmental variables is reduced substantially when such factors moderate their influence on children's behavior (Rahe and Arthur 1978). Among other things, strong coping skills can enable an at-risk child to control his or her stressful environment, modify its meaning in a stress-reducing manner, or alleviate pertinent stress symptoms.

Some observers posit that coping skills provide one with "behavioral flexibility" (Block 1982). Many different competencies contribute to this strength (Kendall, Lerner, and Craighead 1984). Problem-solving ability, achievement skills, and the ability to accurately assess one's environment serve as key protective factors in the face of adversity (Garmezy, Masten, and Tellegen 1984; Nuechterlein 1983; Rolf 1972). Likewise, intelligence, social competence, and self-esteem contribute to a child's ability to cope with highly stressful events (Garmezy 1981). These characteristics interact with the child's environment to shape his or her responses to stressful events (Bryant and Trockel 1976; Rutter 1981). They enable children to modify stressful environments and to alter or adapt crucial aspects of their own behavior.

Both gifted and nongifted children appear equally sensitive to stressful events (Ferguson 1981). However, intelligent children seem more likely to have problem-solving skills that enable them to cope effectively with stressors (Haggerty 1980). Children with high social competence also seem to be relatively invulnerable to stressful situations (Garmezy 1981; Werner and Smith 1982). Among pertinent aspects of social competence are the ability to listen carefully, communicate one's needs to others, and judiciously apply the friendship, advice, and resources of others (Anderson 1977; Andrews, Tennant, Hewson, and Vaillant 1978; Hirsch 1982). Individuals with low self-esteem tend to regard many types of events as threatening (Coyne 1976). This predilection may influence the child's interpretation of events as well as be shaped by them. Adults with low self-esteem suffer from relatively high rates of illness under stress (Kobasa 1979). Analogously, children with low self-esteem manifest more behavior problems than children with high self-esteem (Langner, Gersten, and Eisenberg 1977). Although high self-esteem is characteristic of children who are invulnerable to persistent stress (Garmezy 1981; Werner and Smith 1982), little is known about the relationship between self-esteem and stress.

At intake we queried the Web subjects about coping skills just as they had been asked about environmental risk factors and behavior problems. Among the key coping skills examined in the present study are academic abilities and social competence. We acquired information about academic achievement by means of the subjects' responses to the Wide-Range Achievement Test (Jastak and Jastak 1978). Parents assessed their children's social competence by completing relevant sections of the Achenbach CBCL (1978–1979). Like the behavior problem section of the Checklist, the social competence section is standardized by age and sex. The instrument measures three separate kinds of competence: in activities, in interpersonal relationships,

Figure 12.1.

Frequency Distributions of Social Competence Scores for a General
Population of Children and for the Web Children

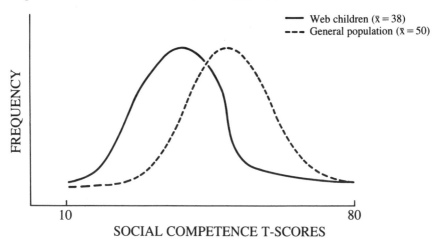

─── Web children ($\bar{x} = 38$)
--- General population ($\bar{x} = 50$)

FREQUENCY

10   80

SOCIAL COMPETENCE T-SCORES

and in school. As with behavior problem scores, we could contrast the
subjects' social competence scores with norms for the general population. In
addition, we acquired information about self-esteem by asking the subjects to
complete a highly abbreviated version of the Coopersmith Self-Esteem
Inventory (1975).

As depicted in figure 12.1, the overall distribution of social competence
scores for Web subjects is skewed positively. The mean score for social
competence is much lower than the mean for the same-age normal population. While varying levels of competence are exhibited by the Web subjects,
it is obvious that the selection criterion for the study (parental mental illness)
yielded a sample of subjects whose mean competence is much lower than
would be expected in a random sample of the normal population. A similarly
skewed distribution appears when the subjects' achievement scores are considered. For example, only 55 subjects attained mathematics achievement
scores that exceed the midpoint on a normal curve (a score of 50), but in a
normal population of the same size, one would expect approximately 153 of
the subjects to earn such scores.

COPING SKILLS AND BEHAVIOR

At the outset, it is germane to determine whether an association exists between the subjects' coping skills and their behavior problems. Specifically,

do at-risk children who have poor coping skills exhibit more problem-ridden behavior than other children? Or are these phenomena unrelated to one another? Our examination of these questions concentrates, in particular, upon academic achievement, social competence, and self-esteem.

Academic Achievement

As noted previously, all subjects completed the Wide-Range Achievement Test (WRAT) at the time of intake. This test yields normed scores for reading, spelling, and mathematics which correlate highly with scores on standard intelligence tests; therefore, they provide an indication not only of the subjects' academic achievement but also of their intelligence. Since the three subscores correlate highly with one another, we report only the sum of the three scores, or the overall WRAT score. In short, we found *no* significant relationship between the subjects' WRAT scores and their behavior problem scores ($r = -.09$). At-risk children who are low achievers do not necessarily behave more poorly than other at-risk children; likewise, at-risk children who are high achievers do not necessarily behave any better.

Social Competence

The subjects' overall social competence exhibits a significant inverse relationship to their CBCL scores ($r = -.33$, $p < .0001$). In short, higher social competence is associated with fewer behavior problems. This does not mean, however, that these phenomena are polar opposites. Children who have serious behavior problems need not necessarily be devoid of social competencies.

Because the three subscores of the social competence measure reveal an interesting pattern of associations with the subjects' behavior, it is informative to examine each one independently. Activity competence refers to the extent and quality of the child's participation in hobbies and sports. Interpersonal competence refers to the child's ability to get along with friends and family members. School competence refers to the child's school-grade performance, derived from parents' reports concerning their children's performance at school. The parents' evaluations are based essentially upon formal and informal reports conveyed to them by school personnel. As such, they are somewhat less objective than the WRAT scores and are shaped to a substantially greater extent by the teachers' global evaluations of the subjects' comportment in the classroom. Surprisingly, perhaps, the data reveal that interpersonal competence bears no relationship to the children's problem behavior. Children with severe behavior problems may or may not have strong interpersonal skills. In contrast, the severity of the subjects' behavior problems is associated inversely with their activity competence ($r = -.34$, $p < .001$) and school competence ($r = -.33$, $p < .001$).

Self-Esteem

A significant relationship does not exist between the children's self-esteem and their behavior problem scores. This may be due, in part, to the fact that self-esteem was measured by means of a much-abbreviated version of the Coopersmith Inventory. Only four items were utilized to represent each of the Inventory's four main dimensions. The small number of items inevitably lowers the instrument's reliability and, therefore, may attenuate the association between self-esteem and behavior problems. Nevertheless, the findings raise the possibility that high self-esteem does not especially help at-risk children cope with stressful life events.

COPING SKILLS AND FAMILY CHARACTERISTICS

The coping skills of the at-risk children are associated in limited fashion with their behavior. Accordingly, it is germane to ascertain whether or not an association also exists between coping skills and basic features of the subjects' families. In particular, we shall examine such variables as family size, current living arrangement, sex, race, socioeconomic status, age of the child, and age of the parents at the time of the child's birth.

Family Size

Family size bears no relationship to the subjects' coping skills—academic achievement, school competence, interpersonal competence, activity competence, or the subjects' self-esteem. When these findings are contrasted with the relationship between family size and problem behavior, we see again that coping skills and maladaptive behavior cannot be regarded merely as polar opposites.

Current Living Arrangement

A significant association exists between the current living arrangement of the at-risk child and his or her respective coping skills (see table 12.1). The most

Table 12.1.

Mean Values for Selected Coping Skills, by Current Living Arrangement of the At-Risk Child

Current Living Arrangement	COPING SKILL			
	Academic Achievement[a]	Activity Competence[b]	Interpersonal Competence[c]	School Competence[d]
Two biological parents ($n = 60$)	47.8	35.2	47.1	42.3
One biological parent and one stepparent ($n = 34$)	43.6	40.4	42.4	42.6
Single biological parent ($n = 132$)	45.7	38.4	43.0	40.6
Alternative family ($n = 69$)	44.2	41.5	40.6	39.9
Group home or institution ($n = 9$)	34.6	30.8	35.0	27.3

[a] $p < .001$, $R^2 = .06$
[b] $p < .01$, $R^2 = .05$
[c] $p < .003$, $R^2 = .04$
[d] $p < .01$, $R^2 = .04$

striking and consistent finding revealed by subsequent t-tests is that children who live in a group home or institution have significantly lower scores on academic achievement ($p < .0001$) and school competence ($p < .004$) than children who live in any other type of setting. Furthermore, children who live in a group home or institution have lower activity competence than children who live with one biological parent and one stepparent ($p < .03$) or who live in an alternative family setting ($p < .01$). They also display lower interpersonal competence than at-risk children who live with only one biological parent ($p < .04$). As might be expected given their high CBCL scores, subjects who reside in a group home or institution tend to have exceptionally poor coping skills. To offset the inadequacies of these children, institutions must offer them far greater environmental protection and less environmental stress than typically appears to be the case.

Children who live with both biological parents have significantly higher scores on academic achievement ($p < .05$) and interpersonal competence ($p < .001$) than children who live in any other setting. Their activity competence is lower than for peers who live in an alternative family ($p < .003$) or with one biological parent and a stepparent ($p < .04$). In general, children who live either with one parent, stepparents, or adoptive or foster parents tend to exhibit social competence and academic achievement scores that fall in the middle ranges.

Except for activity competence, at-risk children who reside with two biological parents tend to have stronger coping skills than children in other living arrangements. Nevertheless, the at-risk children exhibit rather severe behavior problems. The simultaneous presence of relatively strong coping skills and severe behavior problems suggests that the environments of these children subject them to extraordinarily potent stressors. Although their coping skills may permit some degree of resistance to the extant stressors, they obviously are not strong enough to prevail.

The at-risk children who live in alternative family settings exhibit higher scores on activity competence than for other coping skills. Yet, their rather low CBCL scores indicate that they are better able than other at-risk subjects to avoid serious behavior problems. Alternative family settings seem to offer a great deal of environmental protection to the at-risk child. It is evident, then, that placement decisions based solely on a child's putative coping skills may lead authorities to leave the at-risk child with biological parents for a longer than desirable period of time.

Sex

In general, no significant associations appear between the sex of the at-risk child and his or her coping skills. The sole exception pertains to school competence. Girls tend to attain higher scores than boys on this measure ($p < .02$, $r^2 = .02$).

Race

The data reveal several significant associations between the subjects' race and their coping skills (see table 12.2). Such an association exists, for instance, between interpersonal competence and race ($p < .0001$, $r^2 = .06$). White children ($M = 45.1$) have significantly higher scores on interpersonal competence than nonwhite children ($M = 39.1$). However, there are no differences between whites and nonwhites in school or activity competences. In contrast, marked race-related differences are evident in the subjects' academic achievement ($p < .0004$, $r^2 = .04$). White children have significantly higher WRAT scores ($M = 46.7$) than nonwhite children ($M = 42.6$). Nevertheless, the white and nonwhite subjects do not differ significantly in terms of their CBCL scores.

Table 12.2.

Mean Values for Selected Coping Skills, by Race of the At-Risk Child

	COPING SKILL			
Race	Academic Achievement[a]	Activity Competence[b]	Interpersonal Competence[c]	School Competence[d]
White (n = 195)	46.7	37.5	45.1	41.8
Nonwhite (n = 110)	42.7	40.1	39.1	40.0

[a] $p < .0004$, $r^2 = .04$
[b] $p < .07$, $r^2 = .01$
[c] $p < .0001$, $r^2 = .06$
[d] $p < .42$, $r^2 = .002$

Socioeconomic Status

As shown in table 12.3, a significant association exists between the subjects' socioeconomic status and academic achievement ($r = .37$, $p < .0001$) and between SES and interpersonal competence ($r = .31$, $p < .001$). However, SES is not associated with either school competence or activity competence. At first glance, these findings would seem to suggest that children from higher socioeconomic strata are likely to have somewhat stronger coping skills than children from lower socioeconomic strata, but these two coping skills bear no relationship to the subjects' CBCL scores.

Age

The subjects' age is associated inversely with each of the four coping skills except interpersonal competence (see table 12.3). Older children tend to have lower scores in academic achievement ($r = -.30$, $p < .0001$), school competence ($r = -.17$, $p < .01$), and activity competence ($r = -.13$, $p < .05$). These findings are especially notable because the achievement and social competence scores have been normed for age; therefore, under normal circumstances, one would not expect these scores to vary by age. It seems evident that the coping skills of at-risk youngsters can deteriorate over time, especially if subjected to chronic and potent environmental stressors in the absence of countervailing environmental protectors. Systematic longitudinal research is necessary to determine this supposition's validity.

Table 12.3.

Associations among Selected Coping Skills, Age, and Socioeconomic Status
of the At-Risk Child

	COPING SKILL			
	Academic Achievement	Activity Competence	Interpersonal Competence	School Competence
Age	− .30‡	− .13*	− .01	− .17†
SES	.37‡	.03	.31†	.11

*p < .05
†p < .01
‡p < .001

COPING SKILLS AND FAMILY MENTAL HEALTH

The main distinction between the Web subjects and other youngsters is the
mental health of their parents and, to a lesser extent, of their siblings. Web
families differ from other families primarily in terms of the concentration of
mentally ill parents and siblings in the household and how their problems
affect the at-risk child. Accordingly, it is germane to ask whether or not these
factors are linked with the coping skills of the at-risk children.

Proportion of Mentally Ill Family Members

The proportion of mentally ill persons in the family is not associated with the
academic achievement of the at-risk child; however, it is linked with interpersonal competence ($r = .14$, $p < .02$). Perhaps, contrary to expectation but
compatible with our basic model, children from families with higher proportions of mentally ill persons display somewhat greater social and interpersonal competence. Children who develop severe behavior problems are not
necessarily devoid of coping skills. In fact, their coping abilities may sometimes improve in response to the stresses and challenges imposed by their environment. Nonetheless, in the absence of adequate environmental protectors, even youngsters with strong coping skills can become overwhelmed and
subsequently develop severe behavior problems. Indeed, when juxtaposed
with their high C B C L scores, it is obvious that the coping skills of such children are insufficient to prevail against the potent stressors to which they are
exposed.

Type of Parental Mental Illness

Because there are no significant associations between either the father's or the mother's particular type of mental illness and the children's coping skills, one type of parental mental illness does not seem to exert worse effects on the at-risk child than another.

Parents' Ability to Function

The subjects' academic achievement scores are not associated with limitations upon their parents' ability to function because of mental health problems. Even when the parents' functioning is constrained by mental health problems there are no differences in the subjects' academic achievement, interpersonal competence, or activity competence. The sole significant association is between school competence and parents' limitations ($r = -.18$, $p < .03$); more than any other coping skill, school competence seems to be linked with the severity of the mother's mental illness.

COPING SKILLS AND FAMILY PHYSICAL HEALTH

Initially, we presumed that children with serious physical health problems would be rather limited in their ability to cope with parental mental illness; likewise, we assumed that parents with serious physical health problems would be limited in their ability to perform essential childrearing and family support functions. We now examine the validity of these assumptions and their relationship to the children's coping skills.

Children's Physical Health

In brief, we found no significant associations between the children's physical health and any of the coping skills we studied or between allergic conditions and either academic achievement or social competence. Hence, at-risk children with strong coping skills are not necessarily healthier than those with weak coping skills.

Parents' Physical Health

A number of noteworthy findings appear when one examines the parents' physical health and the coping skills of their at-risk children (see table 12.4).

Even though there is no association between the mother's physical limitations and her children's academic achievement or activity competence, there is a significant inverse association between such limitations and the children's interpersonal competence ($p < .01$, $r^2 = .02$) and school competence ($p < .03$, $r^2 = .02$). Interestingly, these trends are nearly reversed when the father's physical limitations are considered. Paternal limitations are inversely associated with the children's scores on academic achievement ($p < .001$, $r^2 = .08$) but not with any of their social competence scores. These findings may be due in part to the parents' respective roles within the family. Since the mother usually spends more time with the child than does the father, she may be more influential in shaping the youngster's social competencies; however, if she is physically limited, her capacity to do so can decline markedly. In contrast, the mother's physical limitations are less likely to impede the academic achievement of the at-risk child because these particular skills can be developed at school and elsewhere. The father's physical limitations, by comparison, may deter his capacity to provide the child with enough economic support to promote optimum academic achievement.

COPING SKILLS AND DISCORD IN FAMILY RELATIONSHIPS

Earlier we discovered that behavior problems on the part of at-risk children are associated with various types of discord in family relationships, especially family discord, mother-child discord, and father-child discord. Thus, it is pertinent to examine the association between such discord and the coping skills of at-risk children. If coping skills and behavior problems are truly independent constructs, they may be associated differentially with discordant family relationships. That is, while behavior problems are linked with discordant family relationships, coping skills may not manifest such a linkage.

Academic Achievement and Discordant Family Relationships

As seen in table 12.5, no significant associations exist between any particular type of discord in the family—family discord, mother-child discord, and father-child discord—and the children's academic achievement (see table 12.5). These findings strongly indicate that academically-oriented coping skills are impervious to discord in the family, and vice versa; similarly, harmonious family relationships do not necessarily assure high academic achievement.

Table 12.4.
Mean Values for Selected Coping Skills, by Physical Health of Parents

	COPING SKILL			
Parental Health	Academic Achievement[a]	Activity Competence[b]	Interpersonal Competence[b]	School Competence[d]
Mother				
No problems ($n = 210$)	45.7	39.1	44.5	41.8
Problems ($n = 72$)	44.9	36.9	40.4	38.6
Father				
No problems ($n = 98$)	46.9	38.2	44.2	41.6
Problems ($n = 37$)	40.4	39.9	42.1	39.5

[a] Mother, NS; Father, $p < .001$, $r^2 = .08$
[b] Mother, NS; Father, NS
[c] Mother, $p < .01$, $r^2 = .02$; Father, NS
[d] Mother, $p < .03$, $r^2 = .02$; Father, NS

Table 12.5.
Associations among Selected Coping Skills and Types of Discord

	COPING SKILL			
Type of Discord	Academic Achievement	Activity Competence	Interpersonal Competence	School Competence
Family ($n = 291$)	.05	−.27†	.02	.05
Mother-Child ($n = 289$)	.00	−.25†	−.11	−.14*
Father-Child ($n = 153$)	−.06	−.19*	.13	−.06

*$p < .05$
†$p < .001$

Social Competence and Discordant Family Relationships

As with academic achievement, there are no significant relationships between spousal discord and the social skills of the at-risk children. Hence, while a discordant relationship between the at-risk child's parents is not associated with the strength of his or her social skills, it is linked with the severity of behavior problems on the child's part. But children reared in families with much spousal discord are no more likely than other youngsters to have severe behavior problems. By themselves, the at-risk children's social skills are seldom strong enough to permit them to avert severe behavior disorders.

Unlike spousal discord, a significant association exists between family discord and the subjects' activity competence ($r = -.27$, $p < .001$). Specifically, at-risk children who live amidst frequent family discord have lower activity competence than other at-risk children, while children who participate extensively in sports and hobbies seem to be less frequently embroiled in family conflict. In part, however, the lack of association between interpersonal competence and discordant family relationships may reflect the measure employed: one question in the social competence measure refers to the subject's ability to get along with other family members, an ability likely to be impaired in families disrupted by frequent discord.

With one exception, mother-child discord is associated with children's social skills in much the same way as family discord. Children who experience frequent mother-child discord have relatively low levels of activity competence ($r = -.25$, $p < .001$). But, unlike family discord, mother-child discord is associated inversely with the at-risk child's school competence ($r = -.14$, $p < .05$). Children who have discordant relationships with their mother tend to do less well at school than other children. Yet, just as discord in the mother-child relationship hinders the child's school performance, poor behavior at school is likely to heighten the discord between mother and child. Again, the crucial nature of the mother-child relationship is highlighted by the fact that these two coping skills are associated more integrally than the others with the severity of the subjects' behavior problems.

Because mother-child discord is associated with school competence but not with academic achievement, it is worthwhile to review the distinction between the two. Children with low scores in school competence may be failing a class, attending school irregularly, or having difficulty in getting along with their peers or teachers. Clearly, they are not in their teachers' best graces whether due to academic performance or social comportment. Yet, the test data show that their achievement in reading, mathematics, and spelling is comparable to that of peers who have a less fractious relationship with teachers and schoolmates. Children who have few hobbies or extracurricular interests, attend school irregularly, or do poorly at school may spend a great deal of nonproductive time at home. This may stimulate the sorts of maternal nagging and coercive family processes that exacerbate the child's maladaptive behavior (cf. Patterson 1982). Indeed, our findings demonstrate that children who do well in school, hobbies, and sports fare better than other youngsters at maintaining a harmonious relationship with their mother. They are also more likely than other children to spend much time in productive activities outside the home.

If maternal role demands substantially influence the relationship between mother-child discord and children's social skills, one might expect somewhat different trends with respect to the relationship between these skills and father-child discord. Fathers usually spend less time at home than mothers, and their socializing relationships with the child revolve around different tasks and activities. Indeed, the only significant association between father-child discord and the subjects' coping skills pertains to activity competence. Children who have low scores on activity competence encounter more frequent discord in the father-child relationship ($r = -.19$, $p < .05$). Thus, the at-risk child's activity competence appears more closely linked to the relationship with the father than are other types of coping skills. Father-child discord, as well as the severity of the father's mental illness, are associated inversely with activity competence but not necessarily with other types of role performance. Since fathers tend to be instrumental in helping their children develop an interest in sports and related activities, discord in the father-child relationship may hinder the development of activity competence, and the child's low activity competence may then exacerbate discord in the father-child relationship. This link is especially important insofar as low activity competence tends to be associated with high CBCL scores.

In sum, then, no form of discord in the family—spousal discord, family discord, mother-child discord, or father-child discord—is associated with systematic variations in the academic achievement of at-risk children. However, mother-child discord is associated inversely with both school competence and activity competence. Moreover, activity competence is the only coping skill associated inversely with each of three different types of discord—family discord, mother-child discord, and father-child discord.

SUMMARY AND DISCUSSION

We have examined two basic types of coping skills in this chapter—academic achievement and social competence. In comparison with children from a normal population, the data show that the Web subjects have rather weak coping skills in both areas. Children with sports skills and extracurricular competencies usually spend relatively large amounts of time outside of the home, acquiring recognition and gratification from such activities. Moreover, they are subjected to less frequent family discord. The data suggest that the parents' ability to perform important childrearing roles is linked closely with the development of relevant social skills on the part of their at-risk children. However, the absence of behavior problems on the part of at-risk children does not necessarily mean they have strong coping skills.

A negative association exists between problem behavior and most coping skills we studied. Thus, children with higher academic achievement, activity competence, or school competence tend to have fewer behavior problems. However, the pertinent correlations are not particularly strong. Many children exhibit severe behavior problems even though they possess strong coping skills whereas other children exhibit few behavior problems even though their coping skills are weak. These seemingly paradoxical findings are entirely consistent with the model of childhood vulnerability in chapter 4: children who possess strong coping skills necessarily must be regarded as victims when they exhibit severe behavior disorders.

The presence or absence of strong coping skills appears linked with several major variables. For instance, children who live in adoptive or foster families have much lower CBCL scores than other children; yet, they are not necessarily more competent than other youngsters. Children who reside with their biological parents display the highest levels of social competence whereas youngsters who live in a group home or institution manifest the lowest. Vis-à-vis other youngsters, the latter are clearly the most deficient in coping skills. Thus, these findings clearly suggest that the protective features of alternative family settings tend to compensate for the deficient coping skills of the at-risk children who reside in them, enhancing the child's capacity to avert severe behavior problems.

Even though the academic achievement and social competence scores of the subjects are normed by age, a significant association exists between these scores and their age. Older children tend to have stronger skills in both areas, which may evolve in part from their increased exposure to constructive social influences outside the home.

No association was found between the subjects' race and problem behavior; yet, there was a significant association between race and social competence. White subjects had consistently higher scores on social competence than nonwhite subjects. These findings may be partly associated with the subjects' differing socioeconomic status since they reflect participation in hobbies and other activities that depend on the family's financial resources. This supposition is supported by the finding that high-SES subjects have higher scores on academic achievement and social competence than low-SES subjects.

Only a limited relationship exists between family mental health and the coping skills of the at-risk children. In contrast with the findings for behavior problems, the data reveal that children from families with a high proportion of mentally ill members have stronger coping skills than other children, especially regarding social competence. These findings again underscore the fact that social competence and behavior problems are not polar opposites; in fact, a given environment can generate either or both phenomena at the same time. At-risk children who live in families with a high concentration of mental illness may develop unique coping skills to deal with their stressful environments. But, depending on the other factors that come into play, these skills may be insufficient to prevail against the extant stressors.

In general, the particular type of mental health problem that afflicts the at-risk child's parent bears little relationship to the presence or absence of the child's coping skills. Such skills are linked, instead, to the parent's ability to perform basic social roles for the family. Limitations in the mother's ability to function are associated inversely with school competence on the part of the at-risk child. Since the mother typically bears much responsibility for her child's performance at school, when mental illness interferes with her ability to shape this competency the child may suffer accordingly. Similar findings obtain with reference to the relationship between coping skills and the physical health of family members. Thus, the mother's physical health is associated with the at-risk child's overall social, interpersonal, and school competence levels. When the mother is unable to function because of physical limitations, these social competencies are less likely to be manifested by her offspring. Likewise, the father's physical health tends to be associated with the child's academic achievement.

Many of the findings regarding family discord also are interpretable in terms of customary parental roles. Poor school competence, for instance, is associated primarily with mother-child discord. Discord in this relationship may deter the mother's ability or desire to promote school competence on her child's part. Conversely, poor school performance may exacerbate the mother-child relationship. Father-child discord is associated only with the activity competence of the at-risk child. Discord in this relationship can militate against the child's acquisition of skills in sports, hobbies, and related activities; likewise, a lack of proficiency in sports and hobbies may exacerbate the father-child relationship.

Significant associations are found most consistently for the subjects' activity competence. Family discord, mother-child discord, and father-child discord are associated inversely with the child's activity competence which seems more susceptible than other coping skills to discordant family relationships. Generally, children with high activity competence spend more time in

extrafamilial activities than other children. Furthermore, a significant association exists between the subjects' overall social competence and both family
and mother-child discord. At-risk children with high social competence tend
to encounter less discord than other youngsters in the mother-child relationship and in the family as a whole.

It is clear that strong coping skills can help the at-risk child avert severe
behavior problems; however, such skills are not by themselves sufficient to
deter all types of disorders. Various factors influence the child's behavior
problems and the quality of his or her individual coping skills. The findings
in this chapter demonstrate that children reared in very similar environments
can develop quite differently; one child may become a victim of parental
mental illness, while the other remains invincible. Moreover, the same environmental factors that foster behavior problems on a child's part may also
promote certain kinds of coping skills. Such interactions among these key
variables are of great importance. Thus far, we have shown, by individual
examination, how each variable of the at-risk child's environment relates to
differing aspects of his or her problem behaviors and coping skills. Now that
we have identified the various threads of the web of mental illness we can
proceed to learn how the threads intertwine to enhance or deter the at-risk
child's vulnerability to a parent's mental illness.

13 A Multivariate Perspective

THUS FAR, WE HAVE IDENTIFIED MANY OF THE MOST CRU-
cial threads in the web of mental illness that appear to play a role
in determining childhood vulnerability. But we have not yet ascertained
which are more important than others and which explain most of the variance
in vulnerability to behavior disorder. Of even greater consequence, we have
not yet discovered how the various threads interact with one another. Does
one variable diminish the importance of any others? Likewise, do the
interactive effects of two or more variables shape childhood vulnerability to a
greater extent than their separate or even cumulative effects? Now that we
have identified the basic elements in the web of mental illness we can
proceed from simple univariate tests to multivariate and interactive analyses.
In this way we will be able to depict the web of mental illness in the most
comprehensive and accurate form.

As discussed in chapter 4, we have posited a social interaction model of
childhood vulnerability. In essence, the relative balance between the at-risk
child's personal coping skills and his or her net environmental stressors and
protectors determines vulnerability and the at-risk child's behavior patterns.
When a child's coping skills clearly surpass his or her net environmental
stressors, the child is likely to be invincible to mental illness (that is, to have
few behavior problems). Conversely, when the net environmental stressors
exceed the child's coping skills, the child is likely to fall victim to mental
illness (that is, to have high CBCL scores). When the net environmental
stressors and the child's coping skills are approximately equal, the child is
likely to be vulnerable to a behavior disorder but not necessarily a victim or
an invincible. However, a modest change either in coping skills or net environmental stressors could generate a marked shift in the at-risk child's
behavior.

The model assumes that even though some children might have poor coping skills, they nonetheless may be able to resist behavior problems if their
net environmental stressors are weak. Analogously, some children with
strong coping skills can fall victim to behavior problems when their net
environmental stressors are extraordinarily potent. It is presumed, therefore,
that childhood vulnerability varies along a continuum reflecting the relative
balance between one's personal coping skills and net environmental stressors

and protectors. We consider this model of childhood vulnerability to accord more readily with the complex dynamics that underlie behavior disorder than many of the simpler models that appear in the literature. While the model assumes the existence of univariate determinants of vulnerability it also posits that the relative balance between coping skills and environmental risk factors is a major determinant of children's behavior. At this juncture, therefore, it is germane to examine the interactive relationships, if any, among the key variables that shape the vulnerability and behavioral outcomes of at-risk children.

In its simplest form, our model is predicated upon the ability to predict a single dependent variable—children's behavior problems—from a set of independent variables that encompasses personal coping skills, environmental stressors, and environmental protectors. Since multiple regression analysis can explain the extent to which each independent variable predicts change in a dependent variable it can illuminate the unique contributions of each factor, or thread, in the web of mental illness. The preceding chapters have identified many independent variables with a potential impact on childhood vulnerability, but, when considered in multivariate fashion, some may prove to be of little predictive value over and above the others. Conversely, while certain variables of theoretical interest initially do not seem to exert a discernible impact on children's behavior, it is possible that existing, more complex relationships are not revealed by univariate models of analysis because predictor variables are usually intercorrelated to some extent in non-experimental research. In the present study, the correlations among key predictors range from −.25 to .22. As noted previously, we hypothesize the existence of multiplicative relationships, or interactions, that may explain additional variance over and above the observed main effects. Since multiple regression takes into account the intercorrelations among predictors and allows for the testing of multiplicative relationships, we employed this mode of analysis to yield a relatively comprehensive and balanced representation of the web of mental illness.

Two major considerations shape our application of multiple regression analysis. First, this form of analysis can accommodate only those cases for which there are no missing data on key variables. Thus, for example, if data are available for 100% of the cases on four variables but merely 50% of the cases on a fifth variable, only 50% of the cases will be entered into the overall multiple regression. In some instances, missing data are inevitable. Fortunately, large numbers of cases are available for the most important variables both in terms of theoretical relevance and previous univariate analyses. Altogether, 42 cases are not reported in table 13.1 because data were missing on at least one of the multiple regression variables. However, a comparison between these cases and the 264 that appear in the analysis reveals no differences between the CBCL scores of the two groups.

Second, we incorporated a substantial number of independent variables into the multiple regression analysis. In all instances, however, we included only those variables that could be linked theoretically to one another or to the dependent variable in a clear and consistent fashion. Although the analyzed variables have been chosen with theoretical care, no a priori order of entry is warranted purely on theoretical grounds. Moreover, the retrospective nature of the study precludes true causal analysis. Therefore, each main effect variable was incorporated into the equation after all other main effects had been entered, yielding a test of their unique contributions to child behavior problems. The hypothesized interactions between discrete coping strengths and environmental factors were then entered as cross-product terms after the main effects (see Cohen and Cohen 1983). The only significant interaction was between activity competence and the proportion of mentally ill persons in the at-risk child's family; therefore, that is the only interaction we retained in the final model.

ENVIRONMENT, COPING, AND BEHAVIOR

As shown in table 13.1, the multiple regression analysis reveals a highly significant relationship ($p < .0001$) between the subjects' behavior and several of the most critical environmental and coping factors that emerged in previous analyses. Two major environmental stressors (the proportion of mentally ill persons in the family and the frequency of discord in the mother-child relationship), two types of personal coping skills (activity competence and school competence), and an interaction (between the proportion of mentally ill family members and activity competence) explain 40% of the variance in the subjects' behavior problems. An adjusted R^2, which accounts for the fit between the number of cases in the analysis and the total number of variables, reveals that this particular combination of predictors accounts for 39% of the variance. Even though this figure is a sizeable one, Abelson (1985) suggests that it may underestimate the actual explained variance since the real effects of these particular variables are cumulative over time and, thus, far more likely to predict long-term behavior patterns than behavioral outcomes examined only once.

When entered into a regression in which each variable lends additional explanatory power to variables already in the analysis, all the cited variables

Table 13.1.

Multiple Regression Analysis of the Cumulative and Interactive
Associations among Important Environmental Factors, Coping Skills,
and Children's Behavior

Source	Degrees of Freedom	Sum of Squares	F Value	Probability	R^2	Adjusted R^2
Model	5	13104.73	34.58	.0001	.40	.39
Error	258	19555.41				
Total	263	32660.15				

Variables	r	Increment in R^2	p
Proportion of mentally ill family members	.28	.07	<.0001
Mother-child discord	.44	.10	<.0001
Activity competence of child	−.37	.06	<.0001
School competence of child	−.31	.04	<.0001
Interaction between activity competence and proportion of mentally ill family members	NA	.02	<.001

NOTE: $n = 264$

explain significant variance in the subjects' behavior. The results reveal a
number of important associations between children's behavior and the predictive variables in the multivariate model. In short, the association between
environmental stressors and children's behavior problems is positive, while
the association between children's coping skills and behavior problems is
negative. Furthermore, a significant interaction emerges between a crucial
coping skill and a major environmental stressor. The results of the analysis
can best be understood by examining the unique predictive contributions of
the separate and interactive variables represented by the reported t-values
that derive from the multiple regression analysis. Such values, denoting both
the significance and the direction of effects, are employed in lieu of beta
weights because interpretations of the latter are confounded by the presence
of interaction effects (see Cohen and Cohen 1983).

Environmental Stressors

As noted above, we examined two environmental stressors in the final model
for the multiple regression analysis—the proportion of mentally ill persons
in the child's family and the frequency of mother-child discord—each of
which plays a unique role in shaping the behavior of at-risk children.

Proportion of Mentally Ill Persons in the Family. In general, children with a higher proportion of mentally ill family members have more behavior problems than children with a lower proportion of mentally ill family members (t = 5.59, p<.0001). This finding is consistent with the results reported in chapter 10. Now, however, we see that this variable also retains its importance when examined in association with other predictors. Moreover, it interacts significantly with the activity competence of the at-risk child to predict the subjects' behavior problem scores (t = −3.20, p<.001). Therefore, the main effect of the proportion of mentally ill family members does not provide all the information necessary to assess its impact upon children's behavior. As seen below, a fuller explanation can be acquired by examining the particular nature of the reported interaction.

Mother-Child Discord. As expected, the greater the frequency of mother-child discord, the higher the behavior problem score of the at-risk child (t = 6.35, p<.0001). However, as noted previously, the association between mother-child discord and children's behavior is far from simple. Children with serious behavior problems are more likely than other youngsters to have a discordant relationship with their mother. Similarly, frequent discord between mother and child is likely to produce a greater likelihood of behavior problems on the child's part. Most probably, therefore, the association between these variables is reciprocal, and the causal relationship between mother-child discord and children's behavior problems is nonrecursive. Nevertheless, the findings indicate that it is possible to make better predictions about the at-risk child's behavior when information is available about both mother-child discord and the proportion of mentally ill family members than when data are available about only one of these variables.

Personal Coping Skills

By means of the multiple regression analysis two important coping skills were identified: school competence and activity competence. These variables, too, play a unique role in shaping the behavior of at-risk children.

School Competence. The school competence of at-risk children is significantly associated with behavior problems. Subjects with high scores on school competence tend to have low behavior problem scores (t = −4.09, p<.0001). Conversely, teachers and parents feel that children with serious behavior problems lack the required competencies for satisfactory school performance.

Activity Competence. In similar fashion, high scores on activity competence are associated with low behavior problem scores (t = −4.93, p<.0001). However, the interaction between activity competence and the proportion of mentally ill persons in the family indicates that this main effect does not convey the information necessary to explain the impact of activity competence on behavior problems.

Interaction Term. A significant interaction (t = −3.20, p<.001) is evident between activity competence and the proportion of mentally ill persons in the at-risk child's family. For illustrative purposes, the nature of this interaction is highlighted by trichotomizing the latter variable into high, medium, and low categories based upon variations of plus or minus one standard deviation (.31) from the mean proportion of mentally ill persons (.44). The significant interaction, in which activity competence and proportion of mentally ill family members predicts the CBCL scores of at-risk children (see figure 13.1), indicates that the relationship between activity competence and behavior problems depends upon the proportion of mentally ill persons in the family. This interaction can also be represented in terms of the relationship between the proportion of mentally ill family members and children's behavior problems and, therefore, as a function of the at-risk child's level of activity competence. In essence, the depicted categories yield a discrete pictorial summary of a fuller array of regression lines defined by the above moderating relationship. As pictured in figure 13.1, the interaction between the environmental stressor (the proportion of mentally ill family members) and the coping skill (the child's activity competence) demonstrates how these variables moderate each other's effects as they predict children's behavior problems. Respectively, the slopes depict how activity competence differentially predicts behavior problems for subjects with either high, medium, or low proportions of mentally ill persons in their family. The regression lines converge toward the high end of scores on the activity competence scale.

When an at-risk child has high activity competence, the proportion of mentally ill persons in his or her family does not seem to affect the extent to which behavior problems are manifested. However, if the child has low activity competence, the proportion of mentally ill family members exerts a strong influence on the extent of his or her behavior problems. Thus, in cases of low activity competence, the proportion of mentally ill persons in the family is strongly linked with behavior problems on the child's part. The difference between the right side of the figure, in which children's competence is high, and the left side, in which it is low, attests to the behavior discrepancy. On the right side there is a clustering of subjects from families with either high, moderate, or low proportions of mentally ill persons. Subjects with high activity competence register very similar scores on the

Figure 13.1.

Behavior Problem Scores as a Function of Activity Competence Scores for Subjects with High, Medium, or Low Proportions of Mentally Ill Family Members ($n = 264$)

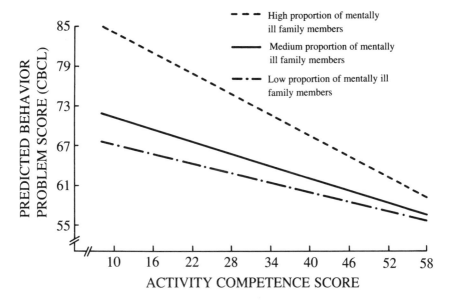

CBCL. But, as depicted on the left side of the figure, if the child's activity competence is low, the extent of his or her behavior problems varies tremendously in accord with the proportion of mentally ill family members. At-risk children who live in a family with a low or moderate proportion of mentally ill persons exhibit considerably lower behavior problem scores than at-risk children who have high proportions of mentally ill persons in their family.

The left side of figure 13.1 also shows that the behavior problem scores of subjects with low activity competence and low proportions of mentally ill family members are similar to those for children with high activity competence and moderate to high proportions of mentally ill family members. This finding is consistent with a social interaction model of childhood vulnerability: children with low activity competence and high proportions of family mental illness tend to have high behavior problem scores. In contrast, as hypothesized, children with low activity competence and low proportions of family mental illness tend to have relatively few behavior problems.

In essence, the three regression lines in figure 13.1 are geometric representations of mathematical equations. First, the equation that characterizes the activity competence/behavior problem relationship for children with a high proportion of mentally ill family members ($n = 51$) takes the form:

$$CBCL' = 90.92 + (- .59) \text{ (Activity Competence)}$$

The slope ($-.59$) indicates that an increment of one point in the activity competence score of the at-risk child yields a decrement of .59 points in his or her predicted CBCL score. The intercept term in the equation (90.92) represents the predicted CBCL score given an activity competence score of zero. However, since the subjects' activity competence scores range from 10 through 55, an activity competence score of zero is purely hypothetical. Hence, the intercept is interpreted as a mathematical constant in the equation, and we can attach no substantive meaning to it.

Second, the equation that characterizes the activity competence/behavior problem relationship for subjects who live in a family with a moderate proportion of mentally ill persons ($n = 170$) takes the form:

$$CBCL' = 74.94 + (- .32) \text{ (Activity Competence)}$$

For these subjects, an increment of one point in activity competence results in a decrement of .32 points in the predicted CBCL score.

Third, the equation that characterizes the activity competence/behavior problem relationship for at-risk children who live in a family with a low proportion of mentally ill persons ($n = 43$) takes the form:

$$CBCL' = 70.86 + (- .29) \text{ (Activity Competence)}$$

An increment of one point in activity competence for these subjects yields a decrement of .29 points in the predicted CBCL score. Clearly, then, activity competence is much less consequential for the at-risk child's behavioral outcomes when he or she resides in a family with few or no mentally ill persons. In such instances, the environmental protectors that affect the child's behavior far outweigh the extant environmental stressors. In contrast, it is especially crucial for an at-risk child to have high activity competence if he or she lives in a family with a high proportion of mentally ill persons.

The findings in this chapter are consonant with the social interaction model set forth in chapter 4: children with strong coping skills have excellent prospects for remaining invincible regardless of the extant environmental forces. But, as the at-risk child's coping skills diminish, he or she is increasingly likely to become a victim of environmental stressors. To remain invincible, at-risk children with weak coping skills must reside in an environment where the extant protectors significantly outweigh the extant stressors. Regardless of environmental stressors, in contrast, children with strong coping skills are far more likely than other youngsters to remain invincible to mental illness. Clearly, then, vulnerability and invulnerability are functions of the at-risk child's environment as well as his or her personal coping skills.

SUMMARY AND DISCUSSION

This chapter's reported findings attest to the power of the multivariate risk model proposed in chapter 4. Children with strong coping skills are often able to resist serious behavior problems even though they are exposed to formidable environmental stressors, but as their coping skills diminish they are increasingly prone to behavior problems. To be relatively free of serious behavior problems, at-risk children with weak coping skills must reside in more protective environments, on balance, than the ones inhabited by children with strong coping skills.

At-risk children who have relatively few behavior problems tend to exhibit two distinct kinds of coping skills: school competence and activity competence. Teachers and parents frequently regard children with high scores on school competence as effective at carrying out their assignments and as responsible in their school comportment. Children with high activity competence participate and tend to excel in a variety of hobbies, clubs, and sports. However, unlike activity competence, school competence does not interact with any of the environmental variables that we studied. Thus, regardless of the proportion of mentally ill persons in the at-risk child's family, school competence is a potent predictor of the extent to which the child exhibits behavior problems. Only the effects of activity competence are moderated by the proportion of mentally ill persons in the child's family. The predictive power of this variable is clearly enhanced when there are high proportions of mentally ill family members.

One presumed coping skill—interpersonal competence—does not significantly predict the behavior of at-risk children. Subjects with differing levels of behavior problems do not necessarily have either more or less friends than one another, nor do they get along better or worse with peers, siblings, or parents. Hence, the main characteristic that distinguishes problem-free children from children with severe behavior disorders is their high performance in such areas of functioning as school and recreational activities. Problem-free youngsters tend to be outgoing and well-rounded children who have multiple interests. While they do not necessarily have more friends than peers who manifest severe behavior problems, they demonstrate greater competence in school and a broad range of other activities.

These findings affirm much of what has been proposed by others who have investigated children's vulnerability to behavior problems; in addition, a key finding has emerged. The empirical evidence attests to the fact that the at-risk child's vulnerability is, at least in part, a function of the interactive relationship between personal coping skills and environmental risk factors. Activity competence, in particular, is of critical importance in determining children's behavior when it is considered in conjunction with a key environmental stressor—the proportion of mentally ill persons in the at-risk child's family. Although we have isolated only a few of the most central variables, multiple regression analysis lends substantial credence to the thesis that the interactive relationships among environmental stressors, environmental protectors, and the at-risk child's personal coping skills determine his or her behavioral outcomes.

The analysis demonstrates further that the behavior of at-risk children is determined in large part by the cumulative effects exerted by mentally ill persons in the family, the child's relationship with his or her mother, and the child's competence in school and activities. Some of these variables are environmental (such as the proportion of mentally ill family members and the frequency of mother-child discord), while others pertain to the at-risk child's coping skills (such as school competence and activity competence). The interactive relationship between his or her activity competence and the proportion of mentally ill persons in the family explains additional variance in the at-risk child's behavior. Each of these variables adds to our understanding of the behavior of at-risk children. Indeed, if the values of at-risk children are known on every one of these variables, 40% of the variance in their CBCL scores can be explained, but, if only a single variable is omitted, the subjects' behavior is predicted with much less accuracy.

The interaction between children's activity competence and the proportion of mentally ill persons in the family clearly reveals the existence of a moderating relationship between these variables. If the at-risk child lives in an extremely dysfunctional environment, personal coping skills are far more important for averting potential behavior problems than if he or she lives in a relatively protective environment. At-risk children who reside in families with a high proportion of mentally ill persons have comparatively little chance of remaining invincible to behavior problems unless they also have strong coping skills. Conversely, children with weak coping skills are unlikely to be invincible unless their family environment is highly protective.

Indeed, it appears that neither coping skills nor environmental forces alone determine a child's vulnerability or invulnerability; rather, the at-risk child's likelihood of manifesting severe behavior problems is a function of the relative balance between his or her personal coping skills and the net environmental stressors and protectors.

14 High-Risk Children versus Low-Risk Children

THUS FAR WE HAVE RESTRICTED OUR ANALYSIS TO YOUNG-
sters deemed at high-risk for behavior problems because of their parents'
mental illness. Some of these youngsters clearly are enmeshed in webs of
mental illness far more destructive and determinate than those in which other
youngsters are enmeshed. While we have been able to identify key strands in
these webs of mental illness, we have not yet ascertained the extent, if any,
to which similar strands exist in the lives of low-risk children whose parents
are not mentally ill. Accordingly, it will be informative to examine how the
environments and personal attributes of the former children differ from the
latter. By so doing we will be able to establish more clearly how children's
lives and behavior are or are not influenced by their parents' mental illness.
Even more, we will learn to what extent the findings cited thus far are or are
not generalizable from high-risk to low-risk subjects.

To strengthen our study in these important respects it is necessary to
contrast the Web subjects with a suitable comparison group of low-risk
subjects. Two main options were available for constituting a comparison
sample. One entails the random selection of youngsters from the general
population. This approach offers the advantage of contrasting the Web subjects with youngsters from a "normal" population, but its main liability inheres in the fact that some youngsters from this type of sample are likely to
live with mentally ill parents and, in this key respect, to be very similar to the
Web subjects. More importantly, because subjects from such a sample are
likely to be of higher socioeconomic status than the Web subjects, the interpretation of findings from this type of sampling procedure could be seriously
confounded by the effects of socioeconomic status.

A second option entails a stratified sampling procedure in which efforts
are made to match the two groups of subjects according to socioeconomic
status and eliminate high-risk subjects from the comparison sample. This
approach greatly reduces the confounds that could be attributed to the subjects' socioeconomic status. Furthermore, it sharpens the distinctions
between the high-risk and low-risk samples by precluding the chance se-

lection of high-risk subjects for the comparison group. Consequently, we selected the second option to create a comparison sample for the Web study. In essence, we sought comparison subjects similar to the Web subjects in socioeconomic status but without mentally ill parents.

Since this aspect of the Web study was not funded by extramural sources, we had to limit the comparison sample to fifty families. To acquire the sample, we expressly targeted the residential areas of the Web subjects by distributing a flyer to every family that lived within a two-block radius of each of the Web subjects. The flyer indicated that our research team was conducting a study of children's growth and development and that we sought interviews with families who had children between the ages of seven and fifteen years. As families called for appointments, we checked the map to assure representative distribution of the comparison subjects. This sampling procedure greatly enhanced the probability that the comparison subjects would be similar to the Web subjects in terms of race, religion, socioeconomic status, and related variables. We excluded late-responding families from the comparison sample if it became obvious that too many children were selected from a particular area, and we excluded one comparison family after the interview indicated that the father might be suffering from a mental health problem. This reduced the comparison sample to forty-nine families.

It should be noted that the difference in size between the Web sample ($n = 306$) and the comparison sample ($n = 49$) poses potential problems of interpretation, and it is especially important to employ inferential statistics conservatively. However, when we examined the variances of the dependent variables we found them to be approximately equal for the Web sample and the comparison sample. Whenever slight differences were evident in the variances of the two groups, the larger variance almost always appeared in the larger sample. The usual mean difference tests (F-tests and t-tests) are quite robust under such circumstances (Milliken and Johnson 1984). As elsewhere, we employed the General Linear Model to assess the mean differences between the two samples. Prior to performing univariate F-tests, we employed a multivariate analysis of variance (MANOVA). This resulted in a significant effect ($p < .003$) based on the Wilks lambda criterion and, as a result, warranted performance of the subsequent "protected" F-tests (Miller 1966, 93).

Analyses of the similarities and differences between the Web subjects and the comparison subjects focused upon a wide range of variables, including basic demographic variables, the children's current living arrangement, the family members' mental and physical health, family discord, the children's behavior problems and social competencies, environmental stressors, family stability, and the family's use of social support systems. Analysis of each of these variables can shed light upon the unique features of the Web subjects and elucidate the ways in which they and their life experiences differ from peers raised by healthy parents. It should be noted at the outset, however, that the requisite statistical tests do not reveal any significant demographic differences between the comparison sample and the Web sample. This is true for such variables as socioeconomic status, race, religion, family size, the subjects' age and sex, and the age of their parents. In many major respects, then, the family backgrounds of the Web subjects and the comparison subjects are very similar; the sampling procedure effectively created a group of comparison subjects who differ very little from the Web subjects in demographic respects that could confound interpretations about the effects of parental mental health.

THE CHILDREN'S ENVIRONMENT

Both the Web subjects and the comparison subjects have been reared in family environments that integrally shape their behavior. But, given the fact that their families do not differ in terms of SES, race, religion, or size, it is gemane to inquire exactly how, if at all, the subjects' families vary from one another.

Current Living Arrangement

The current living arrangements of the Web subjects and comparison subjects are highly dissimilar (chi square = 15.3, p < .004) (see table 14.1). Significantly fewer Web subjects than expected live with either two biological parents or a single biological parent; in contrast, many more comparison subjects than expected live with two biological parents. Larger numbers of subjects from both categories than might ordinarily be expected live with one biological parent and one stepparent. Hence, both groups of children have been subjected to relatively high incidences of marital dissolution and remarriage. The greatest difference between the subjects' current living arrangements is the unusually large numbers of Web subjects who reside in alternative family settings and in group homes or institutions. While sixty-nine Web subjects live in an alternative family setting, only one of the comparison subjects lives in such a setting. The absence of comparison subjects

Table 14.1.

Frequency Distribution of the Current Living Arrangements of Web
Subjects and Comparison Subjects

Current Living Arrangement	WEB SUBJECTS[a]		COMPARISON SUBJECTS[b]	
	Actual	Expected	Actual	Expected
Two biological parents	60	(64.8)	15	(10.2)
One biological parent	133	(139.2)	4	(5.2)
One biological parent and one stepparent	34	(32.8)	28	(21.8)
Alternative family setting	69	(60.5)	1	(9.5)
Group home or institution	10	(8.6)	0	(1.4)

NOTE: Chi square = 15.3, p < .004. Parentheses denote expected frequencies.
[a] $n = 306$
[b] $n = 48$

from a group home or institution is partially attributable to the sampling
procedure we employed.

These findings indicate that the comparison subjects were reared most
frequently in traditional types of family settings. All but one reside with at
least one of their biological parents. Yet, the modal living arrangement of the
comparison subjects is not with two biological parents but rather with one
biological parent and a stepparent; they, too, have been subjected to high
incidences of parental divorce and remarriage. Nevertheless, their behavior
patterns are not clearly associated with these particular experiences. In contrast, the modal living arrangement for the Web subjects is with a single
biological parent. While 31.2% of the comparison subjects live with both
biological parents, only 19.6% of the Web subjects live with both biological
parents. Since 58.3% of the comparison subjects live with a biological parent
and a stepparent, it is evident that the dissolution of their biological parents'
marriage usually results in a reconstituted living arrangement characterized
by the presence of both a male and a female parent. Only 11.1% of the Web
subjects live in such a reconstituted setting. Instead, the dissolution of their
parents' marriage typically results in large numbers of the Web subjects
residing with a single biological parent (43.5%), in an alternative family
setting (22.5%), or in a group home or child care institution (3.3%). Although these variations in the subjects' respective living arrangements may
derive partially from their parents' mental health, they are likely nonetheless
to exert an independent effect on the children's behavior.

Family Mental Health

We designed the sampling procedure to yield comparison subjects without mentally ill mothers or fathers; however, this selection criterion does not necessarily rule out the possibility of mental illness on the part of siblings or other family members. Nonetheless, only one of the comparison subjects has a sibling with any kind of behavior problem. As a result, the proportion of mentally ill members in the families of comparison children ($M = .01$) is markedly lower than for the Web children ($M = .37$). Above and beyond the parents' mental illness, the families of the Web subjects are characterized by much higher concentrations of mental illness than the families of comparison children. While this crucial family characteristic may derive in part from the parents' mental illness, it is probable that it, too, contributes independently to the Web subjects' heightened risk.

Family Physical Health

As noted earlier, much of the mental health literature indicates that families with emotional problems also have a relatively high prevalence of physical health problems. Like the Web parents, therefore, the parents of the comparison subjects were asked whether or not their children had a physical health problem severe enough to limit their functioning. We also asked the parents whether their children had allergies or took medications. In short, the data do not reveal any differences between the Web children and the comparison children in terms of physical health problems, allergies, or use of medications. Whatever their other difficulties, the Web children do not appear at greater risk for a physical health problem than the comparison children. A significant difference is evident, however, in the physical health of the subjects' mothers (chi square $= 8.68$, $p < .003$) and fathers (chi square $= 13.90$, $p < .0002$). In both cases, the parents of the Web children are far more limited by physical problems than are the parents of the comparison children. Hence, they differ markedly from the latter parents in terms of not only mental health problems but also physical problems. Thus, the parents of the high-risk subjects are less able than the comparison parents to perform their childrearing roles both physically and socially or interpersonally. These deficiencies undoubtedly hamper the parents' ability to provide their children with sufficient care and nurturance to minimize the risk for behavior problems.

Table 14.2.
Frequency of Selected Types of Discord for Web Subjects and
Comparison Subjects

	PARENT REPORTS		CHILD REPORTS	
Type of Discord	Web Subjects	Comparison Subjects	Web Subjects	Comparison Subjects
Family[a]	3.3	2.6	2.8	2.4
Mother-Child[b]	2.8	2.4	2.3	1.7
Father-Child[c]	2.6	2.2	2.2	1.9
Spousal[d]	2.9	2.4	NA	NA

[a] Family: parent, $p < .001$, $r^2 = .06$; child, $p < .01$, $r^2 = .02$
[b] Mother-Child: parent, $p < .04$, $r^2 = .01$; child, $p < .001$, $r^2 = .03$
[c] Father-child: parent, $p < .03$, $r^2 = .02$; child, NS
[d] Spousal: parent, NS; child, NA

Discord in Family Relationships

We queried the parents and children in both the Web sample and the comparison sample about the frequency of discord in various types of family relationships. Much similarity characterizes the responses of the children and their parents (see table 14.2). Both parents and children report that mother-child discord and discord within the family as a whole occur with significantly greater frequency in the Web families than in the comparison families. The parents, but not the children, report significantly higher frequencies of father-child discord in the Web families. Data were gathered only from the parents about the frequency of spousal discord, which occurs in Web families no more frequently than in the comparison families.

As stated in previous chapters, spousal discord in the Web families is not linked in any determinate fashion to the behavior of the Web children. Moreover, father-child discord predicts no unique variance in the children's behavior above and beyond the extent of mother-child discord. Aside from the fact of their parents' mental illness, it is evident that the Web subjects are reared in family settings that may exacerbate rather than attenuate their risk status. In comparison with low-risk children, frequent discord marks the interpersonal relationships with their mothers and in the family as a whole. Both the parents and the children attest to these significant differences in the family environments of the two groups of youngsters.

CHILDREN'S BEHAVIOR AND COPING SKILLS

Thus far, we have analyzed key differences in the family environments of the subjects. We have not, however, examined how the Web children and the comparison children differ from one another in terms of behavior patterns and coping skills. In preceding chapters, it is evident that the Web subjects differ considerably on most measures from normative samples reported by the authors of the respective instruments—the Achenbach Child Behavior Checklist, the Wide-Range Achievement Test, and the social competence scales of the Child Behavior Checklist. In all instances, the Web subjects fare worse than children from the normative samples, exhibiting more severe behavior problems and lower scores in mathematics, spelling, reading, and social competence. Nevertheless, these findings hardly prove that the differences are due to the mental health problems of the subjects' parents. Although some investigators might posit that they reflect patterned differences in such factors as the parents' socioeconomic status, race, religion, and age, we have shown that the Web subjects and the comparison subjects are indistinguishable on these dimensions.

Behavior Problems

The Web children have significantly higher CBCL scores ($M = 63.0$) than the comparison subjects ($M = 58.4$) (see table 14.3); therefore, as might be expected, the reported incidence of mental health problems for the former subjects is also significantly higher than for the latter (chi square = 20.4, $p < .0001$). Although 6% of the comparison children had been recently diagnosed as mentally ill or behaviorally disturbed, almost 40% of the Web children had been so diagnosed. Importantly, both the comparison subjects and the Web subjects manifest more severe behavior problems than do subjects from a normative sample, suggesting that their problems may be partially attributable to their similar socioeconomic status. In the case of the comparison subjects, of course, such problems cannot be due to parental mental illness. Regardless of the differences in their parents' mental health, both the Web subjects and the comparison subjects are disproportionately drawn from the lower socioeconomic strata. Evidently, then, the behavior problems of high-risk children are attributable to a broad range of factors—not only the mental illness of their parents but also low socioeconomic status, a high concentration of mental illness in the family, and discordant relationships with their mothers and within the family as a whole. Yet, as we have also noted, such factors can be neutralized in part by the various coping skills of the at-risk child.

Table 14.3.
Mean CBCL Scores and Selected Coping Skill Scores of Web Subjects
and Comparison Subjects

Coping Skill	Web Subjects	Comparison Subjects
CBCL[a]	63.0	58.4
Academic Achievement (WRAT)[b]	45.2	47.4
Interpersonal Competence[c]	43.0	47.2
School Competence[d]	40.7	46.0
Activity Competence[e]	38.4	43.8

NOTE: Web $n = 306$; Comparison $n = 49$.
[a] $p < .009$, $r^2 = .02$
[b] NS
[c] $p < .01$, $r^2 = .02$
[d] $p < .002$, $r^2 = .03$
[e] $p < .002$, $r^2 = .03$

Coping Skills

As noted in chapter 12, two basic types of coping skills have been examined in the present study: the subjects' achievement skills in such academic areas as mathematics, reading, and spelling, and their social competence in three areas (interpersonal competence, school competence, and activity competence). Accordingly, let us examine whether or not the Web children and the comparison children differ significantly with reference to these coping skills.

Academic Achievement. As noted previously, the academic achievement of the Web children is below the norm for the general population, but there are no significant differences between the Web subjects and the comparison subjects in terms of their average scores on the mathematics, spelling, and reading segments of the Wide-Range Achievement Test (see table 14.3). Like the Web children, the comparison children fall below the norm on these measures. Although these findings may be attributable to commonalities in the subjects' demographic backgrounds, it is evident that mental illness on the part of the Web parents does not put their children at undue risk for academic failure. Clearly, the Web children are not inferior to the comparison children in terms of the measured academic coping skills.

Social Competence. The overall social competence measure of the Achenbach CBCL is based upon three subscores—interpersonal competence, school competence, and activity competence. Table 14.3 reveals significant differences between the Web subjects and the comparison subjects on all three of these measures and, therefore, in their overall social competence (p<.0002, $r^2 = .04$). The mean social competence score for the comparison children is 44.3, whereas the comparable score for the Web children is 38.2. Both groups of subjects fall below the mean for a normal population ($M = 50.0$). While the comparison children exhibit lower social competence than children from the general population, their scores are significantly higher than those of the Web subjects. Although their academic achievement is no better than that of the Web children, they seem better able to cope socially and interpersonally. In fact, the Web subjects have significantly lower scores than the comparison subjects on all three measures of social competence (see table 14.3). In general, then, the Web children are less capable than the comparison children in terms of interpersonal skills, school relationships, and social activities and hobbies but not in terms of academic achievement. Their deficits apparently render them more susceptible to the potent stressors found in their families and immediate social environs.

DIFFERENTIAL CHILDHOOD EXPERIENCES

At every age children encounter different kinds of life experiences. Among the most important are stressful life events and major family changes. It is germane, then, to investigate whether or not the Web subjects and comparison subjects differ from one another in terms of these important variables.

Stressful Life Events

Although we have not discovered an association between stressful life events and the behavior of the Web children, it has long been presumed that the presence of a mentally ill parent leads to an increase in the number and/or severity of stressful life events faced by a child. This thesis is supported by the finding that the comparison children are much less likely than the Web children to live in a single parent family, alternative family, group home, or child care institution. To further investigate this question we analyzed differences between the two groups of subjects in terms of the average number of stressful life events to which they were exposed, the average number of such events as weighted by the children themselves, the number of stressful life events experienced by the children during the past year, and the child-weighted stressfulness of the latter events.

The data reveal that the Web children, on the average, experience significantly larger numbers of stressful events each year throughout their lives than do the comparison children (p<.05, $r^2 = .01$). The children's weightings of these events reveal the same trend (p<.03, $r^2 = .01$). Moreover, the Web subjects tend to be bothered more ($M = 2.3$) by these events than the comparison subjects ($M = 1.9$). The subjects also differ significantly with regard to the number of stressful life events experienced during the past year (p<.0001, $r^2 = .07$) and the extent to which they were bothered by them (p<.0001, $r^2 = .04$). On the average, the comparison children experienced only one stressful event during the past year, while the Web children experienced nearly three such events. The latter children reported being bothered two to three times as much as the comparison children by these events. Yet, despite the Web subjects' greater exposure to stressful life events and their higher CBCL scores, the findings from earlier chapters do not reveal a consistent relationship between these two variables. Evidently other factors—such as the subjects' respective environmental protectors and their differential ability to bring coping skills to bear in response to stressful life events—mediate their relationship.

Family Change

Earlier we found that stressful life events are not related to the Web subjects' behavior. Nonetheless, a significant association exists between their behavior and the types of family change patterns to which they are exposed. Furthermore, the Web children and comparison children differ significantly in terms of the total number of family changes to which they have been subjected (p<.0001, $r^2 = .25$). On the average, the former children have experienced 3.3 family changes in their lifetime, while the latter have had only 1.7 changes. This represents a substantial difference in the stability of the subjects' living arrangements. None of the comparison children had ever been removed from their biological family to a group home or child care institution, and only one had ever lived in an alternative family setting. Nearly all had resided continuously with at least one biological parent. Hence, the living arrangements of the Web subjects were very unstable in comparison with those of the comparison subjects (chi square = 32.5, p<.0001). This, too, may heighten their level of risk for significant behavior problems.

FAMILY SUPPORT SYSTEMS

Like the Web families, the comparison families were asked about the presence or absence of major problems during the previous year and their use of formal or informal sources of support to cope with them. As noted before, Web families with higher proportions of mental illness seem less likely to use informal support systems for family problems of a given severity than do Web families with lower proportions of mental illness, suggesting that the former families may be more isolated socially and/or less receptive to assistance from informal sources. Since contrasts with the comparison families can shed further light upon this supposition, we asked both the Web families and the comparison families whether or not they had experienced a major family problem during the past year, the current severity of that problem, the severity of the problem at its worst, how many agencies helped them cope with the problem, how many individuals helped them cope with it, and the helpfulness of those agencies and individuals.

Perhaps contrary to expectation, there are no significant differences between the two samples with reference to either the presence or current severity of family problems. Yet, the problems of the Web families may have been more acute than those of the comparison families since they were significantly more severe at their worst point (respectively, $M = 4.2$ vs. $M = 3.3$; $p < .0001$, $r^2 = .12$). Despite the greater severity of their problems, however, the Web families do not differ from the comparison families with regard to the number of agencies who helped them. Rather, the comparison families seem more prone than the Web families to seek and/or receive support from human service agencies at a less severe stage of dysfunction. Their proclivity to seek help at a less severe phase, perhaps in combination with greater access to sources of support, appears to play a major role in reducing their children's risk for behavior problems.

A significant difference exists between the number of individuals who help the two groups of subjects when they encounter a major family problem ($p < .04$, $r^2 = .04$). The Web families receive help from significantly fewer individuals ($M = 0.6$) than the comparison families ($M = 1.1$). Despite the fact that the Web families tend to have more severe problems at their worst point than those of the comparison families, it is evident that the Web families receive help from fewer individuals and from only the same number of formal agencies. Hence, they seem more socially isolated and less able than the comparison families to seek and/or acquire outside assistance for major problems. When aid is acquired from external sources, however, both groups tend to regard the pertinent individuals and agencies as equally helpful. The comparison families seem to differ most from the Web families not in the helpfulness of their social support networks but in both the size and accessibility of such networks.

CURRENT ENVIRONMENT AND PARENTAL MENTAL ILLNESS

Thus far we have learned that the comparison children have greater social competence, less discord in key family relationships, and fewer behavior problems than the Web children. We also know that low social competence, discordant family relationships, and severe behavior problems on the part of the Web children are linked with the extent of mental illness in their current family. Furthermore, we know that the proportion of mentally ill persons in the family is associated with the behavior of the Web subjects, that the comparison children have virtually no mentally ill family members, and that their behavior is less disordered than that of the Web children. These seemingly disparate findings provide the basis for a tentative examination of the interrelationships among biological and social determinants of childhood behavior disorder and, more specifically, about the mediating effects of the at-risk child's current family.

Of the many Web children who do not currently reside with a mentally ill parent, those who live in an alternative family setting are not exposed to parental mental illness. It is informative, then, to contrast three distinct groups of subjects: Web children who live in an alternative family setting, Web children who live with one or more mentally ill biological parents, and the comparison subjects. By contrasting the latter subjects with the two groups of Web subjects, we can judge how the child's current living arrangement modifies the effects of previous exposure to mentally ill parents.

As might be expected, the data reveal a significant difference between the behavior of the three groups of subjects ($p < .0002$, $r^2 = .05$). The mean CBCL score for the 49 Web subjects who currently live with mentally healthy parents ($M = 58.8$) is virtually identitical with the one for the 49 comparison subjects who live with healthy parents ($M = 58.4$). In contrast, the mean CBCL score for the 242 Web subjects who currently live with a mentally ill parent ($M = 64.0$) is significantly higher than for the other two groups of subjects ($p < .001$ and $< .002$, respectively). These findings strongly suggest that the nature of the at-risk child's current family environment is more influential on his or her behavior than are antecedent factors possibly linked with the behavioral or biogenetic characteristics of parents with whom the child no longer resides.

ASSOCIATIONS AMONG KEY VARIABLES

A number of major differences characterize the Web subjects and comparison subjects; however, we have not yet ascertained whether their effects are

Table 14.4.

Product-Moment Correlations of CBCL Scores with Discordant Family
Relationships and Subjects' Coping Skills

Variable	Web Subjects	Comparison Subjects
Discordant Relationships		
Family Discord	.26‡	.52‡
Mother-Child Discord	.45‡	.41‡
Father-Child Discord	.26‡	.39‡
Coping Skill		
Achievement (WRAT)	− .09	− .35†
Interpersonal Competence	.03	.23
School Competence	− .33‡	− .30*
Activity Competence	− .34‡	− .37†

NOTE: Web n = 306; Comparison n = 48.
* p < .05
† p < .01
‡ p < .001

manifested in relevant associations among the social environments, coping
skills, and behavioral problems of these children. If a child is reared by mentally healthy parents, for instance, are the associations among these variables
discernibly attenuated or modified? To answer this question, each univariate
analysis significantly related to the behavior of the 306 Web subjects was
performed also for the comparison subjects (see table 14.4). Our review of
the pertinent associations will follow the same order of presentation as in the
preceding chapters; respectively, we will examine the subjects' parents, family relationships, social support systems, stressful life events, pattern of living arrangements, and coping skills.

Parents

In chapter 7 we found that the Web subjects have the fewest behavior problems when they live in an alternative family setting, with older parents, or
with a physically healthy mother. The first association is not testable for the
comparison children because nearly all of them live with either or both biological parents, while the latter two associations do not obtain among the
comparison subjects. It seems, then, that the parents' age and the mother's
physical health are especially important mediating factors when a parent is
mentally ill. If the parents' functional abilities are hampered by mental illness, their physical health and age-related experiences become all the more

important for the child's well being, especially in the mother's case. Key stressors or deficits in the child's environment appear especially decisive when the child is already at risk due to a parent's mental illness.

Family Relationships

Chapter 8 scrutinized the families of the high-risk children. We found Web subjects from larger families had fewer behavior problems than Web subjects from smaller families; however, this association does not hold for the comparison subjects. In line with our earlier supposition, it appears that the presence of large numbers of siblings tends to offset the adverse effects of a parent's mental illness, especially when one's siblings tend to be free of mental illness. A relationship between these variables is less apparent, and indeed less important, when the child's parents are problem-free. Consistent with this thesis, we reported in chapter 8 that Web subjects have more severe behavior disorders when large proportions of their siblings display behavior problems. Evidence that this relationship might also exist for the comparison subjects can be inferred from the fact that their mean CBCL score is clearly below the clinical cutting point and that only one comparison subject has a mentally ill sibling.

Previous analyses also revealed that behavior problems on the part of the Web subjects vary in accord with the frequency of mother-child discord, father-child discord, and discord within the family as a whole. In all instances, at-risk children subjected to more frequent discord tend to have more severe behavior problems. The same relationship obtains for the comparison subjects; in their case, however, family discord (r = .52) and father-child discord (r = .39) bear an even stronger relationship to behavior problems (see table 14.4). Perhaps the comparison subjects are less inured to these forms of discord, especially if they occur less frequently in their families, and consequently are affected more adversely by them. Discord in the mother-child relationship greatly affects both the Web subjects and the comparison subjects. Indeed, this type of discord is associated more closely than any other with behavior problems on the part of Web subjects (r = .45). The association between mother-child discord and disturbed behavior is nearly the same for the comparison subjects (r = .41). However, the behavior problems of these subjects are linked even more strongly with family discord (r = .52) than with mother-child discord.

Earlier we noted that behavior problems on the part of Web subjects are predicted on a univariate basis by both mother-child discord and father-child discord. However, further analyses reveal that only mother-child discord significantly predicts the high-risk children's behavior problems. Father-child discord explains no additional variance. Among the comparison subjects, a similar analysis demonstrates that both mother-child discord and father-child discord are of predictive value. Comparison children who have a positive relationship with their mother but a negative one with their father are likely to have poorer behavior than those who have a positive relationship with both. This is not the case for the Web subjects. Regardless of the relationship with their father, mother-child discord exerts a profound impact on the behavior of the Web children; its effects clearly transcend the effects of father-child discord and discord within the family as a whole. The behavior of the comparison subjects may be influenced more readily by the latter types of discord than the behavior of the Web subjects. Indeed, comparison children react more negatively to all three types of discord (mother-child, father-child, and family). However, they are fortunate in that these forms of discord occur with much less frequency in their families than in the Web families.

Social Support Systems

Chapter 9 revealed that the best behavior is displayed by the Web subject who lives in a family free of major problems other than a parent's mental illness. The worst behavior is manifested by the Web subject who lives in a family where additional problems, severe enough to seek outside help, compound the parents' mental illness. Web families with children who have serious behavior problems tend to contact a greater number of human service agencies than other families and to regard them as more helpful than families with relatively problem-free children. Since no such associations appear in the comparison sample, it seems that the added stress of a problem child leads the Web families to seek formal help. But, for the comparison families, this circumstance may not produce enough additional stress to generate help-seeking behavior. The comparison families seem better able to cope with the stress caused by their children's problems; therefore, they may be less inclined to seek formal assistance. Perhaps, also, they are able to obtain informal help more readily than the Web families before the problems of their children or other family members become unduly severe. As a result, they are less likely to need assistance from the formal support systems, called into action only after the family's problems become exceptionally severe or unresponsive to its coping efforts.

Stressful Life Events

Chapter 10 demonstrated that there are no consistent associations between exposure to stressful life events and behavior problems on the part of either the Web children or the comparison subjects. Regardless of the risk status associated with their parents' mental illness, neither the number of stressors to which children are exposed nor the degree to which they are bothered by them seem to make a discernible difference in subsequent behavior.

Pattern of Living Arrangements

The data in chapter 11 reveal that the behavior of the Web subjects is integrally linked with the pattern of their living arrangements: with both biological parents, with at least one biological parent (who may or may not be remarried), with an alternative family, or in a group home or child care institution. The Web subjects who have lived at one point or another in an alternative family setting display by far the best behavior, and those who have lived in a group home or institution exhibit the worst behavior.

Although there are not enough cases in all cells to perform an adequate statistical analysis for the comparison subjects, it seems clear that the trends do not correspond with those observed for the Web subjects. Essentially there are no differences among the CBCL scores of the twenty-four comparison subjects who have lived continuously with both biological parents ($M = 56$), the fifteen who have experienced a change in family composition but nevertheless have always lived with one biological parent ($M = 58.5$), or the three who have lived in an alternative family setting ($M = 59$). Only one comparison child had ever lived in an institution; as expected, that child's CBCL score (67) is considerably higher than for the other subjects.

Unlike the Web subjects, it seems neither particularly beneficial nor especially detrimental to place a low-risk child away from his or her biological parents. Regardless of whether the current parents are biological parents or stepparents, as long as a low-risk child lives in a family setting there is little likelihood of an especially adverse effect upon his or her behavior. But this is not the case for children who live with a mentally ill parent. Web children who left their biological parents to live with relatives, foster parents, or adoptive parents exhibit distinctly better behavior than Web children who remained with their biological parents because the move was from a relatively dysfunctional living situation to a more constructive one. Unlike the Web children, the comparison subjects rarely left their biological parents to live with relatives, foster parents, or adoptive parents. When their living arrangement changed it usually reflected a divorce of their biological parents; subsequently, the spouse with custody of the child remarried. The comparison children who live in reconstituted families exhibit CBCL scores similar to those displayed by youngsters who have never undergone such changes.

These findings have obvious policy implications. The current trend is to retain the at-risk child in his or her biological family if at all possible; however, the foregoing data raise serious questions about the efficacy of this stance. Residence in an alternative family setting does not appear detrimental for children with either mentally healthy parents or mentally ill parents. To the contrary, an alternative family may be distinctly beneficial for the latter children.

Coping Skills

For both the Web subjects and the comparison subjects there is a significant inverse relationship between CBCL scores and two particular coping skills — school competence and activity competence. Hence, regardless of their parents' mental health, children are more likely to exhibit a behavior disorder when their school performance is inadequate and they are unskilled in hobbies, sports, or related activities. In contrast, interpersonal competence is unrelated to CBCL scores both for Web subjects and comparison subjects. Thus, a child with low interpersonal competence can just as well have a low CBCL score as a child with high interpersonal competence.

The two groups of subjects differ primarily with regard to the relationship between academic achievement (WRAT scores) and behavior problems. For the comparison subjects there is an inverse relationship between these two variables ($r = -.35$, $p < .01$). However, in the case of the Web subjects, a discernible relationship does not exist between academic achievement and behavior problems.

As noted in chapter 12, the coping skills of the Web children vary in accord with key features of their social environment. Unlike the comparison subjects, an association exists between the age and coping skills of the Web subjects because they evidently gain increased exposure to positive extrafamilial role models as they become older. This is bound to reduce their susceptibility to the dysfunctional influence of behaviorally disturbed family members. Such an association does not exist among the comparison subjects who live in families characterised by little or no mental illness. Evidently, they are exposed to positive role models within the family at an early age, whereas the Web children are exposed to comparatively negative role models in the family.

The Web children and comparison children are similar in terms of the association between discordant family relationships and coping skills. For both groups, mother-child discord and family discord are associated inversely with activity, interpersonal, and school competences. However, while there is a significant inverse association between discordant family relationships and academic achievement for the Web children, this is not the case for the comparison children. The strong inverse association between discordant family relationships and coping skills for the Web subjects indicates that these relationships may be of greater importance for children with mentally ill parents than for children with mentally healthy parents. Since the Web children encounter many more family problems than the comparison children, they may be in greater need of positive family relationships to develop appropriate coping skills. In contrast, the comparison children have fewer family problems and, therefore, may be able to acquire coping skills even when the social relationships among family members are discordant.

Little association exists between the coping skills of the comparison children and the physical health of either their mothers or fathers. The sole significant association is between the children's interpersonal competence and their mother's physical health. Comparison children with healthy mothers have significantly higher ($p < .03$, $r^2 = .02$) scores on interpersonal competence ($M = 47.9$) than those whose mothers have a physical problem ($M = 39.0$). This finding once again highlights the importance of the mother for the development of the child's social skills. If the mother is physically limited, the child's social development may be hindered regardless of whether she also suffers from a mental illness.

For the comparison subjects, unlike the Web subjects, an association does not exist between stressful life events and social competence. This finding may reflect the fact that the comparison children are exposed to fewer such events than the Web children. Consequently, development of their coping skills may be deterred hardly, if at all, by the comparatively few stressors to which they are exposed. Since the Web children are already burdened with a mentally ill parent, the additional problems imposed by frequent exposure to stressful life events may seriously impede the acquisition of adequate coping skills. In the case of the comparison children, however, the presence of healthy parents apparently diminishes the potential adverse effects of stressful life events upon the development of coping skills.

SUMMARY AND DISCUSSION

This chapter attempts to answer several basic questions about the differences between children who have a mentally ill parent (the Web subjects) and children who have mentally healthy parents (the comparison subjects). Among the variables examined are the subjects' family environments, coping skills, and social behavior. Between the two groups of subjects the data reveal many significant differences that undoubtedly play an important role in shaping their respective levels of risk for behavior problems. Because their parents are physically healthier than those of the Web subjects, the comparison children are exposed less often to the necessity of living with a single parent or of being placed with relatives, foster parents, adoptive parents, or in a group home or child care institution. And, perhaps most importantly, comparison families are plagued less often by mother-child discord, family discord, and severe behavior problems on the part of parents or siblings.

The Web children exhibit less social competence and more severe behavior problems than the comparison children, but they do not differ in terms of academic achievement. They are more behaviorally disturbed than the comparison children, and they possess fewer of the social skills required to offset their behavior problems. Moreover, there are significant differences between the two groups of subjects in terms of the number of stressful life events to which they are exposed and in the extent to which they are bothered by them.

Differences also exist between the Web children and the comparison children in terms of available social support systems. The families of the comparison children have larger support networks even though they encounter fewer problems. Furthermore, the available evidence suggests that they seek help from such networks at an earlier stage of need than do the Web families. Consequently, their approach to family problems seems more proactive than reactive.

The data indicate that the current living arrangement of the at-risk child is a better predictor of his or her behavior than is the mental health of a former parent. Thus, Web subjects who had once lived with a mentally ill parent but who now live in an alternative family setting do not differ in behavior from comparison subjects who have mentally healthy parents. Moreover, the former children exhibit significantly fewer behavior problems than Web children who have remained with both biological parents. This pattern does not obtain for the comparison children for whom separation from their biological parents does not necessarily improve the living situation. Children from either sample who reside in a group home or institution display more severe behavior problems than other youngsters.

In general, Web subjects and comparison subjects who have stronger coping skills, especially school and activity skills, tend to have fewer behavior problems. However, the absence of behavior problems on the part of comparison subjects also seems linked with high academic achievement. This is not the case for the Web subjects who also experience more frequent and severe environmental stressors than the comparison children. Exposure to such stressors tends to be associated with lower competence on their part, whereas this is not the case for the comparison subjects.

In many, if not most, instances it seems that a parent's mental illness is the crucial added burden that potentiates adverse factors which otherwise might remain dormant or unthreatening for the at-risk child. We do not suggest that children with mentally healthy parents are never exposed to such stressors, for in some, but certainly not all, instances they are exposed to the same stressors as the Web children. However, when the environmental stressors and personal deficits which beset the Web children combine with the additional burden of a parent's mental illness, otherwise benign factors may exert powerful adverse effects upon their behavior. In such instances these children become entrapped in a web of mental illness more potent, destructive, and pervasive than that confronting more fortunate youngsters.

15 An Integrated Perspective

W E, LIKE OTHER RESEARCHERS, BEGAN THIS STUDY BY AS-
suming that children who have mentally ill parents are at higher risk
for behavior problems than children who have mentally healthy parents. Although countless studies have yielded this conclusion, our detailed review of
the pertinent literature revealed that the mere fact of a parent's mental illness
does not adequately account for the behavior of the at-risk child. Many difficulties arise when one makes assumptions about the relationship between
behavior disorders manifested by mentally ill parents and their children. If an
at-risk child is expected to exhibit disturbed behavior, there is little assurance
that it will be the same kind displayed by the child's parents. Furthermore,
the literature reveals a need for investigators to distinguish clearly between
the notions of risk and prediction, constructs too often employed inter-
changeably. Prospective estimates about the behavior of a given youth are far
more likely to err than ones that try to predict risk for an entire group of
subjects, thus rendering it difficult to implement effective prevention programs for youngsters at risk for disturbed behavior. From the perspective of
the present study, it is especially important to note that the literature demonstrates parental mental illness as only one of many factors influencing a given
child's level of risk. Unfortunately, few studies have examined the full array
of factors that conduce toward childhood behavior disorder and the extent to
which they either shape, or are shaped by, parental mental illness.

We designed the Web study to contribute to the available body of knowledge about factors that influence the intricate interrelationships between
parental mental illness and the behavior of at-risk children. Its perspective
regarding children's behavior problems is ecological and interactive. Accordingly, throughout the study we have employed a social interaction model
of childhood vulnerability by assuming that the at-risk child and his or her
social environment are engaged in a continuous series of social interactions.
Thus, the child both shapes and is shaped by the environment. Many children
possess important coping skills that enhance their resistance to environmental forces which conduce toward maladaptive behavior. Whether or not these
skills will prevail depends upon the strength and chronicity of the pertinent
forces and on the extent to which they are neutralized by countervailing
environmental protectors. The child's risk status and subsequent behavioral

outcomes are deemed a function of the relative balance between personal coping skills and net environmental stressors and protectors. When the at-risk child's coping skills exceed the net environmental stress, the child is likely to be invincible—free of significant behavior problems; conversely, when the net environmental stress exceeds the available coping skills, the child is likely to fall victim—manifesting severe behavior problems. And, when the child's coping skills and net environmental stress are approximately equivalent, the child is likely to be vulnerable, neither a victim nor an invincible; however, a slight change in coping skills or in the relative balance between environmental stressors and protectors could result in a shift toward either status.

The social interaction model extends substantially beyond previous conceptions of childhood vulnerability by highlighting the fact that parental mental illness is but one of many factors that can shape childhood behavior disorders. Above and beyond the relatively direct effects of a parent's mental illness, a child's risk can be influenced by a virtually infinite array of factors. The model posits that a child's success at resisting adverse environmental forces is not solely a function of his or her unique coping skills. For instance, it recognizes the fact that certain extremely capable youngsters are likely to develop disturbed behavior in the face of relentless environmental pressures. Conversely, some youngsters who possess marginal coping skills may be able to avert severe behavior disorders simply because they reside in settings free of potent environmental stressors or offering a high degree of environmental protection. Rarely does a child's level of risk depend solely upon his or her unique competencies.

The social interaction model provides a framework for the systematic examination of a question central to many investigations of childhood vulnerability: in view of their parents' mental illness, why do children who are exposed to putatively similar levels of risk tend to experience differing behavioral outcomes? In short, why do some at-risk children manifest severe behavior disorders while others appear to be symptom-free? Moreover, why do some youngsters seem to drift in a netherland midway between these extremes? More succinctly, what accounts for the differential tendency of at-risk youngsters to become either victims, vulnerables, or invincibles? The Web study demonstrates that it is not possible to ascertain the true role of parental mental illness in shaping children's behavior unless this variable is considered in conjunction with a broad array of other predictors. Consequently, we have employed an interactive, multivariate, and comparative perspective to examine the subjects' coping skills and the stressful and protective features of their family environments.

ORDERING THE STRANDS

The analyses in the preceding chapters have identified key strands in the web of mental illness. Consequently, we are now in a position to discern the breadth and scope of the web. Our data indicate that the level of risk encountered by the children of mentally ill parents may be much higher than had previously been supposed. Extremely large numbers of the Web subjects had already manifested severe behavior problems by the time of their interview for the study. More than half (53%) had CBCL scores that placed them in the highest decile of scores for same-age children within the general population; by our definition, these children can already be regarded as "victims." Altogether, 90% had CBCL scores beyond the midpoint for a normal population of youths, and only 2% had CBCL scores that would place them in the lowest decile of subjects within the general population. Hence, the prevalence of severe behavior problems among the children of mentally ill parents is substantially higher than for youngsters in the general population.

Our data provide stark evidence of the environmental turmoil experienced by at-risk children. Only 21% of the Web children still lived with both biological parents at the time of the study. Nearly half (43%) resided with a single biological parent, overwhelmingly the mother rather than the father. An affective disorder on the mother's part appears particularly detrimental for the at-risk child because, perhaps more than other types of disorders, it can impede the mother's ability to establish a harmonious relationship with the at-risk child. Consequently, the child is subjected to the most problematic form of discord that can occur in the family—mother-child discord. The extent of mother-child discord is a strong correlate of the at-risk child's behavioral outcomes both in one-parent and two-parent families. In the former family, moreover, the parents' childrearing responsibilities are compounded by the concurrent demands of being the sole breadwinner.

The findings of the Web study reveal that certain clusters of factors— primarily the frequency with which discord occurs between father and child and within the family as a whole—conduce strongly toward behavior problems on the part of at-risk children. Nevertheless, neither of these types of discord accounts for more variance in children's behavior problems than mother-child discord alone explains. The data from parents and children alike attest to this fact. If the mother and child are able to maintain a harmonious relationship, even in instances where the mother is mentally ill, the child is likely to be well protected against behavior problems. This finding is consistent with Rutter's conclusion that a positive relationship with one parent can substantially mitigate a child's risk for disturbed behavior. However, our data suggest that Rutter's conclusion is only partially correct. When the crucial mother-child relationship is marked by frequent discord, its adverse effects are *not* mitigated by a positive relationship between the father and child. In contrast, it appears that a positive relationship between the mother and child can palliate the adverse effects of a discordant father-child relationship. This finding further dramatizes the prepotency of the mother-child relationship, regardless of the sex of the at-risk child. It appears unlikely, then, that the behavior problems of at-risk children are based solely, or even primarily, upon sex-linked identification with their mother.

The maladaptive consequences of mother-child discord can permeate the entire family system. If this form of discord occurs frequently, it is quite likely that discord also exists between the spouses and in the family as a whole. The resulting dysfunctions may weaken the family system and further exacerbate the tenuous situation of the at-risk child. If the mother-child relationship is characterized by frequent discord, the at-risk child's probability of manifesting disturbed behavior is heightened considerably. Perhaps contrary to current rhetoric about maternal and paternal roles, it seems evident—at least in families where a parent is mentally ill—that the mother's relationship with the at-risk child is of paramount importance for the latter's well-being.

The available evidence also indicates that the mother-child relationship is extraordinarily resilient. The bond between mother and child is less susceptible to disruption by mental illness than is the bond between father and child. In fact, mentally ill mothers seem as capable as healthy mothers of maintaining a positive relationship with their at-risk sons and daughters. Moreover, they are able to do so even when faced with the added burden of a mentally ill spouse or no spouse at all. The mother-child relationship appears relatively impervious to factors that tend to disrupt less sturdy relationships. It does not vary, for example, in accord with whether or not the mother is mentally ill, the family is single-parent or two-parent, one parent or both are mentally ill, or the at-risk child is male or female. When this crucial and resilient relationship eventually begins to falter, however, especially deleterious consequences ensue for the at-risk child.

In the Web study we examined the concentration, or density, of mental illness in the at-risk child's family by determining the proportion, or percentage, of mentally ill persons in the household. The at-risk child's likelihood of a behavior disorder increases in accord with the proportion of mentally ill persons in the household. Consistent with this finding is the fact that Web children with CBCL scores in the highest decile of the sample are likely to have more than twice as many siblings with behavior problems as Web children with CBCL scores in the lowest decile. When stated in proportionate rather than absolute terms, the contrast between these two groups of subjects is even more vivid. The proportion of behaviorally disturbed siblings in the family of the former subjects is four times greater than in the families of the latter. In part, these findings might seem to suggest that the behavior problems of at-risk children are determined by their biogenetic background. However, identical trends were also observed when the at-risk child lived with parental surrogates and stepsiblings. Hence, the key determinants of the behavioral outcomes of at-risk children seem to inhere primarily in the psychosocial relationships within their families. The dynamic nature of these relationships is indicated by the association between the proportion of mentally ill persons in the family and the extent of discord within it. For example, family discord is greater when large proportions of mentally ill persons reside in the household, and vice versa.

Our findings suggest that at-risk children can be safeguarded considerably by residing in environments that protect them against seriously debilitating forces. The at-risk child is least likely to manifest severe behavior problems in a family setting relatively devoid of mother-child discord and having only a negligible proportion of mentally ill persons. Unfortunately, however, these important attributes seem relatively scarce in the biological families of at-risk children where a parent's mental illness is usually associated with both frequent discord in the family and severe behavior problems on the part of the at-risk child. These adverse characteristics are much less prevalent in alternative family settings. Hence, there appears to be a need for closer examination of the time-honored imperative that at-risk children be obliged to live with their biological parents at virtually all costs.

Consistent with the social interaction model, our findings demonstrate that the key strands in the web of mental illness—perverse as they sometimes may be—are neither ineluctable nor irreversible determinants of childhood disturbance. The unique coping skills of the at-risk child can palliate the effects of otherwise debilitating forces. Conversely, the coping skills of some children can be overwhelmed by the extant environmental stressors, especially if countervailing environmental protectors are not present. Some family environments demand extremely strong coping skills on the part of the at-risk child, whereas others require only modest ones. In either case, however, personal coping skills alone seldom dictate whether or not a given youngster will become a victim, vulnerable, or invincible. In general, we have found that the formidable environmental stressors encountered by at-risk children require that they possess strong coping skills. Yet, the coping skills of such children are much weaker than those displayed by same-age peers with mentally healthy parents. The former children are comparatively deficient both in terms of academic achievement and social competence. When considered in conjunction with the immense environmental stressors to which they are exposed and the corresponding paucity of their environmental protectors, these findings substantially explain why so many at-risk young-sters become victims or vulnerables rather than invincibles.

As noted above, we examined two basic kinds of coping skills: academic achievement and social competence. And we studied three particular types of social competence: interpersonal, school, and activity. We found the lat-ter two of special importance for the at-risk child because the stronger the child's skills in these areas, the less likely were severe behavior problems. However, these skills tend to be quite weak when frequent discord occurs be-tween the parents and the at-risk child or when there is a high concentration of mentally ill persons in the family. The father's role appears especially influential in shaping the child's activity competence, whereas the mother's role is particularly important for shaping school competence. When discord occurs frequently between the parent and child the relevant coping skill is likely to suffer. Thus, the importance of the parent-child relationship inheres primarily in how it either promotes or deters the development of coping skills and in how it influences crucial aspects of the family's functioning. These dynamics seem to transcend a child's respective race, religion, sex, age, or socioeconomic background.

Although the social competence of at-risk children is associated inversely with behavior problems, there is no relationship between academic achieve-ment and problem behavior. Furthermore, only two of the three social com-petence measures are associated with the subjects' CBCL scores. School competence and activity competence exhibit an inverse relationship with CBCL scores, while interpersonal competence is unrelated to them. Hence, school skills and abilities in sports, hobbies, and related activities may en-able the at-risk child to cope more readily than academic or interpersonal skills.

As expected, the weakest coping skills are displayed by Web subjects who live in a group home or institution, and the strongest are evidenced by subjects who live either with both biological parents or in an alternative family setting. Yet, despite relatively similar abilities, the CBCL scores for these two groups of subjects differ markedly. It appears obvious, then, that factors other than coping skills are of paramount importance in shaping the behavioral outcomes of at-risk children who reside either with both biologi-cal parents or in an alternative family setting. For the most part, these seem to inhere in the differing environmental exposures of the two groups of subjects. At-risk youths who have lived with mentally ill biological parents are far more likely to become victims than peers who have lived with relatives, foster parents, or adoptive parents. These findings, too, attest to the efficacy of a social interaction model of childhood vulnerability that recognizes the interplay between personal coping skills and environmental stressors and protectors.

The data for the Web study also clarify the role of socioeconomic status. We found, for instance, that the academic achievement and interpersonal competence of at-risk children tend to vary in accord with their socioeconomic status. Normally, this would suggest that higher-SES children ought to be less susceptible to behavior problems than lower-SES children. However, these two coping skills do not manifest a clear association with CBCL scores. The coping skills that do manifest such a relationship—school competence and activity competence—do not vary with the subjects' socioeconomic status, indicating that children's vulnerability may be less a function of socioeconomic status than previously supposed.

Unlike the conclusions of earlier studies, we have found that large family size is not a direct correlate of mental health problems on the part of at-risk children. Studies of "normal" families had suggested a direct relationship between these two variables because, as a family increases in size, the parents presumably are less able to socialize each and every child properly. Consequently, their children are at greater risk for disturbed behavior. However, the opposite dynamic seems to obtain in families with a mentally ill parent. When such families are small in size they appear severely hampered in their ability to exert appropriate controls over the at-risk child. If so, the presence of other socializing agents, including older siblings, may exert a particularly beneficial impact on the at-risk child. But family size by itself is of little predictive value with respect to the behavior of at-risk children; indeed, its effects cannot be fully appreciated without knowing about the particular mental health profiles and behavior patterns of the various family members. If their behavior is adaptive, these persons can countervail the adverse influences typically attributed to the mentally ill parent.

Naturally, it is plausible to assume that the dysfunctional consequences of parental mental illness can be averted by assistance from social support networks, either formal or informal, that exist in the family's immediate environs. However, our findings indicate that families with a mentally ill parent do not come by such sources of support very readily. In large part, the availability and utility of support networks depend on the nature of the unique problems that confront the family. Web families encountered a wide variety of serious difficulties above and beyond the mental illness of a parent. In fact, only 10% of the families of the Web subjects regarded the mental illness of a parent as their foremost problem. Nearly 25% of the Web subjects lived in a family where childrearing problems were deemed the paramount problem. Other family problems that affected large numbers of Web subjects were finances, death or severe illness, a recent separation or divorce, and marital difficulties. The problems that the respondents regarded as moderately or very severe tended to be most chronic in nature, and more likely than acute problems to be associated with high CBCL scores on the part of at-risk children.

Whether key family problems devolve in part from a parent's mental illness or, in turn, contribute to it cannot be determined definitively by means of the available data. Regardless, parental mental illness is associated with a broad variety of severe problems, including financial distress and childrearing difficulties. Concurrent with these problems, one of the most salient features of the Web families is their isolation from potential sources of formal and informal support. More than 25% of the Web families with a major problem besides parental mental illness failed to receive assistance from any type of organization or agency. Furthermore, 42% of the Web families received no help from friends, relatives, or neighbors. It appears that these families neither knew how to gain access to support systems nor were motivated to do so. Consequently, the at-risk children within them were enmeshed in a web of mental illness unresponsive to its own plight. Such children ought to be the targets of aggressive outreach programs on the part of human service agencies, but, because of their extreme social isolation, the requisite agencies may never know the plight of many of these children and their families.

Despite the fact that the Web subjects have been buffeted by stressful events throughout their lives, they apparently have adapted to them rather well. Exposure to stressful life events does not seem associated with especially severe behavior problems; instead, such problems appear linked most closely with chronic mother-child discord. Moreover, stressful life events are not associated with one of the key correlates of the children's behavior problems—the proportion of mentally ill persons in the family. This finding suggests that the latter variable exerts its adverse effects not through the stress it engenders in the family but rather by means of other processes such as maladaptive role modeling, dysfunctional patterns of social reinforcement, or discord between parent and child. The number of stressful life events to which at-risk children are exposed, as well as the extent to which they are bothered by them, appears to be an inverse function of socioeconomic status. Yet, the severity of the children's behavior problems appears unrelated to the number of stressful life events to which they are exposed. At first, this finding seems contrary to the general belief that behavior problems are a direct consequence of the stress to which one is subjected, but it is consistent with the social interaction model of childhood vulnerability. To the extent that stress is associated with behavior problems, its effects are likely to be mediated by a variety of factors: foremost among these are the breadth and quality of the child's coping skills and the nature of the available environmental protectors.

In this regard, it should be noted that the particular type of setting in which an at-risk child resides can serve as either a protector or a stressor. At-risk children who live in an alternative family setting have much lower CBCL scores than at-risk children who live with either or both biological parents. This suggests that alternative families are able to provide the children of mentally ill parents with better environmental protectors and/or fewer stressors than their biological families. However, whether the behavior problems of such children actually subside after being transferred from their biological family to an alternative family can be determined with certainty only by means of rigorous longitudinal investigation. At-risk children who live in alternative families are subjected to more disjunctures in their living situations than children who have remained throughout with their biological parents; however, the difficulties engendered by such transitions may be offset by living in a healthier family environment. Our analyses indicate that the beneficial effects of alternative families are associated primarily with the absence of mother-child discord and the relatively small proportions of mentally ill persons who reside in the household.

Mother-child discord occurs most frequently when the at-risk child lives with a single female parent. It is much less prevalent when the child lives with one biological parent and a stepparent in a reconstituted or "blended" family, even though a reconstituted family does not typically yield a reduced concentration of mental illness in the household. In families with a mentally ill parent, the processes of marital dissolution and remarriage seem to result in a form of assortative mating that does not produce appreciable changes in the concentration of mental illness in the child's immediate environment. Rather, the main benefits of the reconstituted family inhere in the fact that the mother acquires sufficient support to sustain a positive relationship with her at-risk child.

LINKING THE STRANDS

In the absence of costly longitudinal research, it is difficult to document the contention that the strands in the web of mental illness interact in a dynamic and ever-changing fashion. Given the design limitations of the Web study, the best procedure for examining the dynamic interrelationships among key variables is multiple regression analysis which utilizes the most potent variables revealed by antecedent univariate analyses. Our analyses have demonstrated that two major environmental stressors (the proportion of mentally ill persons in the family and the frequency of discord in the mother-child relationship), two types of personal coping skills (activity competence and school competence), and an interaction between the proportion of mentally ill family members and activity competence explain 40% of the variance in the subjects' behavior problems. This particular array of variables best identifies which at-risk children are victims and which are invincibles. As had been anticipated, the association between environmental stressors and children's behavior problems was positive, while the association between coping skills and behavior problems was negative. Most importantly, the proportion of mentally ill persons in the at-risk child's family was found to interact with the child's activity competence to predict the severity of behavior problems.

This type of interaction is precisely the kind posited by the social interaction model. It demonstrates that the relationship between activity competence and behavior problems depends upon the proportion of mentally ill persons in the child's family. Similarly, the relationship between the proportion of mentally ill family members and behavior problems is a function of the child's activity competence. When the at-risk child has high activity competence, the proportion of mentally ill persons in the family is linked weakly with the extent of behavior problems. If the child has low activity competence, however, the proportion of mentally ill family members bears a strong and direct relationship to behavior problems. Viewed from another perspective, the CBCL scores of at-risk children with low activity competence and low proportions of mentally ill family members are similar to those for children with high activity competence and relatively high proportions of mentally ill persons in the family. Whereas children with low activity competence and high proportions of family mental illness tend to have rather severe behavior problems, children with low activity competence and low concentrations of family mental illness have comparatively few behavior problems. The activity competence of the at-risk child is much less consequential when the child lives in a family with few or no mentally ill persons. In this instance, the environmental protectors that influence the child's behavior evidently outweigh the extant environmental stressors. In contrast, when an at-risk child lives in a family with a high proportion of mentally ill persons, it is essential for the child to possess high activity competence. Hence, our examination of multiplicative effects reveals that crucial strands in the web of mental illness interact with one another in a highly determinate fashion.

BEYOND THE WEB

To learn more about the web of mental illness, we contrasted the behavior and circumstances of the Web children with those of children reared by mentally healthy parents. The Web subjects exhibited more severe behavior disorders and much weaker coping skills than the comparison subjects. Their scores on interpersonal competence, school competence, and activity competence were especially low. However, they did not differ from the comparison subjects in terms of academic achievement. The Web subjects fared considerably worse than the comparison subjects in terms of the two variables linked most closely with the absence of severe behavior problems—school competence and activity competence.

The Web subjects were also much less likely than the comparison subjects to reside with two biological parents. Their modal living arrangement was with only one biological parent. Large numbers of the Web subjects resided in alternative families and in group homes or institutions. In fact, more lived in an alternative family (with relatives, foster parents, or adoptive parents) than with two biological parents. Like the Web subjects, the comparison children were often subjected to parental divorce. In their case, however, the parent who retained custody of the child was likely to remarry after a comparatively brief period of time. In these instances, the child was reared in a reconstituted family that approximated the traditional model. By contrast, the divorced parents of Web children seldom remarried; only 11.1% of the Web subjects lived in a reconstituted two-parent family. The dissolution of their parents' marriage typically left them to reside with a single biological parent in a living arrangement frequently marked by mother-child discord and other significant stressors such as serious financial problems. In the relatively few instances when a custodial parent did remarry, there was seldom a significant change in the proportion of mentally ill persons in the household. Typically, the at-risk child remained with the mentally ill parent or the child's custodial parent married an individual who was mentally ill. In either case, the new living arrangement tended to yield few benefits for the at-risk child.

The family systems of the Web children and the comparison children differed greatly from one another in key respects. The Web children lived in families marked by high concentrations of mental illness. Also, their mothers and fathers had poorer physical health than the parents of comparison children. These problems may have constrained their ability to impart useful coping skills to the at-risk child. More importantly, mother-child discord, father-child discord, and discord in the family as a whole occurred more frequently in the Web families than the comparison families. In short, the Web subjects were reared in family settings that tended to exacerbate their risk for behavior problems.

The Web children experienced a higher incidence of stressful events each year and were more bothered by such events than were the comparison children. Correspondingly, the two groups differed in terms of the number of stressful events encountered in the year immediately preceding their interview. Nevertheless, these events by themselves do not appear responsible for the Web subjects' behavior problems, and their effects appear to be mediated by other factors such as environmental protectors and the children's differential coping skills.

On the average, the Web subjects resided in twice as many family settings as the comparison subjects; hence, Web living arrangements were much less stable. This instability may have contributed significantly to their behavior problems. Importantly, however, the dysfunctions produced by such changes may largely be neutralized if the at-risk child eventually lives in an alternative family setting. Of the comparison children none had ever been removed from their biological family to a group home or a child care institution, and only one had ever lived in an alternative family. In fact, nearly all had resided continuously with at least one biological parent.

The families of the Web children also differed greatly from the families of the comparison children with respect to their utilization of formal and informal sources of support. The former families experienced more frequent and severe problems than the latter; despite the greater severity of their problems, they did not differ from the comparison families with respect to the number of agencies or organizations from whom they acquired help. Families with mentally healthy parents seemed more prone than the Web families to seek and/or accept formal help for their problems at a less severe stage of dysfunction. Their proclivity to acquire early assistance, perhaps in combination with better access to support systems, may play a major role in helping their children avoid severe behavior problems. The two types of families also differed significantly with regard to the number of informal helpers who provided assistance for major family problems. The Web families received help from significantly fewer individuals than the comparison families even though their problems were more severe. Vis-à-vis families with mentally healthy parents, the Web families were far more isolated and, probably, less capable of seeking or acquiring outside assistance.

The interactions among key strands in the web of mental illness are further illustrated by the effects of family size. Unlike comparison subjects, Web subjects from larger families exhibited fewer behavior problems than Web subjects from smaller families. Hence, it appears that the presence of large numbers of siblings can offset the adverse effects of parental mental illness so long as the siblings' behavior is adaptive. Such a relationship does not exist and, indeed, is of substantially less import when the child's parents are mentally healthy.

Analogous comparisons further highlight the special importance of the mother-child relationship when a parent is mentally ill. For instance, comparison children who have a positive relationship with their mother and a negative one with their father are likely to exhibit somewhat poorer behavior than if they have a positive relationship with both parents, but this is not the case for the Web subjects. Regardless of the nature of the father-child relationship, mother-child discord exerts a profound impact on the behavior of the Web children. Its effects clearly transcend the effects of father-child discord and of discord in the family as a whole. Even though the mother-child relationship is highly resilient, once it begins to falter the consequences are especially problematic for the at-risk child.

All things considered, our data demonstrate that a parent's mental illness constitutes a crucial added burden for a child. It may potentiate adverse factors that otherwise might be of little significance. When environmental stressors and inadequate coping skills beset the at-risk child in concert with a parent's mental illness, otherwise benign factors may exert a powerful adverse impact upon the child's behavior. In such instances at-risk children become trapped in potent, pervasive, and destructive webs of mental illness, unresponsive to potential sources of support. Without extraordinarily strong coping skills, these circumstances are likely to portend a bleak future for the at-risk child.

MODIFYING THE WEB

The web of mental illness is a complex, dynamic, and interactive phenomenon. Indeed, any given youngster can be enmeshed in different kinds of webs at different times. Furthermore, the structures of these webs may change over time and their effects depend in large part upon the ability of the at-risk child to cope with them or even modify their very nature. As we have seen, the behavior of at-risk children is determined primarily by their relationship with their mother, the cumulative effects exerted by mentally ill persons in the family, and their own competence in school and activities. Certain of these variables are environmental (such as the proportion of mentally ill persons in the family and the frequency of mother-child discord), while others pertain to the child's personal coping skills (such as school and activity competence). Unique variance in the at-risk child's behavioral outcomes is explained, among other things, by the interactive relationship between activity competence and the proportion of mentally ill persons in the family. In short, a moderating relationship exists between these two variables. If the at-risk child lives in an extremely maladaptive environment, personal coping skills are far more essential for averting behavior problems than if he or she lives in a protective environment. Conversely, children with weak coping skills are unlikely to be invincible unless their family environment is highly protective. As we have suggested, then, neither coping skills nor environmental forces alone determine a child's vulnerability or invulnerability. Rather, the at-risk child's likelihood of manifesting severe behavior problems is a function of the relative balance between his or her personal coping skills and the net environmental stressors and protectors.

The findings of the Web study demonstrate that efforts to prevent severe behavior problems on the part of at-risk children must recognize the reciprocal relationships between the child and the immediate environs. The behavior of the at-risk child is shaped substantially by the social web in which he or she is enmeshed. In essence, the family of the at-risk child is a small ecosystem where the actions of one person influence the actions and opportunities of others in an endless feedback cycle. This perspective assumes that preventive interventions aimed at a mentally ill mother are likely to exert a meaningful, albeit indirect, impact on the behavior of her at-risk child; similarly, interventions directed toward the child are likely to have an indirect impact on the mother. Therapeutic interventions aimed primarily at the father or siblings of the at-risk child likewise are bound to exert an indirect influence on other persons in the family. To realize maximal benefits for the at-risk child, therefore, preventive interventions must be directed toward all segments of the family system.

The mother-child relationship is one of the most integral components of the family system. Innovative and intensive types of family treatment are necessary to promote or sustain harmony in this relationship and to maximize its beneficial consequences for the at-risk child. Both the mother and the child must learn to recognize and acknowledge each other's basic needs and develop the capacity to improve the quality of their interactions. Therapies based upon a family systems model can indirectly strengthen the mother-child relationship by helping relevant others, including husband and siblings, enhance the extent of harmony between the mother and child by performing their own family roles more efficiently; thus, they diminish potential stresses upon the mother, the at-risk child, and their relationship with one another. It is not sufficient, as has been the case in prior intervention programs, to deal merely with the symptoms or behavioral disturbances of the mentally ill mother. Likewise, preventive efforts directed only at the high-risk child are unlikely to yield optimum outcomes.

The systemic nature of children's vulnerability is illustrated by the fact that their behavioral outcomes also depend upon the proportion of mentally ill persons who reside in the immediate family. To diminish a given child's risk, it is necessary either to reduce the concentration of such persons in the household or to provide more frequent opportunities for the child's escape from the confines of the family by participating in sports, hobbies, work, or play. Participation in such activities may temporarily remove the child from the dysfunctional web in which he or she is enmeshed. The youngster can gain increased exposure to well-adjusted individuals and, most importantly, can improve in activity competence. These strategies recognize the advisability of directing preventive interventions toward the entire family system of the at-risk child. Programs that can improve the behavior and mutual relationships of siblings, parents, and others in the immediate family are likely to exert a positive impact upon the at-risk child. By the same token, behavioral gains on the part of the at-risk child are likely to improve the family climate, generate salutary outcomes for the other family members, and establish a productive feedback loop that yields even further benefits for the at-risk child. Hence, optimum outcomes are likely to be realized when preventive interventions have a multiple focus.

If these strategies cannot be employed productively, it may then be advisable to consider placement of the at-risk child in an alternative family setting.

But, if such placements are to occur on a more proactive basis, it is imperative to improve their quality and availability. It would be tragic indeed if the deficits that prevail in the biological families of at-risk children were also to obtain in their alternative families. Personnel in the latter settings must be screened closely and trained in skills to prevent maladaptive behavior patterns among parents, siblings, the at-risk child, and other persons in the household. Such persons should be regarded as crucial adjuncts to the contemporary mental health system. Hence, vigorous efforts are necessary to professionalize the quality of care in alternative family settings and promote improvements in funding, recruitment, and training.

Similar implications obtain with regard to custody decisions in divorce cases. It is clear, for example, that such decisions should be based primarily upon the nature of the family system in which the at-risk child is expected to reside. Among relevant issues considered are whether or not a stepparent will be involved, the nature of the custodial parent's mental health, and the role to be played by stepsiblings and others in the family. In effect, decision-makers must assess the mental health of the custodial parent and the reconstituted family prior to making a placement decision. This criterion may be of greater significance for the child's well-being than the financial resources of the custodial family. Placement decisions for at-risk children should become increasingly proactive when large proportions of family members are mentally ill, the family is wracked by frequent mother-child discord, and the child's coping skills are severely deficient.

The responsiveness of an at-risk child's family to pertinent interventions will depend, of course, upon its relationship to available helping systems. Since families with a mentally ill parent tend to be highly isolated from formal and informal sources of support, human service agencies must reach out more extensively and intensively to these families. Mental health professionals need to address such central problems as mother-child discord and maladaptive behavior on the part of parents, siblings, and others in the family. Moreover, they must reduce the burden upon target families by helping their members deal with problems regarding physical disabilities, financial strains, and ineffective childrearing. Social service agencies can assist such families by establishing programs that link them more effectively with informal support systems such as neighbors, relatives, and friends. In addition, they can create better coordinated and more efficient referral systems. And, of course, they can strive to improve their own programs both within the agency and in the homes of target families. In short, they can greatly enhance the quality of their preventive services by concentrating upon the entire family system. Without concerted outreach programs the plight of many at-risk children and their families will remain not only ignored but unknown.

Traditional human service agencies can also play an integral and revitalized role in the delivery of prevention programs. The at-risk child's activity competence can be greatly enhanced, for example, by means of appropriate programs at community centers, neighborhood houses, settlement houses, and similar organizations. These agencies can assist large numbers of at-risk children by engaging them in sports, hobbies, and related activities that strengthen their coping skills. Such programs should be offered at a relatively young age to expedite the child's acquisition of crucial skills. Consequently, beneficial side effects may accrue from such programs: enhanced activity competence on the child's part and a significant reduction in mother-child discord. Furthermore, public and private school systems ought to strengthen the school competence of at-risk children by focusing on academic and listening skills, cooperation with teachers and peers, and related abilities.

The fact that environmental variables can moderate the effects of personal coping skills, and vice versa, is of utmost importance from both a theoretical and a practical perspective. Interventions that modify particular strands in the web of mental illness are likely to have important effects upon other strands. By promoting therapeutic gains in one area, the need to intervene in other areas may become less pressing. For example, as the at-risk child's activity competence improves, the concentration of mental illness in the family may be of less concern. Conversely, as the concentration of mental illness in the family is reduced, it may not be as necessary to focus on the child's activity competence. Clearly, however, efforts to diminish a child's level of risk are likely to be maximized when intervention efforts are applied concurrently in both areas.

Some webs of mental illness are more devastating than others. Their social, psychological, and physical characteristics may differ considerably from one another. Furthermore, the particular web that traps a given child at one point may change dramatically in configuration and potency over a period of months or years. Our research has identified only several of the environmental and personal variables that constitute crucial features in the web of mental illness. We acquired the retrospective data for the study at only one point in the subjects' life course. Hence, like an isolated frame from an infinite reel of film, our image of the Web children has been foreshadowed by antecedent events and, in turn, presages subsequent ones.

Future studies will require vast financial, technical, and human resources to fully comprehend the web of mental illness. But they will be predicated upon the realization that childhood vulnerability depends upon the relative balance between individual coping skills and the net environmental stressors and protectors to which the at-risk child is exposed. Prevention programs based upon this understanding can be directed productively at either the at-risk child or the child's immediate environs or both to achieve maximum benefits. In so doing, prevention programs may alter the very nature of the web of mental illness which enmeshes the at-risk child.

APPENDIX:
Research Instruments

Parent Report: pp. 255–267   Child Report: pp. 267–276

Index

CONSTRUCT	ITEM	PAGE
Demographic factors	1–6	256–257
Mental health problems	7–9	258
	20b–20g	262–264
Physical health problems	20a	262
	12–15	268–269
Life events	1–2	256
Family social support	I–III	266–267
Family relationships	10–15	258–259
	17–19	260
Self-esteem	3	276

Code   _ _ _
                                          1 - 4

Form 01

Preliminary Intake Information

1. Would you mind telling me how you found out about our program?
   [Interviewer: note the specific agency or individual.]
   code:
   1 = hospital-private
   2 = hospital-public
   3 = State Division of Family Services
   4 = family service or child mental health agency
   5 = juvenile court
   6 = psychiatrist-private practice
   7 = psychologist-private practice
   8 = social worker-private practice
   9 = Mental Health Association
   10 = friend or neighbor
   11 = relative
   12 = other _____   _ _ _ _
                                                                   8 - 11

2. With whom is (the child) currently living?

   code:
   1 = With both natural parents
   2 = With one natural and one step parent   complete rest of page, then use
   3 = With only one natural parent   the Green Current Family Form

   4 = With adoptive parents
   5 = With a relative _____
                        specify
   6 = With a foster family   go to question #3
   7 = In a group home
   8 = In a treatment facility

                                                                   _
                                                                  16

3. How old is the child? (code in months rounded to nearest year)   _ _ _
                                                                       17 - 19

4. How long has (the child) lived in this current situation?
                  (code in months)   _ _ _
                                                                       20 - 22

   Interviewer:
   a. If more than 1/3 of the child's life
       (1) and the preceding answer was #4, #5, #6   complete rest of page, then use
                                                        the Green and Pink Forms

       (2) and the preceding answer was #7 or #8.   complete rest of page , then
                                                         use Tan, Yellow, and Pink Forms

   b. If less than 1/3 of the child's life   go to questions #5, #6, #7

5. How many families has (the child) had since birth?   _ _
                                                                   23 24

6. How many group homes or institutions has (the child) lived in since
   birth?   _ _
                                                                   25 26

7. With whom has (the child) lived the greatest portion of his/her life?   2⁻7

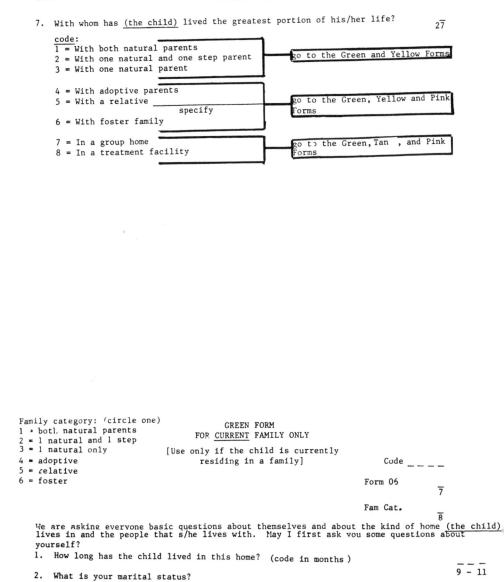

code:
1 = With both natural parents
2 = With one natural and one step parent ⟶ go to the Green and Yellow Forms
3 = With one natural parent

4 = With adoptive parents
5 = With a relative _____ ⟶ go to the Green, Yellow and Pink
                        specify   Forms
6 = With foster family

7 = In a group home ⟶ go to the Green, Tan , and Pink
8 = In a treatment facility   Forms

Family category: (circle one)   GREEN FORM
1 = botl. natural parents   FOR CURRENT FAMILY ONLY
2 = 1 natural and 1 step
3 = 1 natural only   [Use only if the child is currently
4 = adoptive   residing in a family]   Code _ _ _ _
5 = relative
6 = foster   Form 06
                                                              ⁻7

                                                      Fam Cat.
                                                            ⁻8
We are asking everyone basic questions about themselves and about the kind of home (the child)
lives in and the people that s/he lives with. May I first ask you some questions about
yourself?

1. How long has the child lived in this home? (code in months)
                                                              _ _ _
2. What is your marital status?   9 - 11
   code:
   1 = Married
   2 = Separated/divorced
   3 = Widow/widower
   4 = Single
   5 = Living together-unmarried
   6 = Other _____
                                                              _
                                                              12
        [Interviewer: Ask each question for the respondent and
                       then for the respondent's mate . Code "0"
                       for not applicable, don't know and no answer.]

	Female	Male

Race? (Is your spouse of the same race _____?)
code:
1 = Black
2 = White
3 = Hispanic
4 = Asian
5 = American Indian
6 = Other _____

—   —
13   14

Are you a member of any particular religious faith?
code: (Is your spouse? _____)
1 = Protestant
2 = Catholic
3 = Jewish
4 = None
5 = Other

—   —
15   16

What was the last year of school you completed?
(What was the last year of school your spouse completed?)
code:
1 = Less than seventh grade
2 = Ninth grade
3 = Partial high school
4 = High school graduate
5 = Partial college
6 = Standard college or university graduation
7 = Graduate professional training (degree)

—   —
17   18

What was the mother's occupation? (What was the father's occupation?)
code:
1 = Farm laborers/menial service workers
2 = Unskilled workers
3 = Machine operators and semiskilled worker
4 = Smaller business owners (valued less than $40,000)
   skilled manual workers, craftsmen, tenant farmers
5 = Clerical and sales workers, small farm and business owners
   (valued at $40,000-$80,000)
6 = Technicians, semiprofessionals, small business owners
   (valued at $80,000-$125,000)
7 = Small business or farm owners (valued at $125,000-165,000)
   Managers, minor professionals, entertainers and artists
8 = Administrators, lesser professionals, proprietors of
   medium-sized businesses (valued between $165,000-$400,000)
9 = High executives, proprietors of large businesses (valued at
   $400,000) major professionals

[Interviewer: If housewife or retired, leave space blank and write
 e word in]

—   —
19   20

Green Form/Current Family Only   Page 2

7. Were either you or your spouse ever hospitalized for mental
   health reasons?
   <u>code</u>
   1 = yes
   2 = no

(Interviewer: Ask #8 and #9 only if applicable, otherwise go to
#10).

Female	Male
‾21‾	‾22‾

8. What was the starting date of the most recent
   hospitalization? (What was the starting date for your
   spouse's hospitalization?) (month/year)

9. What was the ending date of that hospitalization? (What was
   the ending date of your spouse's hospitalization?)
   (month/year) (code 9999 - if currently in hospital)

Female	Male
‾23‾ ‾/‾ ‾26‾	‾27‾ ‾/‾ ‾30
‾31‾ ‾/‾ ‾34‾	‾35‾ ‾/‾ ‾38

10. Please tell me about your family - that is - how you and
    everyone get along with one another. I will read you five
    sentences and you can tell me which sentence best describes
    your family
    1. We rarely or never have any problems.
    2. We have problems in our family a little of the time.
    3. We have problems in our family some of the time.
    4. We have problems in our family a good part of the time.
    5. We have problems in our family most or all of the time.   ‾39‾

11. Please tell me about (the mother's) relationship with __(the__
    child). I will read you five sentences. Please tell me
    which sentence best describes the mother and (child).
    1. We (or they) rarely or never have any problems.
    2. We (or they) have problems a little of the time.
    3. We (or they) have problems some of the time.
    4. We (or they) have problems a good part of the time.
    5. We (or they) have problems most or all of the time.
    6. We (or they) never see, or hear from, one another.   ‾40‾

12. How about (the father's) relationship with the child?
    1. We (or they) rarely or never have any problems.
    2. We (or they) have problems a little of the time.
    3. We (or they) have problems some of the time.
    4. We (or they) have problems a good part of the time.
    5. We (or they) have problems most or all of the time.
    6. We (or they) never see, or hear from, one another.   ‾41‾

(Interviewer: if the respondent is married or living with someone
ask question #13; otherwise go to #14 & 15)

13. Please tell me about your current relationship with your spouse. I
    will again read you five sentences and you can tell me which
    sentence best describes your relationship.
    1. We rarely or never have any problems.
    2. We have problems a little of the time.
    3. We have problems some of the time.
    4. We have problems a good part of the time.
    5. We have problems most or all of the time.
    6. We never see, or hear from, one another.   ‾42‾

(Interviewer: If the family category is #2 or #3, ask:)

4. Please tell me about your relationship with your former
   spouse. I will again read you five sentences. Please tell
   me which sentence best describes the both of you.
   1. We rarely or never have any problems.
   2. We have problems a little of the time.
   3. We have problems some of the time.
   4. We have problems a good part of the time.
   5. We have problems most or all of the time.
   6. We never see, or hear from, one another. $\overline{43}$

5. How about your former spouse's relationship with the child?
   1. They rarely or never have any problems.
   2. They have problems a little of the time.
   3. They have problems some of the time.
   4. They have problems a good part of the time.
   5. They have problems most or all of the time.
   6. They never see, or hear from, one another. $\overline{44}$

3

Green form   Family History

We would also like to know something about (the child)'s home and all
the people (the child) lives with.

16.   How many people live in the home?
                                                    __ __
                                                    45 46
17.   What are their names, starting with the child?
       [Interviewer: Fill out a column for each person, then ask
       each question in turn, mentioning each family member before
       proceeding to the next question. Do children first; then adults.]

18a.   What is (each family member)'s relationship to (the
       child).

code: code:
       female   male
201=participant   101=participant
202=twin   102=twin
203=sister   103=brother
204=step or ½sister   104=step or ½ bros.
205=cousin   105=cousin
206=not related   106=not related _____
207=natural mother   107=natural father
208=adoptive mother   108=adoptive father
209=step mother   109=step father
210=foster mother/guardian   110=foster father/guardian
2'1=related adult   111=related adult
212=maternal grandmother   112=maternal grandfather
213=paternal grandmother   113=paternal grandfather
214=other_____   114=other_____

[Interviewer: code 18b after the last column response for 18a]

18b.   Which close relatives such as sister, brother,or parent
       no longer live at home? For example, they may be in the
       military service, at college, or in a hospital [Interviewer:
       Continue to fill out a new, separate column for each person.
       Be sure to fill out a column for an absent natural parent.
       Use the same codes as for question 18a. However, code
       females with a 4 and males a 3.]

19.   What is (each family member) 's age? [Get birthdate if possible.]

(1)	(2)		(3)			(4)			(5)
Child	Mother	Father	4	5	6	7	8	9	10
– – – 47 – 49	– – – 9 – 11	– – – 31 – 33	– – – 9 – 11	– – – 31 – 33	– – – 53 – 55	– – – 9 – 11	– – – 31 – 33	– – – 53 – 55	– – – 9 – 11
– – 50 51	– – 12 13	– – 34 35	– – 12 13	– – 34 35	– – 56 57	– – 12 13	– – 34 35	– – 56 57	– – 12 13

Green form   **Problems**

Can you tell me about each person's health in the last six months?

20a. Does (each family member) have any chronic physical or health problem?
      Does the problem affect him/her in anyway?

<u>code</u>:
1 = no problems/no limitations
2 = able to carry on major activity, but limited in other activities
3 = limited in amount or kind of major activity
4 = unable to carry on major activities

20b. Has (each family member)   [If no major problem, code 99 & ask
      had any major behavioral   20e. Then go to next family member.
      or mental health problem   If problem, describe in column (to
      in the last 6 months?   code after interview) & continue
                                       with 20c-20g before going to next
                                       family member?

        Can you describe what types of behavioral problems they are?

        [Interviewer: Optional]:
        Can you give me an example of what (each problem individual) does whe
        the problem occurs?

Name:

(1)	(2)		(3)			(4)			(5)
Child	Mother	Father	4	5	6	7	8	9	10
52	14	36	14	36	58	14	36	58	14
53 —56	15 – 18	37 – 40	15 – 18	37 – 40	59 – 62	15 – 18	37 – 40	59 – 62	15 – 18

Problems
Green form

20c. How old was (each problem individual) when the problem was last noticed?

20d. How old was (each problem individual) when the problem was first noticed?
      code: 99 = first noticed at birth.

20e. Is (each problem individual) being regularly treated ?
      What kind of treatment is it?   How often is it given?
      code: (Choose the nearest appropriate interval.)
      1 = inpatient - hospital   6 = outpatient - 8 times a month onth
      2 = outpatient = less than 1 per   7 = outpatient - 16 times a mos. onth
                       month   8 = outpatient - daily
      3 = outpatient = once a month   9 = no treatment
      4 = outpatient = twice a month
    __5 = outpatient = 4 times a month

20f. Did anyone ever give you an official name or diagnosis for any of the
      problems? If they did, do you remember what it is? [Interviewer: write
      full diagnosis in the column.]

      Can we obtain the official name for this problem from someone?
      name: _____
      address: _____
      telephone: _____

20g. Do the problems affect (each problem individual)'s ability to function in a
      normal work/school setting? Are there any limitations on other activities?

      code:
      1 = no limitations
      2 = able to carry on major activity, but limited in other activities
      3 = limited in amount or kind of major activity
      4 = unable to carry on major activities

Name	(1)	(2)		(3)			(4)			(5)
	Child	Mother	Father	4	5	6	7	8	9	10
	$\overline{57}$ $\overline{58}$	$\overline{19}$ $\overline{20}$	$\overline{41}$ $\overline{42}$	$\overline{19}$ $\overline{20}$	$\overline{41}$ $\overline{42}$	$\overline{63}$ $\overline{64}$	$\overline{19}$ $\overline{20}$	$\overline{41}$ $\overline{42}$	$\overline{63}$ $\overline{64}$	$\overline{19}$ $\overline{20}$
	$\overline{59}$ $\overline{60}$	$\overline{21}$ $\overline{22}$	$\overline{43}$ $\overline{44}$	$\overline{21}$ $\overline{22}$	$\overline{43}$ $\overline{44}$	$\overline{65}$ $\overline{66}$	$\overline{21}$ $\overline{22}$	$\overline{43}$ $\overline{44}$	$\overline{65}$ $\overline{66}$	$\overline{21}$ $\overline{22}$
	$\overline{61}$	$\overline{23}$	$\overline{45}$	$\overline{23}$	$\overline{45}$	$\overline{67}$	$\overline{23}$	$\overline{45}$	$\overline{67}$	$\overline{23}$
	62 – 67	24 – 29	46 – 51	24–29	46–51	68–73	24–29	46 – 51	68 – 73	24 – 29
	$\overline{68}$	$\overline{30}$	$\overline{52}$	$\overline{30}$	$\overline{52}$	$\overline{74}$	$\overline{30}$	$\overline{52}$	$\overline{74}$	$\overline{30}$

Green Form

NETWORK QUESTIONNAIRE

Code ___ ___ ___ ___
                                               1 - 4

Form 07

I. All families have some problems every year. Could you please describe
    the worst problem faced by your family during the past year?

    _____
    _____

    code: presence of problem:
    1 = yes
    2 = no
    [Interviewer: if "no" terminate the Network Questionnaire.]   ___
                                                                                     8

    1. Let's think about this problem for a minute. At its worst, how
        serious was this problem? Would you say:

        code:
        1 = not at all serious?
        2 = a little bit serious?
        3 = fairly serious?
        4 = very serious?
        5 = extremely serious?   ___
                                                                                      9

    2. Currently, how serious is this problem? (Same code as #1)
                                                                                     ___
                                                                                     10

II. Sometimes certain people are able to help us with problems like this,
    for instance, relatives, friends, physicians, clergymen, and others.
    Which people, if any, have been able to help you with the problem that
    you mentioned?

                                                       CODE
                                                       Role: Helpfulness:

    A. Role: _____   ____   ____
    B. Role: _____   ____   ____
    C. Role: _____   ____   ____
    D. Role: _____   ____   ____
    E. Role: _____   ____   ____
                                                       11-15   16-20

                    code: role:
                    code:
                    1 = relative
                    2 = friend
                    3 = neighbor
                    4 = other _____   ___

    1. Let's consider each of these persons for a minute. How helpful would
        you say (each) was? Interviewer: Code this response beside
        the appropriate role.
                    code: helpfulness:
                    1 = not at all helpful?
                    2 = a little bit helpful?
                    3 = fairly helpful?
                    4 = very helpful?
                    5 = extremely helpful?

Green Form

Network Questionnaire

III. Sometimes certain agencies or organizations are able to help us with problems
like this, for instance, social service agencies, job agencies, schools, or
hospitals. Which **agencies**, if any, have been able to help you with this problem?
Type of Agency:

	Agency:	CODE Agency:	Helpfulness:
A. Name:	_____	____	____
B. Name:	_____	____	____
C. Name:	_____	____	____
D. Name:	_____	____	____
E. Name:	_____	____	____
	code: agency:	21-25	26-30

        1 = social service agency
        2 = job agency
        3 = school
        4 = hospital
        5 = financial aid agency
        6 = other _____

1. Let's consider each of these agencies for a second. How helpful
would you say __(each)__ agency was: [Interviewer: Code this
response beside the appropriate agency name.]

    code: Helpfulness:
    1 = not at all helpful?
    2 = a little bit helpful?
    3 = fairly helpful?
    4 = very helpful?
    5 = extremely helpful?

Form for Participant Child

[Interviewer: Address these questions to the child. Code "0"
for don't know, not applicable, or missing information.]

Code Number ____ ____ ____
             1 - 4
Form 02

1. How old are you? _____
When is your birthday? (month/day/year)

__ __/__ __/__ __
 8   -   13

2. Sex: code:
      1 = male
      2 = female

              __
              14

3. Race: code:
        1 = Black
        2 = White
        3 = Hispanic
        4 = Asian
        5 = American Indian
        6 = Other _____

              __
              15

4. Do you have a religion?
   code:
   1 = Protestant
   2 = Catholic
   3 = Jewish
   4 = None
   5 = Other _____

$\overline{16}$

5. What school do you go to?

_____

6. What is the school district?

_____

7. Do you know the address of your school?

_____

8. What grade are you in? _____

$\overline{17}\ \overline{18}$

9. What is your principal's name? _____

10. With which teacher do you spend the most time?

_____

_____

11. What is your counselor's name? _____

12. Are you taking any medicine? _____
    code:
    1 = yes
    2 = no

$\overline{19}$

13. What kinds of medicine?

_____

_____

_____

code:
1 = Sedatives and hypnotics   6 = Stimulants
2 = Anti-convulsants   7 = Anti-anxiety agents
3 = Major tranquilizers   8 = Anti-cholinergics
4 = Minor tranquilizers   9 = Miscellaneous anti-psychotic
5 = Anti-depressants   0 = Other _____

$\overline{20}\ -\ \overline{23}$

Form for Participant Child   Page 2

14. Do you have any allergies?

_____

_____

code:
  = number of allergies
0 = no allergies

$\overline{24}$

How much does the allergy interfere with your activities?

_____

_____

_____

15. Are there any physical or medical reasons for you not to take part
    in some activities?

    _____

    _____

    _____

    code:
    1 = yes
    2 = no   —

16. Who do you live with, and how long have you lived there?   25

    _____

[Interviewer: If the child lives in an institution or group home, go to #20.]

Now I have a few questions about your current family.

17. Please tell me about your family--that is--how you and everyone get
    along with one another. I will read you five sentences. You tell
    me which sentence best describes your family.

    1. We rarely or never have any problems in our family.
    2. We have problems in our family a little of the time.
    3. We have problems in our family some of the time.
    4. We have problems in our family a good part of the time.
    5. We have problems in our family most or all of the time.   —
                                                                    26

18. Please tell me about you and your mother--that is--how you currently get along
    with one another. Once again I'll read five sentences and you tell
    me which one best describes you and your mother.

    1. We rarely or never have any problems.
    2. We have problems a little of the time.
    3. We have problems some of the time.
    4. We have problems a good part of the time.
    5. We have problems most or all of the time.   —
    6. We rarely or never see each other.   27

19. Please tell me about you and your father - that is - how you currently get along
    with one another. Once again I'll read five sentences and you tell me which
    one best describes you and your father.

    1. We rarely or never have any problems.
    2. We have problems a little of the time.
    3. We have problems some of the time.
    4. We have problems a good part of the time.
    5. We have problems most or all of the time.   —
    6. We rarely or never see each other.   28

[Interviewer: If the child has lived in the current family less than one
               third of his/her live ask questions 20-23.]

20a Where did you live for the longest part of your life?

    _____

    _____

20b How long was that? _____

[Interviewer: If the longest living situation was an institution or group
               home go to questions 24 and 25. If it was a family, ask
               questions 21-23.]

Form for Participant Child   Page 3

Can you please tell me something about the family that you used to live with?

21. Please tell me about that <u>family</u>--that is--how you and everyone <u>got</u>
     <u>along</u> with one another. I will read you five sentences. You tell me
     which sentence best describes that <u>family.</u>

     1. We rarely or never had any problems in our family.
     2. We had problems in our family a little of the time.
     3. We had problems in our family some of the time.
     4. We had problems in our family a good part of the time.
     5. We had problems in our family most or all of the time.

                                                                    —
                                                                    29

22. Please tell me about you and the <u>mother</u> of that family--that is--
     how you <u>got along</u> with one another. Once again I'll read you five
     sentences and you tell me which one best describes you and that
     mother.

     1. We rarely or never had any problems.
     2. We had problems a little of the time.
     3. We had problems some of the time.
     4. We had problems a good part of the time.
     5. We had problems most or all of the time.

                                                                    —
                                                                    30

23. Please tell me about you and the <u>father</u> of that family--that is--
     how you <u>got along</u> with one another. Once again I'll read five
     sentences and you tell me which one best describes you and that <u>father</u>.

     1. We rarely or never had any problems.
     2. We had problems a little of the time.
     3. We had problems some of the time.
     4. We had problems a good part of the time.
     5. We had problems most or all of the time.

                                                                    —
                                                                    31

[Interviewer: If the child currently resides in an institution or a group
                home, or has resided in one longer than any place else, ask
                24 and 25.]

24. Please tell me about you and your unit in the institution or group home
     --that is-- how you get (got) along with everyone. I will read you five
     sentences. You tell me which sentence best describes your unit.

     1. We rarely or never have (had) any problems.
     2. We have (had) problems a little of the time.
     3. We have (had) problems some of the time.
     4. We have (had) problems a good part of the time.
     5. We have (had) problems most or all of the time.

                                                                    —
                                                                    32

25. Please tell me about you and the adults in charge of your unit--
     that is--how you get (got) along with one another.

     1. We rarely or never have (had) any problems.
     2. We have (had) problems a little of the time.
     3. We have (had) problems some of the time.
     4. We have (had) problems a good part of the time.
     5. We have (had) problems most or all of the time.

                                                                    —
                                                                    33

272 APPENDIX

Child Report

Child Change/Stress Timeline

structions:

We are interested in some important changes in your life.
Now, I will name several types of things that sometimes happen to children.
ease tell me if these things ever happened to you, how old you were when they happened
and, also, how much they bothered you.

nterviewer: Ask--"Did it ever happen?"   Then ask-- "How old were you?"   Then ask--
"How much would you say that this bothered you?"
ode the age it occurred in the two left hand spaces and the code for bothersomeness
in the right hand space of a three space column.]

code: (in the two left hand spaces
        _ _ = age in years 01 to 15
        00 = under one year old.

Did you ever move:
a. To a new city or town?   How old...?   How bothered...? . . . .
b. To a new home in the same city?   How old...?   How bothered...?
c. To a new school?   How old...?   How bothered...? . . . .

Did you ever have someone you cared for die?   For example:
a. Your mother?   How old...?   How bothered...? . . . .
b. Your father?   How old...?   How bothered...? . . . .
c. A brother or sister?   How old...?   How bothered...? . . . . .
d. A grandparent?   How old...?   How bothered...? . . . . . .
e. Any other close relative?   How old...?   How bothered...? . . .
f. A close friend?   How old...?   How bothered...? . . . . .
g. A special pet?   How old...?   How bothered...? . . . .

Have you ever had any additions to your family?   For example:
[Interviewer: This includes natural or adoptive families only. Cod
a. A new mother?   How old...?   How bothered...? . . . .
b. A new father?   How old...?   How bothered...? . . . .
. A new brother or sister?   How old...?   How bothered...? . . . .
. Other relatives or friends who came to live with you for more than
   one month?   How old....?   How bothered...? . . . .

Code # $\overline{1} - \overline{4}$
Form 04

code: (in the far right space of each column)
1 = didn't bother you at all
2 = bothered you a little
3 = bothered you somewhat
4 = bothered you a lot
5 = bothered you completely
6 = don't know, don't remember, not applicable

				Occurrences						
1st	2nd	3rd	4th	5th	6th	7th	8th	9th	10th	
_ _ _	_ _ _	_ _ _	_ _ _	_ _ _	_ _ _	_ _ _	_ _ _	_ _ _	_ _ _	(1) 9-38
_ _ _	_ _ _	_ _ _	_ _ _	_ _ _	_ _ _	_ _ _	_ _ _	_ _ _	_ _ _	39 - 68
_ _ _	_ _ _	_ _ _	_ _ _	_ _ _	_ _ _	_ _ _	_ _ _	_ _ _	_ _ _	69-80(2)
										9-26

_ _ _	_ _ _			27-32
_ _ _	_ _ _			33-38
_ _ _	_ _ _	_ _ _	_ _ _	39-50
_ _ _	_ _ _	_ _ _	_ _ _	51-62
_ _ _	_ _ _	_ _ _	_ _ _	63-74
_ _ _	_ _ _	_ _ _	_ _ _	75-80 (3) 9-14
_ _ _	_ _ _	_ _ _	_ _ _	15-26

12

tiple people who come at one time as a single occurrence.]

_ _	_ _ _	_ _ _	_ _ _		27-38
_ _ _	_ _ _	_ _ _	_ _ _		39-50
_ _ _	_ _ _	_ _ _	_ _ _	_ _ _	_ _ _	51-68
_ _ _	_ _ _	_ _ _	_ _ _		69-80

Child Report
Child's Life Change Timeline

4. Did you ever have any really bad health problems that kept you at ho
   or in a hospital for more than two weeks? For example:
   a. A serious illness? How old...? How bothered...? . . . . .
   b. A serious injury? How old...? How bothered...? . . . . . .

5. Did you ever go through a period of time when you were separated fro
   your family or parents due to:
   a. Your parent's divorce or separation? How old...? How bothered
   b. Hospitalization of a parent for more than a month? How old...
      How bothered...? . . . .
   c. A parent (or parent substitute) being gone for more than a month
      although not in a hospital? How old...? How bothered...? . .
   d. A sister or brother leaving home (to go to school, get married,
      or for some other reason)? How old...? How bothered ...?.
   e. Your moving to a foster home, group home, or some type of
      institution? How old...? How bothered...? . . . . . .

6. Have there ever been any other really big changes in your life that
   haven't discussed?

   1st (Please describe)_____
   2nd (Please describe)_____
   3rd (Please describe)_____
   4th (Please describe)_____
   5th (Please describe)_____

Now, I would like to ask you a few different types of questions.

7. Did you ever repeat a grade in school? How old...? How bothered

8. Did someone other than a family member ever catch you breaking the
   law? How old...? How bothered...? . . . .

9. Did you ever run away from home? How old...? How bothered...?

10. Has anything else really, really bad happened to you?

    1st (Please describe)_____
    2nd (Please describe)_____
    3rd (Please describe)_____
    4th (Please describe)_____
    5th (Please describe)_____

Page 2.

Occurences:

1st	2nd	3rd	4th	5th	6th	7th	8th	9th	10th
_ _ _	_ _ _	_ _ _	_ _ _	_ _ _	_ _ _	_ _ _	(4) 9-29		
_ _ _	_ _ _	_ _ _	_ _ _	_ _ _	_ _ _	_ _ _	30-50		

1st	2nd	3rd	4th	5th	6th	7th	8th	9th	10th
_ _ _	_ _ _	_ _ _	_ _ _						51-62
_ _ _	_ _ _	_ _ _	_ _ _	_ _ _	_ _ _				6 3-80
_ _ _	_ _ _	_ _ _	_ _ _	_ _ _	_ _ _	_ _ _	_ _ _	_ _ _	_ _ _(5)9-38
_ _ _	_ _ _	_ _ _	_ _ _	_ _ _	_ _ _				39-56
_ _ _	_ _ _	_ _ _	_ _ _	_ _ _	_ _ _	_ _ _	_ _ _	_ _ _	_ _ _ 57-80
									(6) 9-14

_ _ _
_ _ _
_ _ _ 15-29
_ _ _
_ _ _

1st	2nd	3rd	4th
_ _ _	_ _ _	_ _ _	30-38

1st	2nd	3rd	4th	5th	6th	7th	8th	9th	10th
_ _ _	_ _ _	_ _ _	_ _ _	_ _ _	_ _ _	_ _ _	_ _ _	_ _ _	_ _ _ 39-68
_ _ _	_ _ _	_ _ _	_ _ _	_ _ _	_ _ _	_ _ _	_ _ _	_ _ _	_ _ _ 69-80
									(7)9-26

_ _ _
_ _ _
_ _ _ 27-41
_ _ _
_ _ _

3. In general, how often do you:

	RARELY OR NEVER	A LITTLE OF THE TIME	SOME OF THE TIME	A GOOD PART OF THE TIME	MOST OR ALL OF THE TIME	
a. Feel that there are lots of things about yourself that you would change if you could ?	—	—	—	—	—	42
b. Feel that your parents expect too much of you?	—	—	—	—	—	43
c. Feel that kids usually follow your ideas?	—	—	—	—	—	44
d. Feel discouraged in school?	—	—	—	—	—	45

BIBLIOGRAPHY

Abelson, R. P. 1985. A Variance Explanation Paradox: When a Little is a Lot. *Psychological Bulletin* 97: 129–133.

Achenbach, T. M. 1978–79. The Child Behavior Profile: An Empirically Based System for Assessing Children's Behavior Problems and Competencies. *International Journal of Mental Health* 7:24–42.

Achenbach, T. M., and C. S. Edelbrock. 1981. Behavioral Problems and Competencies Reported by Parents of Normal and Disturbed Children Aged 4 Through 16. *Monographs of the Society for Research in Child Development* 46: Serial No. 188.

Alcohol Drug Abuse and Mental Health News. 16 May 1983. 9:1–6.

Amark, C. 1951. A Study in Alcoholism. *Acta Psychiatrica Scandinavica* 70:1–283.

American Psychiatric Association. 1980. *Diagnostic and Statistical Manual of Mental Disorders, III.* Washington, D.C.: American Psychiatric Association.

Anderson, C. 1977. Locus of Control, Coping Behaviors, and Performance in a Stress Setting: A Longitudinal Study. *Journal of Applied Psychology* 63:446–451.

Andrews, G., C. Tennant, D. M. Hewson, and G. E. Vaillant. 1978. Life Event Stress, Social Support, Coping Style, and Risk of Psychological Impairment. *Journal of Nervous and Mental Disorders* 166:307–316.

Anthony, E. J. 1972. The Contagious Subculture of Psychosis. In *Progress in Group and Family Therapy*, ed. C. J. Sager and H. S. Kaplan. 636–658. New York: Brunner/ Mazel.

Anthony, E. J. 1974. A Risk-Vulnerability Intervention Model for Children of Psychotic Parents. In *The Child in His Family: Children at Psychiatric Risk, Vol 3*, ed. E. J. Anthony and C. Koupernik. 99–122. New York: Wiley Interscience.

Anthony, E. J. 1975. Naturalistic Studies of Disturbed Families. *Explorations in Child Psychiatry*, ed. E. J. Anthony. 341–380. New York: Plenum.

Anthony, E. J., and C. Koupernik, eds. 1978. *The Child in His Family: The Vulnerable Child.* New York: John Wiley.

Antonovsky, A. 1979. *Health, Stress, and Coping: New Perspectives on Mental and Physical Well-Being.* San Francisco: Jossey-Bass.

Aronson, H., and A. Gilbert. 1963. Preadolescent Sons of Male Alcoholics. *Archives of General Psychiatry* 8:235–241.

Bandura, A. 1969. Social Learning Theory of Identificatory Processes. In *Handbook of Socialization Theory and Research*, ed. D. Goslin. 213–262. Chicago: Rand McNally.

Bane, M. J. 1976. *Here to Stay: American Families in the Twentieth Century.* New York: Basic Books.

Barnes, J. A. 1975. *Social Networks.* Reading, Mass.: Addison-Wesley.

Bastiansen, S., and E. Kringler. 1973. Children of Two Psychotic Parents: A Preliminary Report. In *Annual Review of the Schizophrenic Syndrome, Vol. 3*, ed. R. Cancro. 349–380. New York: Brunner/Mazel.

Beardslee, W. R. 1984. Familial Influences in Childhood Depression. *Pediatric Annals* 13:32–36.

Beardslee, W. R., J. Bemporad, M. B. Keller, and G. L. Klerman. 1983. Children of Parents with Major Affective Disorder: A Review. *American Journal of Psychiatry* 140:825–832.

Becker, J. V., and P. M. Miller. 1976. Verbal and Nonverbal Marital Interaction Patterns of Alcoholics and Nonalcoholics. *Journal of Studies on Alcohol* 37:1616–1624.

Becker, W. C. 1964. Consequences of Parental Discipline. In *Review of Child Development Research, Vol. 1*, ed. M. L. Hoffman and L. W. Hoffman. 169–208. New York: Russell Sage Foundation.

Beisser, A., N. Glasser, and M. Grant. 1967. Psychosocial Adjustment in Children of Schizophrenic Mothers. *Journal of Nervous and Mental Disease* 145:429–440.

Bell, R. Q. and D. Pearl. 1982. Psychosocial Change in Risk Groups: Implications for Early Identification. *Journal of Prevention in Human Services* 4:45–58.

Bell, N. W., and E. F. Vogel, eds. 1960. *The Family*. New York: Free Press.

Benson, C. S. 1980. Coping and Support among Daughters of Alcoholics. *Dissertation Abstracts International* 41 (5–6):2305-B.

Bleuler, M. 1974. The Offspring of Schizophrenics. *Schizophrenia Bulletin* 8:93–107.

Block, J. 1982. Assimilation, Accommodation, and the Dynamics of Personality Development. *Child Development* 53:281–295.

Bonham, G. S., and L. S. Corder. 1981. *NMCES Household Interview Instruments*. Hyattsville, Md.: U.S. Dept. of HHS, Public Health Service Office of Health Research, Statistics and Technology, National Center for Health Services Research, DHHS Publication No. (PHS) 81–3280.

Boshier, R., and A. Izard. 1972. Do Conservative Parents Use Harsh Child-Rearing Practices? *Psychological Reports* 31:734.

Bott, E. 1971. *Family and Social Network*. London: Tavistock.

Bramwell, S. T., M. Masuda, N. N. Wagner, and T. R. Holmes. 1975. Psychosocial Factors in Athletic Injuries. *Journal of Human Stress* 1:6–20.

Bryant, B., and J. Trockel. 1976. Personal History of Psychological Stress Related to Locus of Control Orientation. *Journal of Consulting and Clinical Psychology* 44:266–271.

Buck, C., and K. Laughton. 1959. Family Patterns of Illness: The Effect of Psychoneurosis in the Parent upon Illness in the Child. *Acta Psychiatrica Neurologica Scandinavica* 34:165–175.

Burke, R., and J. Weir. 1978. Sex Differences in Adolescent Life Stress, Social Support, and Well-Being. *Journal of Psychology* 98:277–288.

Canavan, M., and R. Clark. 1923a. The Mental Health of 581 Offspring of Non-Psychotic Parents. *Mental Hygiene* 7:770–778.

Canavan, M., and R. Clark. 1923b. The Mental Health of 463 Children from Dementia Praecox Stock. *Mental Hygiene* 7:137–148.

Caplan, G. 1974. *Support Systems and Community Mental Health*. New York: Behavioral Publications.

Caplan, G., and M. Killilea. 1976. *Support Systems and Mutual Help: Multidisciplinary Explorations*. New York: Grune and Stratton.

Carter, H., and C. Glick. 1976. *Marriage and Divorce: A Social and Economic Study*. Rev. ed. Cambridge, Mass.: Howard University Press.

Castillo, I. 1980. The Relationship of Stressful Life Events and Adolescent Employment. *Psychological Reports* 47:1195–1198.

Chafetz, M. E., H. T. Blane, and M. J. Hill. 1971. Children of Alcoholics: Observations in a Child Guidance Clinic. *Quarterly Journal of Studies on Alcohol* 32:687–698.

Chandler, L. A. 1981. The Source of Stress Inventory. *Psychology in the Schools* 18: 164–168.

Cicchetti, D. 1984. The Emergence of Developmental Psychopathology. *Child Development* 55:1–7.

Clarke, A. M., and A. D. Clarke, eds. 1976. *Early Experience: Myth and Evidence.* London: Open Books.

Clausen, V. A. 1966. Family Structure: Socialization and Personality. In *Review of Child Development Research Vol. II,* ed. M. L. Hoffmann and L. W. Hoffman. 1–55. New York: Russell Sage Foundation.

Clausen, J. A. 1968. Values, Norms, and the Health Called "Mental": Purposes and Feasibility of Assessment. In *The Definition and Measurement of Mental Health,* S. B. Sells. ed. 115–134. Washington, D.C.: U.S. Department of Health, Education, and Welfare, National Center for Health Statistics.

Clausen, J. A., and C. L. Huffine. 1979. The Impact of Parental Mental Illness on Children. *Research in Community and Mental Health* 5:183–214.

Cloninger, C. R., T. Reich, and R. Wetzel. 1979. Alcoholism and the Affective Disorders: Familial Association and Genetic Models. In *Alcoholism and the Affective Disorders,* ed. D. Goodwin and C. Erickson. 57–86. New York: Spectrum Press.

Coddington, R. D. 1972. The Significance of Life Events as Etiologic Factors in the Diseases of Children: A Study of the Normal Population. *Journal of Psychosomatic Research* 6:205–211.

Coddington, R. D. 1979. Life Events Associated with Adolescent Pregnancies. *Journal of Clinical Psychiatry* 40:180–185.

Cohen, J., and P. Cohen. 1983. *Applied Multiple Regression/Correlation Analysis for the Behavioral Sciences.* 2nd ed. Hillsdale, N.J.: Lawrence Erlbaum Associates.

Collins, A. H., and D. Pancoast. 1976. *Natural Helping Networks.* Washington, D.C.: National Association of Social Workers.

Cooley, E. V., and J. C. Keesey. 1981. Moderator Variables in Life Stress and Illness Relationships. *Journal of Human Stress* 7:35–40.

Cooper, B., and J. Sylph. 1973. Life Events and the Onset of Neurotic Illness: An Investigation in General Practice. *Psychological Medicine* 3:421–435.

Coopersmith, S. 1975. *Coopersmith Self-Esteem Inventory.* Palo Alto, Calif.: Consulting Psychologists.

Cork, R. M. 1969. *Alcoholism and the Family.* Toronto: Addiction Research Foundation.

Coser, L. 1954. *The Functions of Social Conflict.* New York: Free Press.

Cotton, N. S. 1979. The Familial Incidence of Alcoholism. *Journal of Studies on Alcohol* 40:89–116.

Cowie, V. 1961a. Children of Psychotics: A Controlled Study. *Proceedings of the Royal Society of Medicine* 54:675–678.

Cowie, V. 1961b. The Incidence of Neurosis in the Children of Psychotics. *Acta Psychiatrica Scandinavica* 37:37–87.

Coyne, J. L. 1976. Depression and the Response of Others. *Journal of Abnormal Psychology* 85:186–193.

Craig, M. M., and S. J. Glick. 1968. School Behavior Related to Later Delinquency and Nondelinquency. *Criminologica* 5:17–27.

Cummings, E. M., C. Zahn-Waxler, and M. Radke-Yarrow. 1981. Young Children's Responses to Expressions of Anger and Affection by Others in the Family. *Child Development* 52:1274–1282.

DeAlmeida-Filho, N. 1984. Family Variables and Child Mental Disorders in a Third World Urban Area. *Social Psychiatry* 19:23–30.

Doane, J. A., K. L. West, M. J. Goldstein, E. A. Rodnick, and J. E. Jones. 1981. Parental Communication Deviance and Affective Style: Predictors of Subsequent Schizophrenia Spectrum Disorders in Vulnerable Adolescents. *Archives of General Psychiatry* 38:679–685.

Dohrenwend, B. S., L. Krasnoff, A. R. Askenazy, and B. P. Dohrenwend. 1978. Exemplification of a Method for Scaling Life Events: The PERI Life Events Scale. *Journal of Health and Social Behavior* 19:205–229.

Dreikurs, R., and V. Soltz. 1964. *Children: The Challenge.* New York: Duell, Sloan, and Pearce.

Duncan, D. F. 1977. Life Stress as a Precursor to Adolescent Drug Dependence. *International Journal of Addictions* 12:1047–1056.

Elder, G. H., Jr. 1974. *Children of the Great Depression.* Chicago: University of Chicago Press.

El-Guebaly, N., and D. R. Offord. 1977. The Offspring of Alcoholics: A Critical Review. *American Journal of Psychiatry* 134:357–365.

El-Guebaly, N., D. R. Offord, K. T. Sullivan, and G. W. Lynch. 1978. Psychosocial Adjustment of the Offspring of Psychiatric Patients. *Canadian Psychiatric Association Journal* 23:281–289.

Emory, R., S. Weintraub, and J. M. Neale. 1982. Effects of Marital Discord on the School Behavior of Children of Schizophrenic, Affectively Disordered, and Normal Parents. *Journal of Abnormal Child Psychology* 10:215–228.

Erickson, R. C. 1982. Reconsidering Three Dichotomies. *Journal of Religion and Health* 21:115–123.

Erlenmeyer-Kimling, L. 1977. Issues Pertaining to Prevention and Intervention of Genetic Disorders Affecting Human Behavior. In *The Issues: An Overview of Primary Prevention,* ed. G. W. Albee and J. M. Joffe. 68–69. Hanover, N.H.: University Press of New England.

Feldman, R. A. 1978. Delinquent Behavior in the Public Schools: Toward More Accurate Labeling and Effective Intervention. In *School Crime and Disruption,* ed. E. Wenk and N. Harlow. 79–88. Davis, Calif.: Responsible Action.

Ferguson, W. E. 1981. Gifted Adolescents, Stress, and Life Change. *Adolescence* 16:973–985.

Finlay-Jones, R., R. Scott, P. Duncan-Jones, D. Byrne, and S. Henderson. 1981. The Reliability of Reports of Early Separations. *Australian and New Zealand Journal of Psychiatry* 15:27–31.

Fischer, J. C. 1980. Reciprocity, Agreement, and Family Style in Family Systems with a Disturbed and Nondisturbed Adolescent. *Journal of Youth and Adolescence* 9:391–406.

Fish, B., and R. Hagin. 1973. Visual-Motor Disorders in Infants at High-Risk for Schizophrenia. *Archives of General Psychiatry* 28:900–904.

Fisher, L., R. F. Kokes, D. W. Harder, and J. E. Jones. 1980. Child Competence and

Psychiatric Risk. VI.: Summary and Integration of Findings. *Journal of Nervous and Mental Disease* 168:353–355.

Fishman, M. E. 1982. *Ninth Annual Report on the Child And Youth Activities of the National Institute of Mental Health.* Rockville, Md.: Alcohol, Drug Abuse, and Mental Health Administration.

Fowler, R. C., M. T. Tsuang, and R. J. Cadore. 1977. Parental Psychiatric Illness Associated With Schizophrenia in the Siblings of Schizophrenics. *Comprehensive Psychiatry* 18:271–275.

Frances, R., S. Timms, and S. Bucky. 1980. Studies in Familial and Non-Familial Alcoholism: I. Demographic Studies. *Archives of General Psychiatry* 37:564–566.

Freed, D. V., and H. H. Foster. 1969. Divorce American Style. *Annals of the American Academy of Political and Social Science* 383:71–88.

Freeman, H. E., and O. G. Simmons. 1958. Wives, Mothers and the Posthospital Performance of Mental Patients. *Social Forces* 37:153–159.

Friday, P. C., and J. Hage. 1976. Youth Crime in Postindustrial Societies: An Integrated Perspective. *Criminology* 14:347–368.

Friedrich, W. N., R. Ream, and J. Jacobs. 1982. Depression and Suicidal Ideation in Early Adolescence. *Journal of Youth and Adolescence* 11:403–407.

Gamer, E., D. Gallant, H. U. Grunebaum, and B. J. Cohler. 1977. Children of Psychotic Mothers: Performance of Three-Year-Old Children on Tests of Attention. *Archives of General Psychiatry* 34: 592–597.

Gammon, G. D. 1983. Blue Parent, Disturbed Child: Correlation Shown. *Journal of the American Medical Association* 249:11–12.

Garbarino, J. 1977. The Human Ecology of Child Maltreatment. *Child Development* 51:188–198.

Gardner, G. 1967a. The Relationship between Childhood Neurotic Symptomatology and Later Schizophrenia in Males and Females. *Journal of Nervous and Mental Disease* 144:97–100.

Gardner, G. 1967b. Role of Maternal Psychopathology in Male and Female Schizophrenics. *Journal of Consulting Psychology* 31:411–413.

Garmezy, N. 1971. Vulnerability Research and the Issue of Primary Prevention. *American Journal of Orthopsychiatry* 41:101–116.

Garmezy, N. 1974a. The Study of Competence in Children at Risk for Severe Psychopathology. In *The Child in His Family: Children at Psychiatric Risk,* ed. E. J. Anthony and C. Koupernik. 77–97. New York: Wiley Interscience.

Garmezy, N. 1974b. Children at Risk: The Search for the Antecedents of Schizophrenia. Part II: Ongoing Research Programs, Issues, and Intervention. *Schizophrenia Bulletin* 9:65–125.

Garmezy, N. 1981. Children Under Stress: Perspectives on Antecedents and Correlates of Vulnerability and Resistance to Psychopathology. In *Further Explorations in Personality,* ed. A. I. Rabin, J. Aronoff, A. M. Barcai, and R. A. Zucker. 196–269. New York: John Wiley and Sons.

Garmezy, N., A. S. Masten, and A. Tellegen. 1984. The Study of Stress and Competence in Children: A Building Block for Developmental Psychopathology. *Child Development* 55:97–111.

Garmezy, N., and K. H. Nuechterlein. 1972. Invulnerable Children: The Fact and Fiction of Competence and Disadvantage. *American Journal of Orthopsychiatry* 77:328–329.

Gatchill, R. J., M. E. McKinney, and L. F. Koebernick. 1977. Learned Helplessness, Depression, and Psychological Respondence. *Psychophysiology* 14:25–31.

Gershon, E. S., J. Hamovit, J. J. Guroff, E. Dibble, J. F. Leckman, W. Sceery, S. D. Targum, J. I. Nurnberger, Jr., L. R. Goldin, and W. E. Bunney. 1982. A Family Study of Schizoaffective Bipolar I, Bipolar II, Unipolar, and Normal Control Probands. *Archives of General Psychiatry* 39:1157–1167.

Gersten, S. C., T. S. Langner, J. G. Eisenberg, and K. L. Orze. 1974. Child Behavior and Life Events: Undesirable Change or Change Per Se? In *Stressful Life Events: Their Nature and Effects,* ed. B. S. Dohrenwend and B. P. Dohrenwend. 159–170. New York: John Wiley and Sons.

Gibbs, J. T. 1982. Psychosocial Factors Related to Substance Abuse among Delinquent Females: Implications for Prevention and Treatment. *American Journal of Orthopsychiatry* 52:261–270.

Glick, P. C. 1979. The Future of the American Family. *Current Population Reports: Special Studies.* Washington, D.C.: U.S. Census Bureau, Series P-23, 78.

Goldberg, E. L., and G. W. Comstock. 1976. Life Events and Subsequent Illness. *American Journal of Epidemiology* 104:146–158.

Goldston, S. E. 1977. Defining Primary Prevention. In *Primary Prevention of Psychopathology, Vol. 1: The Issues,* ed. G. W. Albee and J. M. Joffe. 18–23. Hanover, N.H.: University Press of New England.

Goodwin, D. W., F. Schulsinger, L. Hermansen, S. B. Guze, and G. Winokur. 1973. Alcohol Problems in Adoptees Raised Apart from Alcoholic Biological Parents. *Archives of General Psychiatry* 28:238–243.

Goodwin, D. W., F. Schulsinger, J. Knop, S. Mednick, and S. B. Guze. 1977a. Alcoholism and Depression in Adopted-out Daughters of Alcoholics. *Archives of General Psychiatry* 34:751–755.

Goodwin, D. W., F. Schulsinger, J. Knop, S. Mednick, and S. Guze. 1977b. Psychopathology in Adopted and Nonadopted Daughters of Alcoholics. *Archives of General Psychiatry* 34:1005–1009.

Goodwin, D. W., F. Schulsinger, N. Moller, L. Hermansen, G. Winokur, and S. B. Guze. 1974. *Archives of General Psychiatry* 31:164–169.

Gottlieb, B. 1975. The Contribution of Natural Support Systems to Primary Prevention among Four Social Subgroups of Adolescents. *Adolescence* 10:207–220.

Gottlieb, B. 1980. The Role of Individual and Social Support in Preventing Child Maltreatment. In *Protecting Children from Abuse and Neglect,* ed. J. Garbarino, S. H. Stocking, and Associates. 37–60. San Francisco: Jossey-Bass.

Haberman, P. W. 1966. Childhood Symptoms in Children of Alcoholics and Comparison Group Parents. *Journal of Marriage and The Family* 28:152–154.

Haggerty, R. J. 1980. Life Stress, Illness, and Social Supports. *Developmental Medicine and Child Neurology* 22:391–400.

Hammer, M. 1963–1964. Influence of Small Social Networks as Factors in Mental Hospital Admission. *Human Organization* 22:243–250.

Hanson, D. R. 1974. *Children of Schizophrenic Mothers and Fathers Compared to Children of Other Psychiatric Controls: Their First Eight Years.* Ph. D. diss., University of Minnesota, Minneapolis.

Heisel, J. A., S. Ream, R. Raitz, M. Rappaport, and R. D. Coddington. 1974. The

Significance of Life Events as Contributing Factors in the Diseases of Children II: A Study of Pediatric Patients. *Journal of Pediatrics* 83:119–121.

Herjanic, B., M. Herjanic, E. Penick, C. Tomellein, and R. Armbruster. 1977. Children of Alcoholics. In *Currents in Alcoholism, Vol. II,* ed. F. Seixas. 445–455. New York: Grune and Stratton.

Heston, L. L. 1966. Psychiatric Disorders in Foster Home Reared Children of Schizophrenic Mothers. *British Journal of Psychiatry* 112:819–825.

Higgins, J. 1976. Effects of Child Rearing By Schizophrenic Mothers: A Follow-Up. *Journal of Psychiatric Research* 13:1–9.

Hirsch, B. J. 1982. Coping And Adaptation in High-Risk Populations: Toward an Integration Model. *Schizophrenia Bulletin* 8:164–172.

Hollingshead, A. B. 1974. *Four Factor Index of Social Status: Working Paper.* New Haven, Conn.: Yale University.

Holmes, T. H., and M. Masuda. 1974. Life Change and Illness Susceptibility. In *Stressful Life Events,* ed. B. S. Dohrenwend and B. P. Dohrenwend. 45–85. New York: John Wiley.

Holmes, T. H. , and R. H. Rahe. 1967. The Social Readjustment Rating Scale. *Journal of Psychosomatic Research* 11:213–218.

Houston, K., L. Bloom, T. Burnish, and E. Cummings. 1978. Positive Evaluation of Stressful Experience. *Journal of Personality* 46:205–214.

Hudgens, R. W., E. Robins, and W. B. Delong. 1970. The Reporting of Recent Stress in the Lives of Psychiatric Patients. *British Journal of Psychiatry* 117:635–643.

Hudson, W. W. 1982. *The Clinical Measurement Package: A Field Manual.* Homewood, Ill.: Dorsey.

Humphries, I., M. Kinsbourne, and J. Swansen. 1978. Stimulant Effects on Cooperative and Social Interaction Between Hyperactive Children and Their Mothers. *Journal of Child Psychology and Psychiatry* 19:13–22.

Husaini, B. A., and J. A. Neff. 1978. Characteristics of Life Events and Psychiatric Impairment in Rural Communities. *Journal of Nervous and Mental Disorders* 87:49–74.

Ilfeld, F. W., Jr. 1977. Current Social Stressors and Symptoms of Depression. *American Journal of Psychiatry* 134:161–166.

Imboden, J. B., A. Canter, and L. E. Cluff. 1963. Separation Experiences and Health Records in a Group of Normal Adults. *Psychosomatic Medicine* 25:433–440.

Inbar, M. 1976. The Vulnerable Age Phenomenon. *Social Science Frontiers, No. 8.* New York: Russell Sage Foundation.

Jacob, T., A. Favorini, S. S. Meisel, and C. M. Anderson. 1978. The Alcoholic's Spouse, Children, and Family Interactions. *Journal of Studies on Alcohol* 39:1231–1251.

Jacobs, J., and E. Charles. 1980. Life Events and the Occurence of Cancer in Children. *Psychosomatic Medicine* 42:11–23.

Jacobs, M. A., Z. Spilken, and M. M. Norman. 1971. Patterns of Maladaptation and Respiratory Illness. *Journal of Psychosomatic Research* 15:63–72.

Jacobs, S., and J. Myers. 1976. Recent Life Events and Acute Schizophrenic Psychosis: A Controlled Study. *Journal of Nervous and Mental Diseases* 162:75–87.

Jastak, J. F., and S. Jastak. 1978. *WRAT Manual: Wide Range Achievement Test.* Wilmington, Del.: Jastak Associates.

Jenkins, C. D. 1979. Psychosocial Modifiers of Response to Stress. *Journal of Human Stress* 5:13–15.

Johnson, J. H., I. G. Sarason, and J. M. Siegel. 1979. Arousal-Seeking as a Moderator of Life Stress. *Perceptual Motor Skills* 49:667–676.

Jonsson, G. 1967. Delinquent Boys, Their Parents, And Grandparents. *Acta Psychiatrica Scandinavica* 195:Supplement.

Kalverboer, A. F., and W. H. Brouwer. 1983. Visuo-Motor Behavior in Pre-School Children in Relation to Sex and Neurological Status: An Experimental Study on the Effect of "Time-Pressure." *Journal of Child Psychology and Psychiatry and Allied Disciplines* 24:65–88.

Kammeier, M. L. 1971. Adolescents from Families With and Without Alcohol Problems. *Quarterly Journal of Studies of Alcoholism* 32:361–372.

Kandel, D., ed. 1978. *Longitudinal Research in Drug Use: Empirical Findings and Methodological Issues.* Washington, D.C.: Hemisphere.

Kaplan, H. B. 1980. *Deviant Behavior in Defense of Self.* New York: Academic Press.

Kaplan, H. B., and A. D. Pokorny. 1976. Self Attitudes and Suicidal Behavior. *Suicide and Life Threatening Behavior* 6:23–35.

Kaplan, S. L., B. Lander, C. Weinhold, and I. R. Shenker. 1984. Adverse Health Behaviors and Depressive Symptomatology in Adolescents. *Journal of the American Academy of Child Psychiatry* 23:595–601.

Karlsson, J. L. 1968. "Genealogic Studies of Schizophrenia." In *The Transmission of Schizophrenia,* ed. D. Rosenthal and S. S. Kety. 85–94. Oxford: Pergamon Press, Ltd.

Kauffman, C., H. Grunebaum, B. Cohler, and E. Gamer. 1979. Superkids: Competent Children of Psychotic Mothers. *American Journal of Psychiatry* 136:1398–1402.

Kendall, P., R. M. Lerner, and W. E. Craighead. 1984. Human Development and Intervention in Childhood Psychopathology. *Child Development* 55:71–82.

Kety, S. S., D. Rosenthal, P. H. Wender, F. Schulsinger, and B. Jacobsen. 1975. Mental Illness in the Biological and Adoptive Families of Adopted Individuals Who Have Become Schizophrenic: A Preliminary Report. In *Genetic Research in Psychiatry,* ed. R. Fieve, D. Rosenthal, and H. Brill. 147–165. Baltimore: Johns Hopkins University Press.

Klein, M., and S. Shulman. 1980. Behavior Problems of Children in Relation to Parental Instrumentality-Expressivity and Marital Adjustment. *Psychological Reports* 47:11–14.

Kobasa, R. P. 1979. Stressful Life Events, Personality and Health: An Inquiry Into Hardiness. *Journal of Personality and Social Psychology* 37:1–11.

Kohn, M. L. 1969. *Class and Conformity: A Study in Values.* Homewood, Ill.: Dorsey Press.

Kohn, M. L. 1973. Social Class and Schizophrenia: A Critical Review and a Reformulation. *Schizophrenia Bulletin* 7:60–79.

Kokes, R. F., D. W. Harder, L. Fisher, and J. S. Strauss. 1980. Child Competence and Psychiatric Risk. V: Sex of Patient Parent and Dimensions of Psychopathology. *Journal of Nervous and Mental Disease* 168:348–352.

Kreitman, N. 1968. Married Couples Admitted to a Mental Hospital. *British Journal of Psychiatry* 114:699–718.

Lander, H. S., E. J. Anthony, L. Cass, L. Franklin, and L. Bass. 1978. A Measure of

Vulnerability to the Risk of Parental Psychosis. In *The Child in His Family, Vol 4: Vulnerable Children*, ed. E. J. Anthony and C. Koupernik. 325–333. New York: Wiley Interscience.

Langner, T. S., J. C. Gersten, and J. G. Eisenberg. 1977. The Epidemiology of Mental Disorder in Children: Implications for Community Psychiatry. In *New Trends of Psychiatry in the Community*, ed. G. Serban. 69–110. Cambridge, Mass.: Ballinger.

Lee, E. E. 1983. Survey of Knowledge, Attitudes, and Practices of Fifth and Eighth Grade Students Regarding Alcoholic Beverages in Urban Parochial Schools. *Journal of Alcohol and Drug Education* 28:73–84.

Lei, H., and H. H. Skinner. 1980. A Psychosomatic Study of Life Events and Social Readjustment. *Journal of Psychosomatic Research* 24:57–66.

Lewis, J. M., W. B. Beavers, J. T. Gossett, and V. A. Phillips. 1976. *No Single Thread: Psychological Health in Family Systems*. New York: Brunner/Mazel.

Lidz, T. 1970. The Family as the Developmental Setting. In *The Child in His Family: International Yearbook for Child Psychiatry and Allied Disciplines. Vol I*. ed. E. J. Anthony and C. Koupernik. 19–40. New York: Wiley Interscience.

Lin, N., A. Dean, and W. M. Ensel. 1981. Social Support Scales: A Methodological Note. *Schizophrenia Bulletin* 7:73–89.

Linden, E., and J. C. Hackler. 1973. Affective Ties and Delinquency. *Pacific Sociological Review* 16:26–46.

Lord, D. B. 1983. Parental Alcoholism and the Mental Health of Children: A Bibliography and Brief Observations. *Journal of Alcohol and Drug Education* 29:1–11.

MacCrimmon, D. J., J. M. Cleghorn, R. F. Asarnow, and R. A. Steffy. 1980. Children at Risk for Schizophrenia: Clinical and Attentional Characteristics. *Archives of General Psychiatry* 37:671–674.

Marcus, J. 1974. Cerebral Function in Offspring of Schizophrenics: Possible Genetic Factors. *International Journal of Mental Health* 3:57–73.

Maroribanks, K. 1981. Sibling and Environmental Correlates of Children's Achievement: Sex Group Differences. *Social Biology* 28:96–101.

Markush, R. E., and R. V. Favero. 1974. Epidemiologic Assessment of Stressful Life Events, Depressed Mood, and Psychophysiological Symptoms: A Preliminary Report. In *Stressful Life Events: Their Nature and Effects*, ed. B. S. Dohrenwend and B. P. Dohrenwend. 171–190. New York: John Wiley.

Marsella, A. J., and L. L. Snyder, 1981. Stress, Social Supports and Schizophrenic Disorders: Toward an Interactional Model. *Schizophrenia Bulletin* 7:152–163.

McCord, J., and W. McCord. 1957. The Effects of Parental Role Model on Criminality. *Journal of Social Issues* 13:66–75.

McFarlane, A. H., K. A. Neale, G. R. Norman, R. G. Roy, and D. L. Streiner. 1981. Methodological Issues in Developing a Scale to Measure Social Support. *Schizophrenia Bulletin* 7:90–100.

McLachlan, J. F. C., R. L. Walderman, and S. Thomas. 1973. *A Study of Teenagers with Alcoholic Parents*. Monograph No. 3. Toronto: Donwood Institute Research.

Mechanic, D. 1976. Stress, Illness, and Illness Behavior. *Journal of Human Stress* 2: 2–6.

Mednick, S. 1970. Breakdowns in Individuals at High Risk for Schizophrenia: Possible Predispositional Perinatal Factors. *Mental Hygiene* 54:50–63.

Mednick, S., and F. Schulsinger. 1968. Some Premorbid Characteristics Related to

Breakdown in Children with Schizophrenic Mothers. In *The Transmission of Schizophrenia,* ed. D. Rosenthal and S. Kety. 267–291. Oxford: Pergamon Press.

Mednick, S. A., F. Schulsinger, and R. Cudeck. 1980. Copenhagen High-Risk Project. Paper presented at the Risk Research Consortium Plenary Conference, San Juan.

Mik, G. 1970. Sons of Alcoholic Fathers. *British Journal of the Addictions* 65:305–315.

Miller, A., and E. Cooley. 1981. Moderator Variables for the Relationship between Life Change and Disorder. *Journal of General Psychology* 104:223–233.

Miller, D., G. Challas, and S. Gee. 1972. Children of Deviants: A Fifteen-Year Follow-Up Study of Schizophrenic Mothers, Welfare Mothers, Matched Controls, and Random Urban Families. San Francisco: Scientific Analysis Corporation. Mimeo.

Miller, D., and M. Jang. 1977. Children of Alcoholics: A 20 Year Longitudinal Study. *Social Work Research and Abstracts* 13:23–29.

Miller, L. C. , E. Hampe, C. Barrett, and H. Noble. 1971. Children's Deviant Behavior within the General Population. *Journal of Consulting and Clinical Psychology* 37:16–22.

Miller, R. P. 1966. *Simultaneous Statistical Inferences.* New York: McGraw-Hill.

Milliken, G., and D. Johnson. 1984. *Analysis of Messy Data. Vol. I.* Belmont, Calif.: Wadsworth.

Mills, M., C. Puckering, A. Pound, and A. Cox. 1985. What Is It about Depressed Mothers That Influences Their Children's Functioning? In *Recent Research in Developmental Psychopathology. Journal of Child Psychology and Psychiatry Book Supplement No. 4,* ed. J. Stevenson. 11–17. Oxford: Pergamon Press.

Mitchell, J. C. 1969. The Concept and Use of Social Networks. In *Social Networks in Urban Situations,* ed. J. C. Mitchell. 1–50. Manchester, England: Manchester University Press.

Molholm, L. H., and S. Denitz. 1972. Female Mental Patients and Their Normal Controls. *Archives of General Psychiatry* 26:606–610.

Morehouse, E. 1979. Working in the Schools with Children of Alcoholic Parents. *Health and Social Work* 4:144–162.

Morris, A. M., J. M. Williams, A. E. Atwater, and J. H. Wilmore. 1982. Age and Sex Differences in Motor Performance of 3 Through 6 Year Old Children. *Research Quarterly for Exercise and Sport* 53:214–221.

Moskalenko, V. D. 1972. A Comparative Study of Families with One or Both Schizophrenic Parents. *Zhurnal Neuropatologii i Psikhiatrii* 72:86–92.

Murphy, L., and A. Moriarty. 1976. *Vulnerability, Coping and Growth from Infancy to Adolescence.* New Haven, Conn.: Yale University Press.

Myers, J. K., J. J. Lindenthal, M. P. Pepper, and D. R. Ostrander. 1972. Life Events and Mental Status: A Longitudinal Study. *Journal of Health and Social Behavior* 13:398–406.

Nardi, P. M. 1981. Children of Alcoholics: A Role-Theoretical Perspective. *Journal of Social Psychology* 115:237–245.

Newcomb, M. D., G. J. Huba, and P. Bentler. 1983. Mothers' Influence on the Drug Use of Their Children: Confirmatory Tests of Direct Modeling and Mediational Theories. *Developmental Psychology* 19:714–726.

Nuechterlein, K. H. 1983. Signal Detection in Vigilance Tasks and Behavioral Attributes among Offspring of Schizophrenic Mothers and among Hyperactive Children. *Journal of Abnormal Psychology* 92:4–28.

O'Gorman, P. A. 1975. Self-Concept, Locus of Control, and Perception of Father in Adolescents from Homes with and without Severe Drinking Problems. Ph.D. diss., Fordham University, New York.

Orvaschel, H. S., S. Mednick, F. Schulsinger, and D. Rock. 1979. The Children of Psychiatrically Disturbed Parents: Differences as a Function of the Sex of the Sick Parent. *Archives of General Psychiatry* 36:691–695.

Pancoast, D. L. 1980. Finding and Enlisting Neighbors to Support Families. In *Protecting Children from Abuse and Neglect: Developing and Maintaining Effective Support Systems for Families,* ed. J. Garbarino, S. H. Stocking, and Associates. 109–132. San Francisco: Jossey-Bass.

Parsons, T. 1965. The Normal American Family. In *Man and Civilization: The Family's Search for Survival,* ed. S. Farber, P. Mustacchi, and R. H. Wilson. 31–50. New York: McGraw-Hill.

Patterson, G. R. 1982. *A Social Learning Approach. Vol. 3: Coercive Family Processes.* Eugene, Ore.: Castalia Publishing Co.

Paykel, E. S. 1978. Contribution of Life Events to Causation of Psychiatric Illness. *Psychological Medicine* 8:245–254.

Paykel, E. S., J. K. Myers, M. N. Dienelt, G. L. Klerman, J. J. Lindenthal, and M. P. Pepper. 1969. Life Events and Depression: A Controlled Study. *Archives of General Psychiatry* 21:753–760.

Pearlin, L., and J. Johnson. 1977. Marital Status, Life Strains, and Depression. *American Sociological Review* 42: 704–715.

Pearlin, L. S., and C. Schooler. 1978. The Structure of Coping. *Journal of Health and Social Behavior* 19:2–21.

Pedhazur, E. J. 1982. *Multiple Regression in Behavioral Research: Explanation and Prediction.* 2nd ed. New York: Holt, Rinehart, and Winston.

Phillips, S. L. 1981. Network Characteristics Related to the Well-Being of Normals: A Comparative Base. *Schizophrenia Bulletin* 7:117–124.

Pines, M. 1979. Superkids. *Psychology Today,* Jan.: 53–63.

Polansky, N. A., M. A. Chalmos, E. Buttenweiser, and D. P. Williams. 1981. *Damaged Parents: An Anatomy of Child Neglect.* Chicago: University of Chicago Press.

Potvin, R. H., and C. F. Lee. 1980. Multistage Path Models of Adolescent Alcohol and Drug Use: Age Variations. *Journal of Studies on Alcohol* 41:531–542.

Pound, A., A. Cox, C. Puckering, and M. Mills. 1985. The Impact of Maternal Depression on Young Children. In *Recent Research in Developmental Psychopathology. Journal of Child Psychology and Psychiatry Monograph Supplement No. 4,* ed. J. Stevenson. 3–10. Oxford: Pergamon Press, Ltd.

President's Commission on Mental Health. 1978. *Task Panel Reports Submitted to the President's Commission on Mental Health.* Washington, D.C.: U.S. Government Printing Office.

Prinz, R. J., S. Weintraub, and J. M. Neale. 1975. Peer Evaluations of Children Vulnerable to Psychopathology. In *Children at Environmental and Genetic Risk: New Data Amid Speculation,* chaired by J. E. Rolf and J. E. Hasaji. Symposium presented at the meeting of the American Psychological Association, Chicago.

Quinton, D., M. Rutter, and O. Rowlands. 1976. An Evaluation of an Interview Assessment of Marriage. *Psychological Medicine* 6:577–586.

Rahe, R. H. 1981. Life Change Events and Mental Illness: An Overview. *Journal of Human Stress* 7:2–10.

Rahe, R. H., and R. J. Arthur. 1978. Life Change and Illness Studies: Past History and Future Directions. *Journal of Human Stress* 4:3–15.

Rice, E. P., M. C. Ekdale, and L. Miller. 1971. *Children of Mentally Ill Patients: Problems in Child Care.* New York: Behavioral Publications.

Robins, L. N. 1975. Arrest and Delinquency in Two Generations. In *Annual Progress in Child Psychiatry and Child Development,* ed. S. Chess and A. Thomas. 125–140. New York: Brunner/Mazel.

Robins, L. N., W. M. Bates, and P. O'Neal. 1962. Adult Drinking Problems of Former Problem Children. In *Society, Culture, and Drinking Patterns,* ed. D. J. Pittman and C. R. Snyder. 395–412. New York: John Wiley and Sons.

Robins, L. N., J. E. Helzer, M. M. Weissman, H. Orvaschel, E. Gruenberg, J. D. Burke, Jr., and D. A. Regier. 1984. Lifetime Prevalence of Specific Psychiatric disorders in Three Sites. *Archives of General Psychiatry* 41:949–958.

Robins, L. N., and R. G. Lewis. 1966. The Role of the Antisocial Family in School Completion and Delinquency: A Three-Generation Study. *Sociological Quarterly* 7:500–514.

Robins, L. N., S. P. Schoenberg, S. J. Holmes, K. S. Ratcliff, A. Benham, and J. Works. 1985. Early Home Environment and Retrospective Recall: A Test for Concordance between Siblings with and without Psychiatric Disorders. *American Journal of Orthopsychiatry* 55:27–41.

Robins, L. N., P. A. West, and B. L. Herjanic. 1975. Arrests and Delinquency in Two Generations: A Study of Black Urban Families and Their Children. *Journal of Child Psychology and Psychiatry* 16:125–140.

Rolf, J. 1972. The Social and Academic Competence of Children Vulnerable to Schizophrenia and Other Behavior Pathologies. *Journal of Abnormal Psychology* 80:225–243.

Rolf, J. E., and N. Garmezy. 1974. The School Performance of Children Vulnerable to Behavior Pathology. In *Life History Research in Psychopathology. Vol. 3,* ed. D. F. Ricks, A. Thomas, and M. Roff, 87–107. Minneapolis: University of Minnesota Press.

Rolf, J., and P. B. Read. 1984. Programs Advancing Developmental Psychopathology. *Child Development* 55:8–16.

Rosenman, R. H., C. Brant, and E. Jenkins. 1976. Multivariate Predictors of Coronary Heart Disease. *American Journal of Cardiology* 37:903–910.

Rotter, J. B. 1975. Some Problems and Misconceptions Related to the Construct of Internal Vs. External Control of Reinforcement. *Journal of Consulting and Clinical Psychology* 43:56–67.

Rouse, B. A., P. F. Waller, and J. A. Ewing. 1973. Adolescents' Stress Levels, Coping Activities, and Father's Drinking Behavior. *Proceedings of the American Psychological Association* 81:681–682.

Russell, M., C. Henderson, and S. B. Blume. 1985. *Children of Alcoholics: A Review of the Literature.* New York: Children of Alcoholics Foundation, Inc.

Rutter, M. 1966. *Children of Sick Parents: An Environmental and Psychiatric Study.* Monograph No. 16. London: Maudsley.

Rutter, M. 1970. Sex Differences in Children's Responses to Family Stress. In *The Child in His Family,* eds. E. J. Anthony and C. Koupernik. 165–196. New York: Wiley Interscience.

Rutter, M. 1974. Epidemiological Strategies and Psychiatric Concepts in Research on the Vulnerable Child. In *The Child In His Family: Children at Psychiatric Risk. Vol. 3,* ed. E. J. Anthony and C. Koupernik. 167–179. New York: Wiley Interscience.

Rutter, M. 1977. Other Family Approaches. In *Child Psychiatry: Modern Approaches,* ed. M. Rutter and L. Hersov. 74–108. London: Blackwell Scientific Publications.

Rutter, M. 1980. *Changing Youth in a Changing Society.* Cambridge, Mass.: Harvard University Press.

Rutter, M. 1981. The City and the Child. *American Journal of Orthopsychiatry* 51:610–625.

Rutter, M., and G. Brown. 1966. The Reliability and Validity of Measures of Family Life and Relationships in Families Containing a Psychiatric Patient. *Social Psychiatry* 1:38–53.

Rutter, M., and N. Madge. 1976. *Cycles of Disadvantage: A Review of Research.* London: Heinemann.

Rutter, M., and D. Quinton. 1984. Parental Psychiatric Disorder: Effects on Children. *Psychological Medicine* 14:853–880.

Rutter, M., D. Quinton, and W. Yule. 1977. *Family Pathology and Disorder in Children.* London: John Wiley.

Rutter, M., B. Yule, D. Quinton, O. Rowlands, W. Yule, and M. Berger. 1975. Attainment and Adjustment in Two Geographical Areas. III: Some Factors Accounting for Area Differences. *British Journal of Psychiatry* 126:520–533.

Sameroff, A. J., and R. Seifer. 1981. The Transmission of Incompetence: The Offspring of Mentally Ill Women. In *The Uncommon Child,* ed. M. Lewis and L. A. Rosenblum. 259–280. New York: Plenum Press.

Sameroff, A. J., R. Seifer, and M. Zax. 1982. Early Development of Children at Risk for Emotional Disorder. *Monographs of the Society for Research in Child Development* 47: Serial No. 199.

Sandler, I. N., and M. Block. 1979. Life Stress and Maladaptation of Children. *American Journal of Community Psychology* 7:425–440.

Sandler, I. N., and T. B. Ramsey. 1980. Dimensional Analysis of Children's Stressful Life Events. *American Journal of Community Psychology* 8:285–302.

Satir, V. 1972. *Peoplemaking.* Palo Alto, Calif.: Science and Behavior Books.

Scanzoni, J. H. 1977. *The Black Family in Modern Society: Patterns of Stability and Security.* Chicago: University of Chicago Press.

Schuckit, M. A. 1982. The Importance of Family History of Affective Disorder in a Group of Young Men. *Journal of Nervous and Mental Disease* 170:530–535.

Schuckit, M. A., and J. A. Chiles. 1978. Family History as a Diagnostic Aid in Two Samples of Adolescents. *Journal of Nervous and Mental Disease* 166:165–176.

Schuckit, M. A., D. Goodwin, and G. Winokur. 1972. A Study of Alcoholism in Half-Siblings. *American Journal of Psychiatry* 128:122–125.

Schulsinger, H. 1976. A Ten-Year Follow-Up of Children of Schizophrenic Mothers: Clinical Assessment. *Acta Psychiatrica Scandinavica* 53:371–386.

Segal, J., and H. Yahraes. 1978. *A Child's Journey: Forces That Shape the Lives of Our Young.* New York: McGraw-Hill.

Skolnick, A. S., and J. H. Skolnick, comp. 1977. *Family in Transition: Rethinking Marriage, Sexuality, Child Rearing, and Family Organization.* 2nd ed. Boston: Little, Brown, & Co.

Sobel, D. E. 1961. Children of Schizophrenic Parents: Preliminary Observations of Early Development. *American Journal of Psychiatry* 118:512.

Sokolovsky, J., and C. I. Cohen. 1981. Toward a Resolution of Methodological Dilemmas in Network Mapping. *Schizophrenia Bulletin* 7:109–116.

Solomon, J., and M. Hanson. 1982. Alcoholism and Sociopathy. In *Alcoholism and Clinical Psychiatry,* ed. J. Solomon. 111–127. New York: Plenum Medical Book Co.

Spivack, G., and M. B. Shure. 1977. Preventively Oriented Cognitive Education of Preschoolers. In *Primary Prevention: An Idea Whose Time Has Come,* ed. D. C. Klein and S. E. Goldston. 79–82. Washington, D.C.: U.S. Government Printing Office.

Spring, B., and J. Zubin. 1977. Vulnerability to Schizophrenic Episodes and Their Prevention in Adults. In *The Issues: An Overview of Primary Prevention,* ed. G. W. Albee and J. M. Joffe. 254–284. Hanover, NH: University Press of New England.

Sroufe, L. A., and M. Rutter. 1984. The Domain of Developmental Psychopathology. *Child Development* 55:17–29.

Staples, R., ed. 1971. *The Black Family: Essays and Studies.* Belmont, Calif.: Wadsworth Publishing Co.

Statistical Abstracts of the United States: 1982–1983. 103rd ed. 1983. Washington, D.C.: U.S. Department of Commerce.

Stiffman, A. R., J. G. Orme, D. A. Evans, R. A. Feldman, and P. A. Keeney. 1984. A Brief Measure of Children's Behavior Problems: The Behavior Rating Index for Children. *Measurement and Evaluation in Counseling and Development* 17:83–90.

Suls, J., and B. Mullen. 1981. Life Events, Perceived Control and Illness: The Role of Uncertainty. *Journal of Human Stress* 7:30–34.

Teuting, P., S. H. Koslow, and R. M. A. Hirschfeld. 1981. *Special Report on Depression Research.* Rockville, Md.: National Institute of Mental Health.

Touliatos, J., and B. Lindholm. 1980. Birth Order, Family Size, and Children's Mental Health. *Psychological Reports* 46:1097.

Uhlenhuth, E. H., R. S. Lipman, and M. B. Balter, 1974. Symptom Intensity and Life-Stress in the City. *Archives of General Psychiatry* 31:759–764.

United States National Center for Health Statistics. 1985. Advance Report of Final Divorce Statistics, 1982. *Monthly Vital Statistics Report* 33 (11).

United States National Center for Health Statistics. 1986. Births, Marriages, Divorces, and Deaths for 1985. *Monthly Vital Statistics Report* 34 (12).

Vaillant, G. E. 1983. Natural History of Male Alcoholism: V. Is Alcoholism the Cart or the Horse to Sociopathy? *British Journal of the Addictions* 78:317–326.

Vaux, A., and M. Ruggiero. 1983. Stressful Life Change and Delinquent Behavior. *Adolescence* 18:169–183.

Vincent, K. R., and H. A. Rosenstock. 1979. The Relationship between Stressful Life Events and Hospitalized Adolescent Psychiatric Patients. *Journal of Clinical Psychiatry* 40: 28–31.

Wallerstein, J. S., and J. B. Kelly. 1980. *Surviving the Breakup: How Children and Parents Cope with Divorce.* New York: Basic Books.

Walters, J., and N. Stinnett. 1971. Parent-Child Relationships: A Decade Review of Research. In *A Decade of Family Research and Action,* ed. C. Broderick. 99–140. Washington, D.C.: National Council on Family Relations.

Warheit, C. J. 1979. Life Events, Coping, Stress, and Depressive Symptomatology. *American Journal of Psychiatry* 136:502–507.

Waring, M., and D. G. Ricks. 1965. Family Patterns of Children Who Became Adult Schizophrenics. *Journal of Nervous and Mental Disease* 140:351–364.

Weinberg, S. K., and R. M. Weinberg. 1982. Family and Peer Relations in the Onset of Schizophrenia. *International Journal of Sociology of the Family* 12:229–240.

Weintraub, S., and J. M. Neale. 1984. The Stony Brook High-Risk Project. In *Children at Risk for Schizophrenia: A Longitudinal Perspective,* ed. N. F. Watt, E. J. Anthony, L. C. Wynne, and J. E. Rolf. 243–263. New York: Cambridge University Press.

Weintraub, S., J. M. Neale, and D. E. Liebert. 1975. Teacher Ratings of Children Vulnerable to Psychopathology. *American Journal of Orthopsychiatry* 45:838–845.

Weintraub, S., R. J. Prinz, and H. M. Neale. 1978. Peer Evaluations of the Competence of Children Vulnerable to Psychopathology. *Journal of Abnormal Child Psychology* 6:461–473.

Weissman, M. 1984. Alcoholism and Depression: Separate Entities? Seventh Annual Alcohoism Symposium of the Cambridge Hospital. Boston, Mass.

Weissman, M. M., J. K. Myers, and P. S. Harding. 1978. Psychiatric Disorders in a U.S. Urban Community: 1975–1976. *American Journal of Psychiatry* 135:459–462.

Weissman, M. M., E. S. Paykel, and G. L. Klerman. 1972. The Depressed Woman as a Mother. *Social Psychiatry* 7:98–108.

Welner, Z., A. Welner, M. D. McGary, and M. A. Leanard. 1977. Psychopathology in Children of Inpatients with Depression: A Controlled Study. *Journal of Nervous and Mental Disease* 164:408–413.

Werner, E. E., and R. S. Smith. 1982. *Vulnerable But Invincible: A Longitudinal Study of Resilient Children and Youth.* New York: McGraw-Hill.

West, D. J., and D. P. Farrington. 1973. *Who Becomes Delinquent?* London: Heinemann.

Wilson, C., and J. Orford. 1978. Children of Alcoholics: Report of a Preliminary Study and Comments on the Literature. *Journal of Studies on Alcohol* 39:121–142.

Winokur, G. 1974. The Division of Depressive Illness into Depression Spectrum Disease and Pure Depressive Disease. *International Pharmacopsychiatry* 9:5–13.

Winokur, G., T. Reich, J. Rimmer, and F. N. Pitts. 1970. Alcoholism: III. Diagnoses and Familial Psychiatric Illness in 259 Alcoholic Probands. *Archives of General Psychiatry* 23:104–111.

Wolfe, A. W., and H. R. Huessy. 1981. Stress, Social Support, and Schizophrenia: Two Discussions. *Schizophrenia Bulletin* 7:173–180.

Wolff, H. G. 1968. *Stress and Disease.* Springfield, Ill.: Thomas.

Worland, J., H. Lander, and V. Hesselbrock. 1979. Psychological Evaluation of Clinical Disturbance in Children at Risk for Psychopathology. *Journal of Abnormal Psychology* 88:13–26.

Yeaworth, R., J. York, M. A. Hussey, M. Ingle, and T. Goodwin. 1980. The Development of an Adolescent Life Change Event Scale. *Adolescence* 57:91–97.

Zegiob, L. E., and R. Forehand. 1975. Maternal Interactive Behavior as a Function of Race, Socioeconomic Status, and Sex of the Child. *Child Development* 46:564–568.

Zuckerman, M., E. A. Kolin, L. Price, and I. Zoob. 1964. Development of a Sensation-Seeking Scale. *Journal of Consulting and Clinical Psychology* 28:477–482.

INDEX

(Page numbers in italics indicate tabular material.)

academic achievement: as a coping skill, 189; discord in family and, 196
accidents, 6
Achenbach, T., 58
Achenbach Child Behavior Checklist (CBCL). *See* Child Behavior Checklist (CBCL)
achievement scores, 188
activity competence, 90, 208–210, 212. *See also* coping skills and coping behavior
adults: good relationship with at least one, 51; importance of healthy and supportive, 185. *See also* parents; significant others
affective disorders, 11–13, 28–29; effects on children of parents with schizophrenia vs. parents with, 13–19
age: of child at onset of parent's illness, 15, 16; coping skills and, 193, *194*
alcoholism: affective disorders and, 28–29; among children of alcoholics, 22; antisocial personality disorders and, 29–30; behavioral influences of, 23; and children, 21–30; depression and, 28–29; factors associated with parental, 28; family dynamics and, 24–28; genetic relationships and, 21–23
Ambruster, R., 29
Anderson, C. M., 23
Anthony, E. J., 39–40
antisocial personality disorders: alcoholism and, 29–30; childhood risk and parents', 19–21
apathy-futility syndrome, 18
Asarnow, R. F., 9
attention, impairment of, 6, 9

Beardslee, W. R., 12–13
Becker, J. V., 24
behavior: changes in, 59; coping skills and, 188–190; establishment of maladaptive, 18; family discord and children's, 134–141; family mental health and discord and children's, 139–141; family problems and children's, 151–152; help-seeking, 153; parental mental illness, social support, and children's, 154–158; social support and children's, 152–154; stressful events and children's, 165–168

behavioral disorders of children, 58–59; environmental factors and, 60–61; family size and, 121–123; parental mental illness and, 5–8, 9, 13, 21–30, 39, 108–111, 112–113, 114. *See also* mental illness
Behavioral Rating Index for Children (BRIC), 102
behavior problems, 15; activity competence and, 210; alternative family settings and, 180, 182–183, 192, 242, 248–249; children invulnerable to, 2, 15, 38–51, 51–54, 56; children victimized by, 67–69; chronic stress and, 152, 156, 158, 171, 241; classroom, 14; interpersonal skills and, 189–190; living arrangements and, 178–179, 180–183; mother-child relationship and, 136–137, 138, 180, 236–237, 241, 242; mother's mental health and child's, 112; nature of family problems and children's, 156; predictors of children's, 8, 32, 117–118, 140–141, 243; preventing, 2, 42, 70, 247–248; research instruments and, 81–83, 152; social support networks and, 156–157
behavior problem scores, Web study and, 95–97, 100–104
Beisser, A., 7
Bemporad, J., 12–13
Benson, C. S., 27
blacks, 17; delinquency-resistant children among, 20; effects of maternal and paternal delinquency among, 20. *See also* race
Blane, H. T., 24
Bleuler, M., 5
Blume, S. B., 25, 28
Buttenweiser, E., 18

Canavan, M., 5
case illustrations: invincible child, 71–72; victimized child, 66–69; vulnerable child, 65–67
CBCL. *See* Child Behavior Checklist
Chafetz, M. E., 24
Challas, G., 7–8
Chalmos, M. A., 18
child abuse, 148

Child Behavior Checklist (CBCL), 58, 81–83, 90, 91, 93; activity competence and, 210; of children in Web study, 94, 95–97, 100–104, 105; chronic problems and, 152; factors with inverse relationship to, 230; family discord and scores on, *135*, 231; family problems and, 151–152; living arrangements and, 178–179, 180–182; medications and, 104; mother-child discord and, 180; parental characteristics and scores on, *110*; parental mental illness and, *115*; sex of mentally ill parents and of child and scores on, *124*

childhood risk (of mental illness): affective disorders and, 11–13; from family disturbances, 19; neurotic depression of parents and, 17; parent's antisocial personality disorder and, 19–21; schizophrenic disorders and, 4–10; variables associated with, 31–32. *See also* vulnerability to mental illness

Child Life-Change Timeline, 162, 167

child rearing problems, 154. *See also* family problems (Web study)

children: of alcoholics, 21–30; with both parents mentally ill, 12; with both parents schizophrenic, 9; close involvement with psychotic parents by vulnerable, 39; critical factors in development of, 185; custody of, 249; of depressed mothers, 8, 12; of depressed parents, 11; determinants of behavior of at-risk, 212; family histories of, 80–81; in foster homes, 9, 116; illegitimate, 164; in institutions, 8, 116; outstanding, 54; of parents with psychoses, 14; prediction of behavioral outcome of, 8, 18, 85, 117–118, 125, 140–142, 243; predictive temperamental features of, 47; of psychoneurotic mothers, 7; safeguarding at-risk, 238; of schizophrenic vs. affective-disordered parents, 13–19; of schizophrenic mothers, 5–8; of schizophrenic parents, 16; of schizophrenic parents but reared by nonschizophrenic parents, 8–10; separated from mentally ill parents, 10, 116; superphrenic, 54; vulnerable to mental illness, 64–67; of welfare mothers, 5–8

Chiles, J. A., 30

Clark, R., 5

Clausen, J. A., 16

Cleghorn, J. M., 9

clumsiness, 6

Cohler, B. J., 6, 52–53

communication between parent and child, 16

competence: criteria of childhood, 42; as indicator of invulnerable child, 41; invulnerability and, 49

Coopersmith Self-Esteem Inventory, 188

coping skills and coping behavior, 56, 186–190, 205–213; age and, 193, *194*; of children of alcoholic fathers, 27; current living arrangements and, 190–191; discord in family and, 196–199; environmental stressors and, 43–45, 49, 61; exhaustion of (Web families), 155; family characteristics and, 190–195; family mental health and, 194; family physical health and, 195–196; institutional or group living and, 191; race and, 192, *193*; SES and, 193, *194*; summary and discussion of, 199–202; two kinds of, 239; and weaknesses, 89–91

Cork, R. M., 28

Cotton, N. S., 21–22

critical periods, 46, 166; development and, 84

Cudeck, R., 8

custody decisions, 249

data analysis in Web study, 92–94, 204–205, 243

death, 163–164

delinquency (juvenile): parental criminality and, 19–21; parental mental illness and child's, 15

delusions, credulity about parental, 39

demographic factors (Web study), 84–85

depression, 11–13; among alcoholics, 28–29; among children of alcoholics, 22–23, 25; impact of material, 17–18, 53; socioenvironmental factors in development of, 17–18

desertions, 173

destructiveness, 7

diagnosis of childhood behavior disorders, 58–60

Diagnostic and Statistical Manual (DSM) of Mental Disorders (American Psychiatric Association, 1980), 11, 100

discord: children's assessments of, 130–131; children's behavior and family, 134–136, 139–141; children's behavior and father-child, 137–138; children's behavior and mother-child, 136–137, 140–141, 227, 236; children's behavior and parental, 138–139; family, 19, 27, 46, 88–89, 127–132, 134–141, 180, 238; marital, 27; most problematic form of, 236; mother-child, 136–137, 138, 180, 236–237, 241, 242; parental assessments of, 130, 132; sibling mental illness and family, 134

divorce and separation, 27, 107, 146, 151–152, 164, 173, 176; custody decisions in, 249

drugs, abuse of, 27. *See also* alcoholism; substance abuse disorders

DSM. *See* Diagnostic and Statistical Manual (DSM) of Mental Disorders (American Psychiatric Association, 1980)

Edelbrock, C., 58

educational attainment of child, factors influencing, 16

environment, 9; childhood, 57; critical factors in, 205–207, 208, 212, 216–219; protective-to-stressful continuum of, 60

environmental protectors against mental illness, 60–61; research instruments (Web study) and, 83–89

environmental stressors: major, 50; personal coping skills and, 43–45, 49, 61; research instruments (Web study) and, 83–89

epidemiological perspective and strategies, 45, 46

Erlenmeyer-Kimling, L., 10

extracurricular activities, 211–212, 248; coping skills and, 199

families: alcoholic, 23; alternative, 175–176, 182–183; children's behavior problems and mental health of, 125–126; coping skills and characteristics of, 190–195, 196–199; definitions of, 174; discord in, 19, 28, 46–47, 88–89, 127–132, 134–141, 180, 219, 238; dissolution of, 173; importance of climate of, 27; infants in single-child, 17; instability of, 5, 80; major changes in (Web study), 164; mental health of, 218; multiproblem, 26; physical health of, 218; proportion of mentally ill persons in, 113–114, 126, 142, 169, 182–183, 194, 212, 237, 243; research on influence of, 119; results of changes in, 107; with schizophrenic mother or father, 5, 54; single-parent, 114, 173; size of, 109, 113, 121–123, 126, 190, 240; social support for, 27, 28, 145–148, 149, 150, 240, 241, 249; sources of stress in alcoholic, 28; tension in, 28; two-parent, 173

family problems (Web study): acute but short-lived, 148, 152, 155; children's behavior and, 151–152; chronic, 152, 155, 158, 171, 241;

financial, 146; most frequent, 145–146; severity of, 147–148; support systems and, 145–151; types of, 145–147, 240–241

family settings: alternative, 180, 182–183, 192, 238, 242, 248–249; departures from traditional, 184

fathers: ages of, 109; bond between children and, 133; child's discord with, 137–138; daughters of alcoholic, 27; delinquent black, 20; mental health problems of, 117; stressful life events and health of, 171

Favorini, A., 23

financial problems, 40–41, 146, 154, 156

foster care, 8, 9, 108, 116; placing a child in (Missouri law), 164

friends as source of help, *149*, 150, 151, 155, 156

Gallant, D., 6

Gamer, E., 6, 52–53

Gammon, G. D., 11

Gardner, G., 10

Garmezy, N., 40–45

Gee, S., 7–8

gender: coping skills and, 192; influence of, 15, 33, 46–47, 192; Web study and, 98–99

genetic influences, mental illness and, 9

Gibbs, J. T., 29

Glasser, N., 7

Goodwin, D., 22–23

Grant, M., 7

group homes, 108, 116; coping skills and living in, 191, 239

Grunebaum, H. U., 6, 52–53

Guse, S. B., 22–23

Haberman, P. W., 23

help seeking, 152–153, 156–157. *See also* social support

Henderson, C., 25, 28

Herjanic, B., 20, 29

Herjanic, M., 29

Hesselbrock, V., 14

Heston, L. L., 9

Higgins, J., 7

high risk children: changes in living arrangements of, 174–179; family change and living arrangements of, 172–174; longitudinal (ten-year) study of, 5–6

Hill, M. J., 24

Hirschfeld, R.M.A., 18

hospitals as source of social support, *149*, 151, 156

Huffine, C. L., 16

incest, 148

institutions, 176, 177, 180; coping skills and living in, 191, 239

intelligence/achievement, 91

intervention, 250; preventive, 2, 42, 70, 242–248; priorities in, 73; social interaction model and, 73; social skills and, 155; therapeutic, 247–248

interview procedure and problems (Web study), 76, 77–80, 80–81, 87

invulnerability, 2, 15, 38–51; case illustration of, 71–72; competence and, 49; conceptualization of, 42; environmental stressors and personal coping skills and, 43–45; epidemiological approach to study of, 45; risk status and, 37–38. *See also* superkids

Jacob, T., 23

Jang, M., 25–27

juvenile delinquency. *See* delinquency (juvenile)

Kammeier, M. L., 24

Kauai (Hawaii) Longitudinal Study, 50

Kauffman, C., 52–53

Keller, M. B., 12–13

Klerman, G. L., 12–13

Knop, J., 22–23

Koslow, S. H., 18

Lander, H., 14

Liebert, D. E., 14

life-change events, 86–88, 159–160

life events, weighting, 161. *See also* stressful life events

living arrangements: changes in, 174–179; children's behavior and current, 180–183; coping skills and current, 190–191; effects on low-risk children of, 229–230; family change and, 172-174; institutional, 176, 177, 180; most disruptive, 180; of Web study participants, 88, 116, 179–180, 183–185, 216–217

MacCrimmon, D. J., 9

McLachlan, J.F.C., 25

Masten, A. S., 42–43

Mednick, S. A., 5–6, 8, 22–23

Meisel, S. S., 23

mental health status: changes in, 59; child's, *43*; measuring family, 125; parents', 111–116; research about childhood, 120

mental illness: alternative family settings and low incidence of, 182–183; childbearing patterns and, 123; children vulnerable to, 64–67; concentration in family, 141; current environment and parental, 225; environmental model of childhood, 56; factors protecting children from impact of parent's, 39, 56; in families of Web subjects, 85; family discord and, 132–134; intervention and social interaction model and, 63–64; maternal, 133; parental diagnosis and childhood, 8; parental (as family problem), 145, 146, 154; paternal, 133; prevention of, 2, 42, 70, 234; research implications of social interaction model for, 63–64; sex-linked transmission of, 85; social interaction model of childhood, 56–74; social interaction model of vulnerability to, 3, *59*; social support, children's behavior, and parental, 154–158; stressful life events and proportion of family members with, 169; trait model of childhood, 56. *See also* behavioral disorders of children; behavior problems; invulnerability; vulnerability to mental illness; *names of specific types of mental illness*

Miller, D., 7–8, 25–27

Miller, P. M., 24

Morehouse, E., 28

Moriarity, A., 62

mothers: ages of, 109; bond between children and, 133; children of depressed, 8, 17; children of psychoneurotic, 7; children of schizophrenic, 5–8; children of welfare, 5–8; child's discord with, 136–137, 138, 180, 241, 242; delinquent black, 20; with depressive disorders, 11, 17–18, 53; influence of, 52; mental health of, 117; neglectful, 18; physical health of, 116–117; psychosocial adjustment of adult children of schizophrenic, 9; of schizophrenic children, 10; supportive involvement with child by mentally ill, 53. *See also* parents

Murphy, L., 62

Nardi, P. M., 27

National Institute of Mental Health (NIMH) Laboratory of Developmental Psychology, 17–18

Neale, H. M., 8
Neale, J. M., 10, 14
neighbors as source of help, *149*, 150, 151
neurological dysfunctions, 6

Orford, J., 27, 28
Orvaschel, H. S., 6

parental delinquency or criminality, childhood
  conduct disorders and juvenile delinquency
  and, 19–21, 32
parental expectations, confused and inconsistent, 27
parental mental illness: childhood risk and,
  30–33; influence of type of, 195; mediation
  of impact on children of severe, 27; sex-based
  linkages between child's behavior and, 10
parent-child relationship, 46, 52, 53, 127–128
parents: ability to function, 195; adoptive, 107,
  108, 177; age of, 109, 116; alcoholic, 21–30;
  at-risk children and characteristics of, 108–
  111; biological, 106–108, 173, 175, 191–
  192; children with psychiatrically disturbed,
  6; children reared by schizophrenic, 5–8, 9;
  children's behavior and discord between,
  138–140; children's behavior and health of,
  111–116; children's behavior and mental
  health of, 112–113, 114–116; children's
  coping skills and physical health of, *197*;
  children's disorders and diagnosis of, 19;
  competence-inducing, 40; cost of caring for
  mentally ill, 146; criminal, 19, 20–21; delinquent black, 20; discord between, 16, 18, 27,
  138–139; divorce of, 164; foster, 107–108;
  hospitalization of, 113; hostile behavior of,
  18; imitation of behavior of, 13; importance
  of good relationship with one, 46; inability to
  control children, 145–146; interviews with,
  79; of invulnerable children, 44; irritability toward child by, 16; mediating factors with
  mental illness of, 226; mentally ill, 18, 108,
  114–116, 236; with personality disorder, 16,
  18; religion of, 109, 116; risk to children of
  mentally ill, 236; separation from, 46, 108;
  separation or divorce of, 27, 106, 146,
  151–152, 173; severity of psychopathology
  of, 7; sex of affected, 16, 124–125; social interactions between children and schizophrenic, 8; step-, 106, 107, 164; substance
  abuse disorders and, 21–31. *See also* father;
  mother

Paykel, E. S., 12
Penick, E., 29
physical health problems: in families of Web
  subjects, 85–86; of parents, 111
Pines, M., 51
Polansky, N. A., 18
prediction of behavior problems, 8, 18, 85,
  140–142, 243; factors useful for, 117–118,
  125; variables and, 204
preventive intervention, 2, 42, 70, 247–248;
  difficulty with, 234
Prinz, R. J., 8, 10
protective factors, 187. *See also* coping skills
  and coping behavior
psychiatric disturbances, important factors in
  children's, 18, 47

Quinton, D., 15–16, 18–19

race, 17, 20; Web study and, 99, 110
recreational activities, 211–212
relatives: children living with, 177; as source of
  help, *149*, 150, 151, 156
religion, Web study and, 99–100, 109, 116
remarriage, 183
research: difficulties in, 78; epidemiological,
  5–6; on influence of the family on child's
  mental health, 119–120; mechanisms for
  sharing problems of, 35; weakness in, 16. *See
  also* Web study
research instruments (tests, checklists, etc.),
  253; for behavior problems, 81–83; BRIC,
  102, 105; CBCL, 58, 81–83, 90, 91, 93, 94,
  95–97, 99, 100–104, 105, *110, 115, 124,
  135,* 151–152, 187; Child Life-Event Timeline, 87; for environmental stressors and protectors, 83–89; Likert scale, 87, 88, 89, 91;
  multiple respondent interview procedures as,
  87; for self-esteem, 188; used in Web study,
  81–91; WRAT, 91, 187
residences and residential factors. *See* living
  arrangements
risk factors, 50, 59
risk status, 41; defining, 57; factors shaping, 73;
  ranking of, 73
Robins, L. N., 20
role models, 53; alcoholic parents as, 23;
  dysfunctional, 125
Rolf, D., 6
Russell, M., 25, 28
Rutter, M., 8, 14–16, 18–19, 45–47

Sameroff, A. J., 8, 17

schizophrenia: child's mental illness and maternal, 10; difficulty with studies of, 8; family stress and onset of, 9–10; genetic predisposition for, 9; peak risk period for, 8, 10; sex role identification and, 10

schizophrenic mothers, 5–8

schizophrenic parents, 4–10; effects on children of parents with affective disorder vs., 13–19; risk to offspring and separation from, 10

school: behavior in, 14, 91; mother's mental illness and competence of child in, 195; parents' social status and children's performance in, 16; predictive value of competence in, 211; as source of social support, *149*, 151, 156

Schuckit, M. A., 22–23, 29, 30

Schulsinger, F., 5–6, 8

Segal, J., 34

Seifer, R., 8, 17

self-esteem, 90–91, 187, 188; as a coping factor, 190

separation from parents, 46, 108

SES. *See* socioeconomic status

sex. *See* gender

sex role identification, etiology of schizophrenia and, 10

siblings: with behavior problems (Web study), 126, 142; conflict between, 7; family discord and mental illness of, 134; influence of number of, 123–124; mentally ill, 85; new, 164; proportion with behavior problems, 142; stress and, 163

significant others, child's risk and, 31

single-parent families, 114

sleep interruption, 7

Smith, R. S., 50–51

Sobel, D. E., 9

social competence, 53, 89–90, 187; behavior problems and, 239; as a coping skill, 189; distribution of scores on test of, *188*; family discord and, 197–199; parental alcoholism and, 25–26

social interaction model of childhood mental illness, 3, 9, 56–57, 235; childhood behavior disorders and, 58–60; environmental stressors and protectors and, 60–61; interactions between coping skills and environmental factors and, *59*, 63; invincible children and, 61, *59*, 69–72; main features of, *59*; personal coping skills and, 61–62, 69–72; summary and discussion of, 72–74; victimized children

and, *59*, 67–69; vulnerable children and, *59*, 64–67

social service agencies, as source of help, *149*, 151, 156, 249

social support, 27, 28, 240, 241; children's behavior and extent of network for, 157; family problems and, 145–148; formal systems of, 149–150; gender and effective use of, 144; helpfulness of networks of, 150–151; informal, 150, 249; most useful networks of, 144; parental mental illness and children's behavior and, 154–158; source of, *149*; for stress caused by mental illness, 143. *See also* help seeking

socioeconomic status (SES), 7, 16; CBCL scores and, 111; of depressed mothers, 17–18; number of stressful life events of at-risk children and, 169, 241; one-child families and high, 17; role of, 240

sports, coping and, 199, 248

Spring, B., 47–50

statistical studies, 92–94, 204–205, 243

stealing, 7

Steffy, R. A., 9

stress: changes in level of, 166–167; children's severe behavior problems and chronic family, 156; chronic, 152, 155, 158, 171, 241; depression and, 18; examining children's, 161; exogenous factors that help children remain invulnerable to, 44; in family, 9–10, 28, 152, 156, 158, 171, 241; illness and, 159–160; parent impairment or unavailability and, 13; prolonged family, 156, 158, 171, 241; social support for mental illness-caused, 143; sources of (in alcoholic families), 28

stressful life events: of at-risk children, 162–165; behavior of at-risk children and, 165–168; changes in living arrangements as, 177; effects of, 159–160; families of children in Web study and, 168–171; research about, 160–162; and risk status, 48; vulnerability and, *48*

stress-resistant children, 38, 56. *See also* invulnerability; superkids

study. *See* Web study

substance abuse disorders: childhood risk and parents', 21–30; delinquent personality type and, 29–30

suicide, 6

superkids, 2, 38, 51–54. *See also* invulnerability

superphrenics, 2, 54
support systems. *See* social support

tactile sensitivity, 6
Tellegen, A., 42–43
temper tantrums, 7
Teuting, P., 18
therapeutic intervention, 247–248
Thomas, S., 25
Tomellein, C., 29

variables: children's CBCL scores and family, *122*; that enable invulnerables to resist stress, 46; environmental, 35, 44; exogenous and endogenous, 37–38; importance of social support, 27; interactions and relationships among, 32, 34, 63, 119, 225–231; moderating, 212; predictive, 8, 117–118; shaping vulnerability, 50; statistical approaches to study of, 204
victimized children, 67–69
vulnerability to mental illness: case illustration of, 65–67; close involvement and identification with psychotic parent and, 39; critical periods in, 84; epidemiology of childhood, 47; factors in, 73; Garmezy's model of, 42–43; key finding about, 212; life event stressors and, *48*; models for, 56–57; multivariate model of, 203–213; peak periods of, 32; risk status and, 36–37; social interaction model of childhood, 3, 56–74; variables shaping, 50
Vulnerable But Invincible: A Study of Resilient Children (Werner and Smith), 50

Walderman, R. L., 25
Web study, 1, 2–3; activity competence and, 90; behavioral characteristics and problems of children in, 100–104, 220; comparison (control) sample in, 214–216, 225–226, 232–233, 244–246; coping strengths and weaknesses and, 89–91, 155, 221–222; data analysis in, 92–94, 204–205, 243; demographic factors and, 84–85; environmental stressors and protectors and, 60–61; family change and, 223; family discord and, 88–89, 219; family instability and, 106–107; family mental health problems and, 85, 218; family problems and, 145–147; family social report data in, 88, 223–224; high and low risk subjects in, 75–76; intake interview, 76; intake process, 77–80; intelligence and achievement and, 91; interviews, 76, 77–80, 80–81, 87; life-change events and, 86–88, 159–160; living arrangements and, 88, 106–108, 174–179, 179–183; medications used by subjects in, 103–104; most common family problems in, 145–146; personal coping skills and, 61–62; physical health problems and, 85–86, 103–104, 218; race of children in, 99; referral to, 76, 77; religion and, 99–100; research instruments in, 81–91, *253*; sample in, 75, 104–105; school behavior and, 91; school performance and, 104; self-esteem and, 90–91; sex of children in, 98–99; social competence and, 89–90; social isolation of families in, 224; treatment status of children in, 101; subjects with fewest behavior problems, 226; subjects with most behavior problems, 228; WRAT in, 91, 187
Weinberg, R. M., 9
Weinberg, S. K., 9
Weintraub, S., 8, 10, 14
Weissman, M. M., 12
Werner, F. E., 50–51
West, P. A., 20
Wide-Range Achievement Test (WRAT): behavior problem scores and scores on, 189; stressful life events recall and, 171; in Web study, 91, 187
Williams, D. P., 18
Wilson, C., 27, 28
Worland, J., 14

Yahraes, H., 34
Yule, B., 15–16

Zax, M., 8, 17
Zubin, J., 47–50